SO-CFF-868

The Professional Cosmetologist

Third Edition*

*Written to assist students taking state or national licensing tests written by individual states, the National Interstate Council of State Boards of Cosmetology, or Educational Testing Service.

The Professional Cosmetologist

Third Edition

John W. Dalton

Ann Music Streetman
Editor

Artwork developed by
Scientific Illustrators

West Publishing Company

St. Paul   New York   Los Angeles   San Francisco

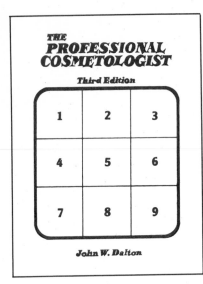

COVER PHOTOS:

Numbers 1, 3, 5, 7, and 9

Courtesy of Plum Studio
St. Paul, Minnesota

Number 2

Belvedere First Lady "Mondo" All Purpose Hairstyling Chair
and Belvedere "Columbia" Styling Station with Belvedere's
Cameo Shampoo Bowl.

Numbers 4 and 6

Tools and supplies provided by
Cassidy Inc., St. Paul,
Minnesota

Number 8

The Nail Bar is the Belvedere Cosmos Nail Bar
and Mondo Seating Chairs.

Permanent Hair Color Comparison Chart
courtesy of LAMAUR Incorporated.

COPYRIGHT © 1976 BY WEST PUBLISHING CO.
COPYRIGHT © 1979 BY WEST PUBLISHING CO.
COPYRIGHT © 1985 BY WEST PUBLISHING CO.,
                     50 West Kellogg Boulevard
                     P.O. Box 43526
                     St. Paul, Minnesota 55164

All rights reserved

Printed in the United States of America

Library of Congress Cataloging in Publication Data

Dalton, John W., 1942–
    The professional cosmetologist.

    Bibliography: p.
    Includes index.
        1. Beauty culture. I. Title.
TT957.D27 1984   646.7'26   83-25974
ISBN 0-314-77877-2   2nd Reprint—1987
ISBN 0-314-77878-0 (pbk.)   4th Reprint—1987

To my wife Judy
for her patience,
support,
and love.

Contents

Introduction

"INTRODUCTION" OR "TO THE STUDENT"

This is the second revision of The Professional Cosmetologist (TPC), which is consistent with the author's promise to respective State Boards of Cosmetology and school instructors/owners to revise and update TPC. (The State Board Review Questions were revised in 1978 and in 1979.) The paragraphs that follow will:

1. identify some of the major changes of the TPC text and Study Guide;
2. provide statements from students and instructors now using TPC;
3. explain "The Professional Cosmetologist's MASTER PLAN" for "Performance-Based Learning"; and
4. express the author's appreciation to individuals and companies for various forms of support.

This new edition has grown from recommendations by State Board Members, instructors, and school owners. Their helpful changes will make learning easier for students, teaching easier for instructors, and ensure even greater chances of success for students when they are taking their State Board Examinations.

FIRST of all, the Table of Contents in the front of the book has been redesigned to make topics or subjects easier to find at a glance. NEXT, we have added new illustrations, and replaced others. For your convenience, SELECTED SAMPLE QUESTIONS have also been added to the end of each chapter. A speedy-reference answer key for these selected questions can be found after the Questions at the bottom of the page. The performance objective (what you "do" for a particular job) PAGES HAVE BEEN SHADED with a tint screen. This tint will automatically permit you to find the steps for a certain task (job), and gives you a quick visual way to locate the beginning and end of each chapter.

The STUDY GUIDE for The Professional Cosmetologist has also been revised. New to this edition are the Cosmetology Worksheets and Hair Color Layout sheets.

To the Student

INTRODUCTION FOR THE TPC LEARNING SYSTEM

The short section which follows will help you use "performance-based learning" effectively. Designed around a series of questions you might ask, this introduction:

1. defines important terms;
2. identifies the resources in this system;
3. gives hints for preparing for State Board exams; and
4. details the MASTER PLAN for using these resources

Practiced successfully for many years in schools and training facilities throughout the country, the MASTER PLAN provides the key to effective use of THE PROFESSIONAL COSMETOLOGIST'S LEARNING SYSTEM.

WHAT IS A PERFORMANCE-BASED LEARNING SYSTEM?

We call it "performance-based" because the skills you learn are the ones you must "do" on-the-job as a cosmetologist. Studies done by beauty schools, State Boards of Cosmetology, universities, and the author reveal which services a successful cosmetologist performs.

Notice we called this a "learning system"—not just a textbook. A textbook is one of many resources that you will use in learning cosmetology. Other resources include:

→ the instructor
→ fellow classmates
→ audio-visual materials
→ workbooks
→ study guides
→ lectures/demonstrations

All these resources combine to form a "learning system" designed carefully to help you learn the "performance" required in cosmetology.

WHAT RESOURCES MAKE UP THE PROFESSIONAL COSMETOLOGIST LEARNING SYSTEM?

The major resources making up the learning system you are now beginning are:

→ you, the student
→ this textbook
→ your instructor
→ the Study Guide
→ the State Board Review Questions
→ Dalton's Professional Guide to Cosmetology

Since these resources are a "system" for learning, they are used together (as shown below) in the following way:

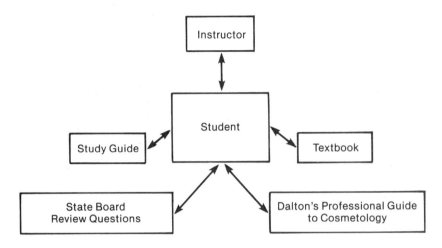

Let's look at each part of this learning system in a bit more detail:

You are the center of this sytem. You are the best resource for mastering cosmetology skills. Apply yourself by using TPC resources effectively, and you will learn successfully.

> Student

The instructor is the manager of your instruction. He/she shares the wisdom of years of experience to assist you by:
1. teaching successful techniques;
2. pinpointing and solving learning problems;
3. helping review and practice.

> Textbook

Your instruction must be reinforced and strengthened periodically by activities. The TPC Study Guide lists the way your performance will be evaluated, and provides a chart for you to keep track of your progress.

> Study Guide

This booklet helps you practice your question answering skills, and review the content for the State Board Examinations.

> State Board
> Review Questions

This booklet is an evaluation instrument which measures what the student actually knows about the practical skills—What to do, When to do it, and Why to do it. The problems in it are "real life" applications of the theory *and* practice of cosmetology.

> Dalton's Professional Guide
> to Cosmetology

HOW DO I USE ALL THE TPC RESOURCES TO LEARN COSMETOLOGY?

Step 1— Turn to the Table of Contents in the front of the book—the "bold print" chapter headings list the skills and knowledge you will learn in order to be a cosmetologist. Look this list over carefully.

Step 2—Pick any chapter in the Contents, and read through the listing of performances written in small letters. After instruction and practice, you will be required to "know" and be able to "do" these activities to show HOW WELL you can perform each SKILL. These performances are called "subobjectives," and will act as "stepping stones" for you to learn each skill.

Step 3—Page through the text, glancing at the illustrations and discovering the basic layout of the instruction.

WHAT IS THE MASTER PLAN?

MOTIVATE YOURSELF =

Successful use of this system requires your active, interested participation. Make up your mind from the beginning to concentrate, work hard, and use all available resources. Renew this self-motivation at the beginning of each chapter and whenever you need a little attitude boost. Start every chapter by reading the title and purpose carefully. These items tell WHY you are studying the chapter and how important it is.

ANALYZE =

1. Read and study each major objective. This learning tool tells exactly what you must "do" at the END of instruction and practice to learn the skill.
2. Analyze the Level of Acceptability statement carefully. It identifies the conditions under which you must do the "major objective," and at least HOW WELL you must perform it for mastery.
3. Read and study the Knowing and Doing Subobjectives. They tell you the exact steps you must take to perform the Major Objective. Accomplishing these subobjectives will become the main part of your instruction in each chapter. Your instructor may add information or examples to these subobjectives.

STUDY =

Once you have analyzed the introductory material in each chapter, begin study to achieve each subobjective.

1. Read the instruction in the Knowing Subobjectives carefully. **Notice each subobjective is printed conveniently in the margin at**

the beginning of instruction. Refer back to this statement whenever necessary, so you always know what performance you are working to master.

2. Look up unfamiliar words in the Glossary at the end of each chapter.
3. Do the Study Guide activities for the Knowing Subobjectives when you have studied the instruction in the book carefully. Check your answers immediately and ask necessary questions.
4. Read the instruction in the Doing Subobjectives. Study the procedures carefully.
5. Complete the Study Guide activities for the Doing Subobjectives. Again check your answers immediately and clear up any questions keeping in mind your instructor will have the "most right answer."

TAKE TIME =

Clarify any confusion or misunderstanding about the skill you are learning.

1. Ask the instructor for help in problem areas.
2. Review the procedures for the Doing Subobjectives.
3. Read over "Performance/Product Checklist" for this skill in the Study Guide. This checklist tells you **at least** how well you must do a particular job.
4. Gather your necessary supplies in preparation to practice this skill.

EMPHASIZE PRACTICE =

1. Walk through the step-by-step procedure using your text.
2. Ask the instructor for clarification and assistance.
3. Refer to the "Performance/Product Checklist."
4. Try doing the performance with little or no help from text, instructor, or other resources.
5. Perform task (job) for evaluation with **no** resources.

REVIEW =

Once you complete each performance to the Level of Acceptability, review the entire chapter.

1. Do the "Cosmetology Worksheets" and "Hair Color Worksheets" in the TPC Study Guide to reinforce your knowledge.
2. Try answering the TPC State Board Review Quesions in the booklet with this learning system.
3. Write answers to the "selected study questions" on the shaded pages at the end of each chapter. Teaming up with a few of your classmates to ask each other study questions will also provide a good review.

4. Answer performance questions in Dalton's Professional Guide to Cosmetology.

This simple TPC MASTER PLAN is the key to your successful use of this learning system!

HOW SHOULD I PREPARE FOR THE STATE BOARD EXAMS?

Here are a few suggestions for preparing for your licensing examinations:

→ Use this entire learning system as described in the MASTER PLAN.
→ Review all Study Guide activities for Knowing and Doing Subobjectives.
→ Study criteria listed in "performance/product checklists" of Study Guide.
→ Review "study questions" on the shaded pages at the end of each chapter. Look up answers where necessary.
→ Answer sample items in State Board Review Questions booklet which is part of this system and review questions in Dalton's Professional Guide to Cosmetology.
→ Follow directions given by your instructor "to the letter."

PUTTING IT ALL TOGETHER

You are about to benefit from the use of a "performance-based learning system." Each skill is divided into specific performances or activities you must complete to become a successful cosmetologist. Instruction is organized into a "learning system" composed of various resources. You, the student, are the center of this system as illustrated below:

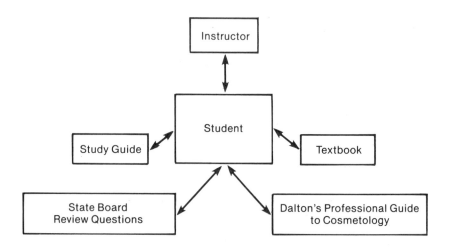

As the center of this learning system, YOU must use the TPC system effectively. So let's quickly review how the TPC MASTER PLAN will guide you to success:

MOTIVATE YOURSELF

→ Take charge of your own learning
→ Begin each chapter by reading Title and Purpose.

ANALYZE

→ Major Objective.
→ Level of Acceptability.
→ Knowing and Doing Subobjectives.

STUDY

→ Knowing Subobjective instruction and Study Guide activities.
→ Doing Subobjective instruction and Study Guide activities.

TAKE TIME

→ Clarify all problem areas.
→ Question instructor.
→ Review doing procedures in textbook.
→ Gather supplies ready for practice.

EMPHASIZE PRACTICE

→ Walk through procedures in The Professional Cosmetologist.
→ Ask instructor assistance where necessary.
→ Refer to Performance/Product Checklist in Study Guide.
→ Do performance with minimal help from resources.
→ Do performance with **no** help from resources.

REVIEW

→ Look over chapter.
→ Do Cosmetology Worksheets and Hair Color Worksheets in Study Guide.
→ Answer State Board Review Questions.
→ Try Study Questions on shaded pages of text.
→ Answer questions in Dalton's Professional Guide to Cosmetology.

Following the MASTER PLAN for The Professional Cosmetologist Learning System will guide you to mastering the skills of a licensed cosmetologist. GOOD LEARNING!!

REFERENCE LIST

Anthony, Catherine P., and Thibadeau, Gray A. *Structure and Function of the Body*. 6th Ed. Saint Louis: The C. V. Mosby Co., 1980.

Bogert, L. Jean. *Fundamentals of Chemistry*. 8th ed. Philadelphia: W. B. Saunders Co., 1958.

Burns, R. W. *New Approach to Behavioral Objectives*. Dubuque: William C. Brown Co., Publisher, 1973.

The Cosmetic, Toiletry and Fragrance Association. *CTFA Cosmetic Ingredient Dictionary.* Washington, D.C.: The Cosmetic, Toiletry and Fragrance Association, Inc., 1973.

Diehl, H. S. and Dalrymple, Willard. *Healthful Living*. 9th ed. New York: McGraw-Hill Book Co., 1973.

Gordon, Myron J., and Shillinglaw, Gordon. *Accounting—A Management Approach*. Illinois: Richard D. Irwin, Inc., 1969.

Gray, Henry. *Anatony of the Human Body.* 27th ed. Edited by Charles Mayo Goss. Philadelphia: Lea & Febiger, 1959.

Greenstone, Arthur W.; Harris, Sidney, P. *Concepts in Chemistry*. 3rd ed. New York: Harcourt Brace Jovanovich, Inc., 1975.

Hall-Smith, P.; Cairns, R. J.; and Beare, R. L. *Dermatology*. New York: Grune & Stratton, Inc., 1973.

Kilgour, O. F. G., and McGarry, Marguerite. *An Introduction to Science and Hygiene for Hairdressers*. New York: Funk & Wagnalls, Inc., 1964.

Leftwich, R. H. *The Price System and Resource Allocation*. New York: Holt, Rinehart and Winston, 1966.

Mager, Robert F. *Preparing Instructional Objectives*. Belmont, Calif.: Fearon Publishers, 1962.

Mager, Robert F., and Beach, Kenneth M., Jr. *Developing Vocational Instruction*. Belmont, Calif.: Fearon Publishers, 1974.

Miller, Benjamin E., and Keane, Claire Brackman. *Encyclopedia and Dictionary of Medicine and Nursing*. Philadelphia: W. B. Saunders Co. 1972.

Morris, William, ed. *The Xerox Intermediate Dictionary*. New York: Grossett & Dunlap, Inc., 1973.

Nass, Gisela. *The Molecules of Life*. New York: McGraw-Hill Book Co., 1970.

Pillsbury, D. M.; Shelley, W. B.; and Kligman, A. M. *Dermatology.* Philadelphia: W. B. Saunders Co., 1968.

Pucel, David J. and Knaak, William C. *Individualizing Vocational and Technical Instruction*. Columbus, Ohio: Charles E. Merrill Publishing Compnay, 1975.

Sauer, G. C. *Manual of Skin Diseases*. 4th ed. Philadelphia: J. B. Lippincott Co., 1980.

Shelley, W. B. *Consultations in Dermatology II with Walter B. Shelley*. Philadelphia: W. B. Saunders Co., 1974.

Smith, L. Y., and Roberson, G. G. *Business Law*. UCC 5th ed. Saint Paul: West Publishing Co., 1982.

Stedman's Medical Dictionary. 22nd ed. Baltimore: The Williams & Wilkins Co., 1972.

Stewart, F. S. *Bacteriology and Immunology for Students of Medicine*. 9th ed. Baltimore: The Williams & Wilkins Co., 1968.

Turner, C. E. *Personal and Community Health*. 14th rev. ed. Saint Louis: The C. V. Mosby Co., 1971.

Whitmore, Charles W., and Young, William H. *A Complete Guide to Skin and Hair for the Cosmetologist*. Lynchburg, Va.: Education and Research Foundation for the Health and Beauty Care of Skin, Hair, and Nails, Inc., 1972.

Acknowledgments

The author would like to express his thanks to special people who worked with him to make this book possible—Karol Goebel, Ann Streetman, Gary Wilkes, and Linda Ford.

A sincere thanks to the following for various forms of support, advice, and assistance to Aurie Gosnell, Joel Mumphrey, Hamilton Wilson, Edna West, and Del Baker. Special thanks also to Dr. Charles Whitmore, Robert Mager, Ted Dragoo, Leon Duke, Florian Harvat, Rosalyn Duncan, Fred Laurino, and Carol Shaw.

Careers in Cosmetology 1

As a beginning student in cosmetology, you have probably thought about your career as something in the distant future. Actually that career is not very far away. You have already taken the first step, and before you know it, a wide range of exciting and challenging opportunities will be yours.

Cosmetology is the art and science of beauty care. A person who is licensed to perform these services is a **cosmetologist**. One of a cluster of health-related occupations, cosmetology involves care of the skin, hair, scalp, and nails.

One of the reasons you will have such a wide variety of opportunities before you as a cosmetologist is that cosmetology is both an art and a science—as well as a business. If you have a flair for the artistic, you will be able to find positions that emphasize these talents. If your interest is in the sciences, there are positions that emphasize this kind of skill. Also, there are many business opportunities available to experienced cosmetologists.

As a beginning student, you may not have thought this far ahead. Although a background in science, business, and art can be helpful, it is not necessary for a career in cosmetology. At this point you may not have even thought about a highly specialized career—you may simply be interested in serving people as a practicing cosmetologist. On the other hand, it can be nice to know that opportunities are available if you wish to advance.

This chapter explains the basic requirements for different careers in cosmetology and gives a number of suggestions that will help to make your student life successful. The chart on page 2 diagrams some of the various career options open to you as a cosmetologist.

General Requirements

Several personal qualities are especially desirable for all people working in cosmetology. Some of them might seem rather obvious, but you should keep them in mind.

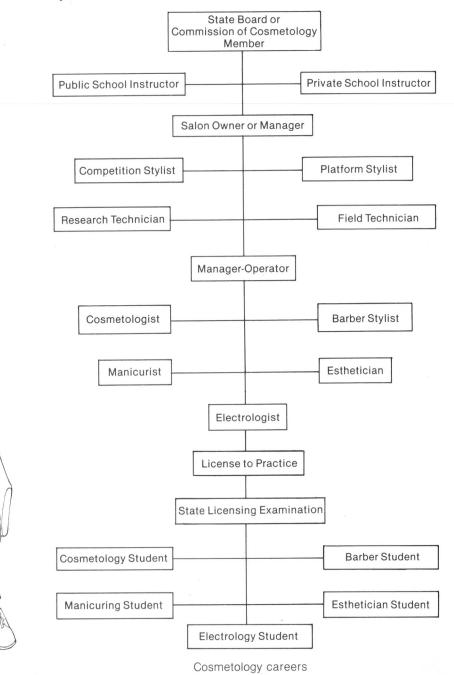

Cosmetology careers

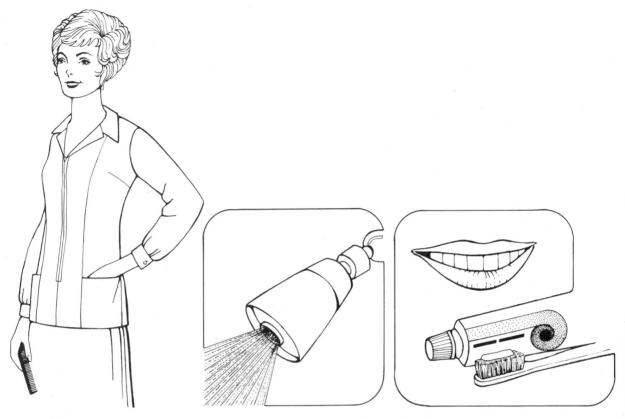

Personal grooming   Personal hygiene

Personal Grooming Personal grooming refers to one's daily appearance and cleanliness. Your clothing should be freshly laundered, your shoes should be polished, your nails should be neatly manicured, your skin should be properly cleansed and cared for, and your hair should be arranged neatly. Cosmetologists deal directly with the public every day, and good appearance is very important. While people shouldn't be judged by appearances, a person's first impressions can be powerful and difficult to change.

Personal Hygiene A good daily personal hygiene schedule is as important to you as it is to your clients. You probably know about the basic parts of personal hygiene, such as bathing or showering and brushing and flossing your teeth and using a mouthwash every day to prevent **halitosis** (hal-eh-TOH-siss), or bad breath. However, there are many other aspects of personal hygiene that many people do not practice. They are very important, and you should remember them. A good place to start is with a working definition. Personal hygiene is the daily routine you follow to preserve and promote your health.

In these days of fast-food restaurants, we often fail to eat properly. We have a cup of coffee and a roll for breakfast, grab a cheeseburger and french fries for lunch, and have fried chicken for dinner. This kind of **nutrition** (noo-TRISH-en) will keep you from performing at your peak level. Good nutrition depends on the **balance** as well as the **amount** of food you eat. A proper balance of meat, fish, eggs, fruits and vegetables, milk, and cereal will make you look better, feel better, and work better. If you are uncertain about your diet, ask your doctor or a nutritionist.

All of us work hard to get ahead. However, sometimes our own hard work can be our worst enemy. Sometimes we work too hard. Exercise, relaxation, and sufficient sleep are necessary for everyone.

Physical Exercise   **Vigorous physical exercise** is one of the most important parts of good health. Exercise provides a fast, continuous pumping of blood through the heart and lungs; and it refreshes the entire body.

We also need sufficient sleep and relaxation. **Everyone's mind** and **body** need sleep. Most people need seven or eight hours of sleep to feel refreshed and relaxed. Without it we become fatigued and cannot function properly. Sleep helps us relieve the frustrations and tensions of everyday activity.

Relaxation   "Getting away from it all" is also very important. Relaxing doesn't mean collapsing into a deep sleep, although short naps can be relaxing. We all need a change of pace. It might be reading a good book, watching television, or going for a walk. Whatever it is, get some kind of relaxation to provide a change of pace for both mind and body.

Good Posture   As a cosmetologist, you will be on your feet much of the time. You should have good body posture and take good care of your feet. If you do not, you will feel a great deal of strain in your back, legs, and feet.

In addition to getting the proper exercise, you can follow a few simple **rules to maintain good posture.** Keep your head up. Your chin should be level with the floor. Your shoulders should be relaxed, and your stomach and lower abdomen should be flat.

Some of your customers will be taller than you are; others will be shorter. Never stoop when you are working. Keep this rule in mind: let the customer come to you whenever possible. If your customer is shorter than you are, do not bend over. **Raise the chair.** If your customer is taller than you are, do not reach up. **Lower the chair.** This is true for all cosmetology services you perform: always maintain correct posture, erect but relaxed.

It is also important to take good care of your feet. This is particularly a problem for female cosmetologists. If you wear heels, they should be low and broad. Low, broad heels will give your body good, natural support. High, skinny heels will cause foot strain. If you have any special problems, consult a foot doctor.

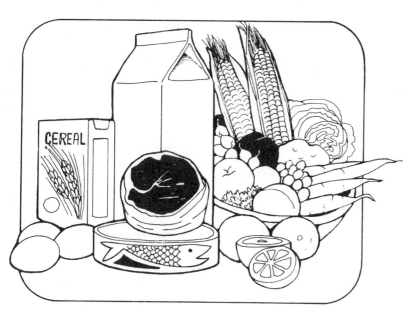

Eat a balanced diet

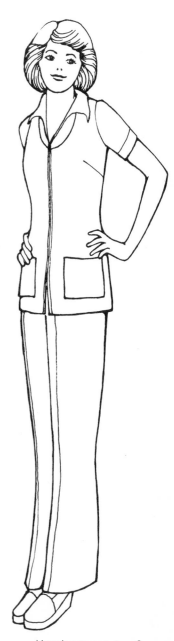

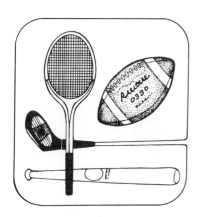

Exercise is important

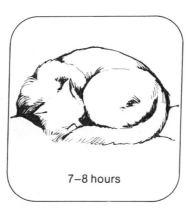

7–8 hours

Do you get enough sleep?

How is your posture?

Communicating with Others

Because careers in cosmetology are people-oriented, they require good communications techniques—the ability to convey one's thoughts and attitudes, both verbal and nonverbal, in a pleasant manner.

Verbal Communication **Verbal communication** concerns what is said and **how** it is said. A client will always appreciate a courteous response or question much more than an impolite answer.

A good rule of thumb is an old saying: many times **how** you say something is much more important than **what** you say. A cheerful tone and proper inflection (emphasis) in your voice let a client know that you are enthusiastic and ready to help. Speak distinctly when you answer the telephone. Remember: a cheerful "May I help you?" when answering a client in person or on the telephone doesn't cost a thing, and it often means the difference between success and failure.

Nonverbal Communication You have probably experienced nonverbal communication, though you may not have realized it at the time. Have you ever walked up to a counter in a store where two clerks were standing? One slinks over to you, slouches, looks all around the store, and then finally asks you what you want. The other walks directly over to you, stands erect but relaxed, looks you straight in the eye, and asks the same question.

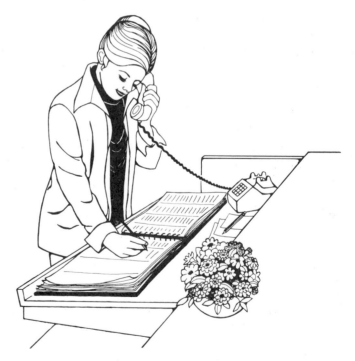

Verbal communications are very important for a successful salon

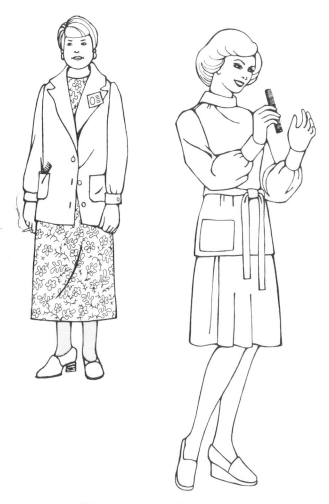

Where are you in this picture?

Both clerks communicated an attitude to you before they spoke a word. You probably felt that the first clerk couldn't care less and that the second clerk was interested in serving you. They may have said exactly the same words in the same tone of voice. The first clerk, in fact, may have been much more anxious than the second clerk to serve you, but that attitude wasn't communicated.

This is important to remember. Nonverbal communication, sometimes called **body language**, tells a client that you are interested even before you speak. One point to remember is that much of **nonverbal communication involves being a good listener;** eye contact is very important. By looking directly at the client when you are speaking and listening, you show that you are interested in what he or she has to say.

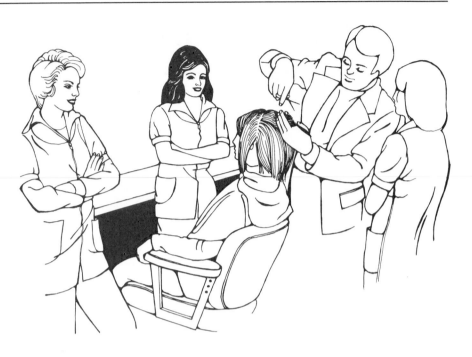

Requirements for a Student

You have just begun your life as a cosmetology student, so you are probably familiar with the general requirements for enrolling in a school of cosmetology in your state. However, some of the information in this section will help you to make your student days successful and will give you an idea of what other cosmetology students are like.

While a person usually can enter a cosmetology program at any age, most state boards (or commissions) of cosmetology (or beauty culture) require that a student be sixteen or seventeen years old before applying for the state's written and demonstration examinations. **But remember:** your state's requirements may be different.

Whatever your age, you will be well on your way to success if you try to work on several personal characteristics. Learning to get along with people and being reliable will make you an attractive student and, later, a good cosmetologist.

Educational requirements vary from state to state, but generally a student must have at least an eighth-grade education. Although courses in science (anatomy, physiology, chemistry, biology), business (economics, accounting, law), and art are not required, they are helpful. Additional education, later in life as well as now, is often needed to progress.

You probably had to have a complete health examination by a doctor before you were accepted as a student, so you know about this requirement. It is good practice to have a checkup every six months. In addition to maintaining general good health, you should ask your doctor to focus on two particular points.

Allergy   You will be exposed to cosmetics, such as shampoo, rouge, lipstick, and hair spray. People who are extremely sensitive to cosmetics may suffer severe reactions to them or become ill if they breathe the fumes from cosmetics in the beauty school or salon.

Color Blindness   **Color blindness** is a partial or total inability to see colors. Some types of color blindness will keep a person from becoming a cosmetologist. While blindness to reds and greens is permitted, blindness to **browns** and **blonds** could keep the student from performing hair-coloring tasks. You can be tested for color blindness by your family eye doctor (see color plate 1).

Cosmetologists are more concerned than the average person about allergies and color blindness. If you specifically ask your doctor to watch for problems in these areas, you will have made him alert to your special interests, and he will be sure to watch for any signs of trouble. This is especially important since you can develop an allergy suddenly, even though you have never had one in the past.

Since a cosmetologist should not work while having a contagious disease such as influenza or strep throat, **it pays to stay healthy.** Be sure to ask your doctor whenever you are in doubt about your health.

Cosmetology students cannot earn money, except tips, from their experience in a school or salon. If you need financial aid, your instructor should be able to help you get the necessary information.

A licensed or registered cosmetologist has successfully completed the written and practical examination given by the state. A variety of terms is used to describe this person. Some of them are:

Requirements for a Licensed or Registered Cosmetologist

Licensed Cosmetologist, L.C.
Registered Cosmetologist, R.C.
Registered Beauty Culturist, R.B.C.
Hairstylist
Operator
Coiffeur (male cosmetologist)
Coiffeuse (female cosmetologist)
Hairdresser

Hair fashions change as rapidly as clothing fashions. Thus, most cosmetologists find it necessary to attend local workshops and seminars to keep pace with the ever-changing hairstyles and technology of new products. These seminars are sponsored by the **Hair America (Official Hair Fashion Committee),** which is the educational arm of the **National Hairdressers and Cosmetologists Association.** Private and public cosmetology schools also offer seminars that should be attended whenever possible. Full-service beauty supply dealers and manufacturers also conduct educational seminars that feature current hairstyles, hairstyling techniques, and new products.

Experienced cosmetologists earn money in proportion to the volume and type of services rendered for their clientele. However, the new graduate hasn't developed a clientele yet, so he or she **must** be paid the minimum hourly rate as required by State or Federal Law.

For example, a newly licensed cosmetologist begins working for My Fair Lady Beauty Salon as a full-time employee. He or she could expect to make the minimum wage times ($\times$) 40 hours per week. If the **Hourly Minimum Wage** were (for example) $4.00 per hour, the employee would figure $4.00 $\times$ 40 hours equals $160.00 per week.

The weekly rate of $160.00 would continue until the employee's receipts (the amount the employee brings into the salon) double. Another way to explain this is that the salon owner's break-even point occurs when the new employee brings in an amount of money for service that is **twice** as much as the employee is being paid at an hourly rate. So in the example, the employee would have to bring into the salon two times (2 $\times$) $160.00, or $320.00. Up until the $320.00 has been brought in per week, the salon owner is **losing money**. This is true because the new employee is paid the $160.00 whether the person does zero clients, or five or ten. Oftentimes, if the employee hasn't developed at least a basic clientele in 3–6 months, he or she should consider additional training.

Guarantee   The "guarantee," as it is sometimes referred to in the salon, is usually an amount of money the salon owner **must** pay the full-time employee **(40 hours per week)**, which is required by a State or Federal **Minimum Wage Law**. For example, if the minimum wage law requires the employer to pay at least $5.00 per hour to all full-time employees of the salon, then the salon MUST pay the person at least $5.00 $\times$ 40 hours = $200.00 — even if the person only is booked with 2 appointments for the entire week.

Commission   An experienced hairdresser with an established clientele usually receives a commission. This **Commission** is a percentage (%) of the money taken into the salon for the services performed by the employee. So, for example, if the employee has agreed to work in the salon for a 50% commission and has brought in $600.00 during the week, he or she would get 50% $\times$ $600.00 = $300.00.

The usual job steps for the newly licensed hairdresser would be to work in a salon for the minimum wage and develop a clientele. When he or she brings in money for services that is twice as much as the **Guarantee**, then, the employee receives the commission on money that is **over** the guarantee.

As an operator's clientele increases, it is reasonably easy to exceed the base pay. As with other jobs, skills and salesmanship in cosmetology increase with experience, and an increase in these abilities will produce a larger clientele.

Barber Stylist

The barber stylist is a person who has graduated from an approved school of barbering and successfully passed a licensing test. The duties of a barber stylist are difficult to define because individual states have such different laws which regulate the practice of this license. For example, some states license barbers and cosmetologists together. Other states have a "cross-over" licensing arrangement, which permits a licensed barber or cosmetologist to obtain the other license with a minimum of additional school, or in some cases, no school. In one state the barber stylist isn't licensed to give permanent waves or manicures, while another state will permit the person to perform all services. But there does seem to be a tendency toward some sort of a merging of the function of these two boards. This process has started in some states, and more changes will probably occur in the next 10 years. The term **tonsorial** is sometimes used for that which pertains to a barber or barbering.

Manicurist

The manicuring business is more popular today than it has ever been. Many states have a separate license for a manicurist. Manicuring became "big business" with the introduction of new products and services for the manicurist to offer their clients. Among these new products are services to strengthen and beautify the fingernails, and in some cases, the toenails. Nail wrapping and the application of artificial nails has greatly increased the number of various services in the beauty salon, and also the barber salon (in some cases where permitted by law). Many states also license manicuring salons as a separate and different business from the beauty salon.

Esthetician

Esthetics is a profession in which a person specializes in **preservation** and **beautification of the face and neck of the client**. This also is a very lucrative business in many areas of the world, particularly, with the emphasis today on exercise and everyone wanting to look young "forever." The practice involves specially formulated products, vitamins, facial procedures, facial appliances to clean, stimulate, and supposedly preserve the skin. Facial salons have been very successful in many areas of the country.

Electrologist

The electrologist practices the art of electrology. The electrologist uses different kinds of electrical current that travels through a very fine needle to permanently **remove unwanted facial and body hair** for the client. Once again, fashion conscious clients who want to look their best all the time pay the electrologist to remove unwanted hair permanently. Licensing laws vary considerably from state to state, and in fact some states don't license electrologists at all. There is some speculation that with the on-going political pressure to "protect the consumer," more and more areas of the world will license electrologists to insure that the consumer (client) will receive a service from a competent person who practices as an electrologist. Currently, electrology is taught by the manufacturer in most instances, rather than a licensed school with a curricula.

Research and Field Technicians

The **research technician** works for a cosmetics manufacturer. The technician usually works in the research salon and tests new products and com-

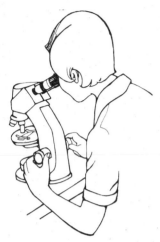

Research technician

pares them to determine their quality, safety, cost, and marketability. The research technician works on clients who come to the salon for *free* quality services. These clients are required to sign release forms because of the experimental nature of the work performed.

The **field technician** travels extensively throughout an area (one of several states) and demonstrates a manufacturer's products in salons, schools, and educational seminars.

Research and field technicians must be of legal age, eighteen to twenty-one years old, depending on the state in which they work. They should be mature, poised, and observant. They should be able to speak effectively before small or large groups of people.

Most state laws require that any technician who is practicing cosmetic sciences on another living person must be a licensed or registered cosmetologist. Manufacturers may also require one or two years of experience in a salon.

The base salary for both a research technician and a field technician is usually between the salary of the average salon operator and that of a manager-operator in a given area. The salary of the research technician is usually increased at six-month intervals, while salary increases for the field technician are often based on a bonus program that reflects an increase in dollar volume of sales for the territory worked by the individual. The field technician's traveling expenses are also paid by the company.

Competition and Platform Hairstylists

Hairstylists who have a creative flair and enjoy the challenge of competing or performing before large audiences often become either **competition** or **platform hairstylists** in addition to working in a salon.

A hairstyling contest is an event in which cosmetologists challenge each other's hairdressing skills. Hairstyles are judged for originality, execution, adaptability, and trend. **Originality** refers to the general design of the style. **Execution** refers to how well the design was set and combed into the hair. **Adaptability** refers to the suitability of the hairstyle: did the hairstyle improve the appearance of the model? **Trend** is the basic silhouette and design from which the contestants work. Most contests have their own special rules that are distributed before each contest.

Contests are sponsored by the National Hairdressers and Cosmetologists Association or one of its local affiliates as well as manufacturers and beauty supply dealers. Newly licensed or registered cosmetologists as well as very experienced practitioners enter contests. Many also encourage student competition on the local, state, and national levels.

Trophies, plaques, cups, and cash prizes are awarded. Many different types of contests may be entered: student, novice, women's daytime, evening, and fantasy hairstyling as well as air waving and men's hairstyling.

Often, cosmetologists who repeatedly win these contests are offered jobs to conduct **platform demonstrations** at educational seminars for manufacturers. These demonstrations usually take place on Sundays and Mondays

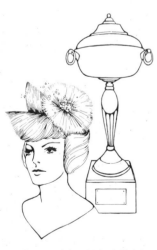

Competition hairstylist

in the fall and spring. These seminars can vary in size from five to two hundred persons. Platform artists are paid a daily rate in addition to all expenses for travel, meals, and lodging. The favorable publicity that contestants and platform stylists receive can help increase their clientele.

In some salons the **manager-operator** only supervises the work of other operators, while in others he or she also serves clients. In either case the manager-operator usually must be legally an adult and have received a manager-operator's license from the state board (commission) of cosmetology. Licensing requirements vary from state to state.

Manager-Operator

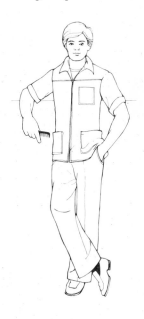

A manager-operator needs several special skills. In addition to being a registered cosmetologist who has a basic education and is skilled in all of the salon's basic services, the effective manager of an average salon (three or four operators) should have two or three years' work experience. He or she should be able to assist the owner in managing the salon. He or she also must have the personality and patience to supervise workers. Bookkeeping training and knowledge of other management tasks, such as purchasing supplies and attending management seminars on the MBO (Management by Objectives) system, also can be helpful.

The pay range for a manager-operator varies from salon to salon. Some of the usual methods of compensation are: (a) an additional weekly commission of 5 percent over the operator's commission (for a total of 55 percent); (b) an additional commission of 5 percent at the end of the year; or (c) an additional percentage above the total dollar figure for the salon.

The knowledge that a manager-operator gains can prepare him or her for salon ownership.

A **salon owner** usually is a working cosmetologist who has developed **business** as well as professional skills. He or she should be an expert technician who has developed a large clientele. The owner also has developed the personal qualities necessary for dealing with a wide variety of customers and employees.

Salon Owner

Although a person can become a salon owner as soon as he or she is legally an adult, most salon owners have had at least one year's experience as a manager-operator. This experience is very helpful for operating one's own business—for everything from advertising to bookkeeping.

An owner can—and should—take advantage of other educational opportunities. Seminars on management and staff-training programs are available and helpful.

The working salon owner gets a 58 percent commission on the work he or she performs. (This percentage equals the operator's 50 percent, a manager-operator's 5 percent, plus another 3 percent.) Of course, he or she gets a profit (money left over after expenses have been paid). The salon owner takes all of the financial risk (the owner must have an excellent credit rating

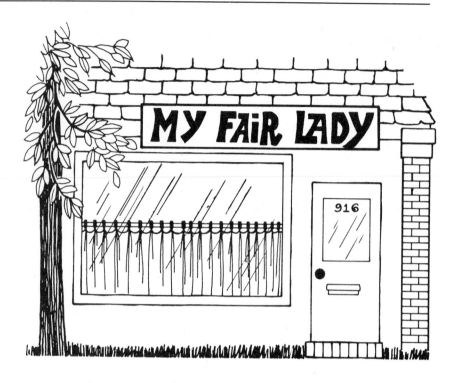

and make a down payment for the purchase of supplies, equipment, and salaries to open the salon), but in the long run a successful owner makes more money than an operator.

Public and Private School Instructors

Instructors are licensed, registered, or certified to teach by the state board (commission) of cosmetology and the state's department of education. Some state departments of education require college courses including human relations, philosophy of vocational education, teaching methods and practices, tests and measurements, and course construction. State boards (commissions) of cosmetology require successful completion of a written and practical exam. Some states require instructors to take yearly physicals. The instructor is generally an expert in most phases of cosmetology. Although age requirements vary with states, cosmetologists usually do not become instructors until they are about twenty-six years old.

The successful instructor has exceptional patience and an interest in the student as an individual and a potential professional. At times he or she must be like a counselor, friend, or parent to students. Salaries range anywhere from $7,500 to $35,000 a year. The actual salary would depend on the instructor's salon experience and education.

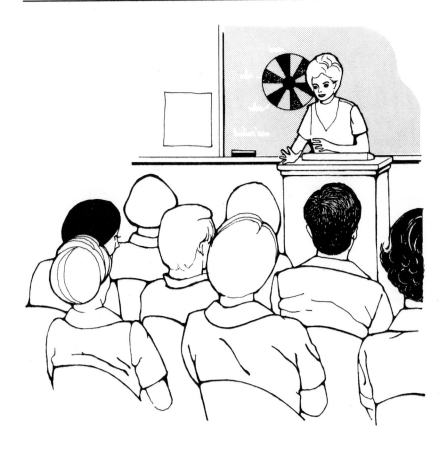

Allergy Extreme sensitivity to a factor or substance in the environment.

Barber stylist A person who has graduated from an approved school of barbering and successfully passed a licensing test.

Body language Communication through eye contact, facial expression, posture, and other nonverbal means.

Color blindness A partial or total inability to see or differentiate colors.

Commission A percentage of money taken into the salon for the services performed by the employee.

Competition hairstylist A hairstylist who enters hairstyling contests to win trophies, plaques, cups, or cash prizes.

Cosmetologist A person who is licensed to perform the services of cosmetology.

Cosmetology The art and science of beauty care involving care of the skin, hair, scalp, and nails.

Electrologist A person who uses different kinds of electrical current that travels through a very fine needle to permanently remove unwanted facial and body hair.

GLOSSARY

Esthetician The practitioner who specializes in the preservation and beautification of the face and neck.

Esthetics The specialization in preservation and beautification of the face and neck.

Field technician A cosmetologist who travels extensively throughout an area and demonstrates a manufacturer's products in salons, schools, and educational seminars.

Good posture A way of holding the body so that the head is up, the chin is level with the floor, the shoulders are relaxed, and the stomach and lower abdomen are flat.

Guarantee The amount of money a salon owner must pay a full-time employee, which is required by a state or federal minimum wage law.

Halitosis (hal-eh-TOH-siss) Stale or foul-smelling breath.

Manager-operator A legal adult who is a registered cosmetologist and is licensed to manage and operate a salon.

Manicurist The practitioner who specializes in the care of hands and fingernails; sometimes feet and toenails also.

Nonverbal communication Communication of one's thoughts and attitudes nonverbally; body language.

Nutrition (noo-TRISH-en) The process of maintaining good health by eating a proper balance and amount of food.

Personal grooming One's appearance of attractiveness, cleanliness, and good health.

Personal hygiene The daily routine followed to preserve and promote health and cleanliness.

Platform hairstylist A hairstylist who is paid to conduct demonstrations before an audience, such as at educational seminars.

Research technician A cosmetologist who works for a cosmetics manufacturer testing new products and comparing them to determine their quality, safety, cost, and marketability.

Salon owner A working cosmetologist who has developed business as well as professional skills and owns a beauty salon.

Tonsorial Pertaining to a barber (as a tonsorial artist) or barbering.

Verbal communication Communication of thoughts and attitudes through what is spoken and the tone and inflection used to say it.

QUESTIONS

1. Define cosmetology.
2. Name three general areas in which the cosmetologist is licensed to perform services.
3. Define personal hygiene.
4. Does good posture have anything to do with taking care of your feet?
5. What is it called when a client has a reaction to a cosmetic product used in the salon?

6. According to law, what is the least amount of money that is paid to a full-time beginning cosmetologist?
7. To be considered a full-time employee, how many hours per week must you work?
8. A licensed person who specializes in preservation and beautification is called what?
9. What is the technical name for the person who permanently removes hair, using an electrical device?
10. What is halitosis?

ANSWERS

1. Cosmetology is the art and science of beauty care. 2. The cosmetologist is licensed to perform services on the hair, skin, and nails. 3. Personal hygiene deals with care of the individual. 4. Yes. 5. Allergy, or an allergic reaction. 6. The minimum wage. 7. Forty hours per week. 8. Esthetician. 9. Electrologist. 10. Bad breath.

Sanitizing Implements and Equipment 2

Purpose

Promoting and protecting good health in the community is called **public hygiene** or **sanitation** (san-eh-TAY-shun). Everyone who provides services to the public has a responsibility to help protect the health of the community. As a cosmetologist you will perform services on the hair, scalp, and other parts of a client's body, so you must keep the salon clean and sanitary by following certain procedures to destroy harmful germs that can contaminate working implements and equipment and spread disease.

Major Objective

With the sanitation supplies pictured, use chemical agents and ultraviolet rays to sanitize implements and equipment in the salon. Use the proper steps to sanitize the setting, combing, and cutting implements contained in your implement kit within 20 minutes.

Level of Acceptability

Score 75 percent or better on a multiple-choice exam on the information in this chapter.

Knowing Subobjectives

1. Define the terms used to describe and classify bacteria.
2. Describe five methods of sanitation.
3. Describe the measures used to sanitize the service area.
4. Describe safety measures for school/salon-chemical storage, fire safety, and first aid.

Doing Subobjectives

5. Sanitize the setting, combing, and cutting implements and other equipment in the salon.

KNOWING SUBOBJECTIVE 1

Define the terms used to describe and classify bacteria.

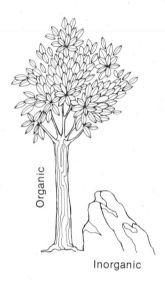

Organic

Inorganic

A bright, sunny day makes you feel happy to be alive. Everything seems to be bursting with life—the birds in the air, the trees and flowers—even the rocks seem to be alive. Of course, you know perfectly well that rocks aren't alive. But all of those things have at least one thing in common: they are **matter**. Matter is anything that takes up space and has weight.

Scientists talk about two kinds of matter. One kind is **inorganic** matter. It has never been alive. The other kind is **organic** (awr-GAN-ik) matter. It includes all things that are living or have been alive in the past. A living tree is organic matter, but so is a dead tree. Unlike inorganic matter, organic matter can be food for other living things after it dies. (For instance, when leaves die and fall from a tree, they provide food for the tree and the grass around the tree.)

Organic matter comes in many shapes and sizes. The basic units of organic matter are called **cells**. (There are smaller units, but you don't need to be concerned about them here.) Any independent group of cells is called an **organism**. We see many organisms around us every day. Some of them are rather simple, while others are very complicated and are described by complicated scientific formulas. But there is another kind of organism that some people don't even realize exists. They look right at it everyday, but they don't see it. These are **microorganisms** (migh-kroh-OR-gehn-iz-uhmz). Humans can see microorganisms only by using a microscope. Some of them are made up of only a few—or even one—cell.

One kind of microorganism that cosmetologists must know about is **bacteria** (bak-TIR-ee-ah). The scientific study of bacteria is called **bacteriology**. Bacteria are one-celled microorganisms, sometimes called microbes (MIGH-krobs). They are everywhere—in the air, on the ground, and even inside of us. Scientists only discovered them a little more than a hundred years ago. Before that time, people lived in constant fear of diseases and epidemics like the Black Death, which killed over one-third of all the people living in Europe six hundred years ago. Although people today sometimes talk about "epidemics," no one living in a modern country like the United States needs to worry about an epidemic like the Black Death unless he or she ignores the rules of good personal and public hygiene.

Safety Tip

The reason for this difference is very simple: public health, or sanitation. After scientists discovered that some bacteria cause disease (pathogens [PATH-ah-jenz], or **pathogenic** [path-ah-JEN-ik] bacteria), governments could make and enforce laws to improve sanitation and thus protect the health of the community. This is why knowledge of bacteria and sanitation is so important for the cosmetologist.

There are two basic kinds of bacteria: **pathogens** and **nonpathogens**. **Pathogenic bacteria** can **cause disease**. They are commonly called **germs**. **Nonpathogenic bacteria** do not cause disease. Actually most of them are very helpful (one particular type—**saprophytes** [SAP-roh-fightz]—causes

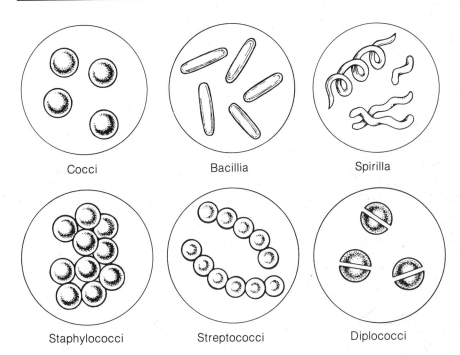

Cocci   Bacillia   Spirilla

Staphylococci   Streptococci   Diplococci

dead organic matter to decay and thus helps enrich the soil). The bacteria in yeast cause bread to rise, and other bacteria create the alcohol in wine.

Pathogenic bacteria are divided into three types: **cocci**, (KOK-sigh), **spirilla** (spigh-RIL-ah), and **bacilli** (bah-SIL-igh). Each has a different **shape**, which can be seen through a microscope. Cocci have **round** shapes, spirilla have **spiral** shapes, and bacilli are shaped like **rods**.

Cocci (round) usually cause pus-forming diseases such as boils, abscesses, and pustules. There are three forms of cocci: staphylococci (staf-eh-low-KOK-sigh), streptococci (strep-tah-KOK-sigh), and diplococci (dip-low-KOK-sigh).

Staphylococci, which usually grow in clusters, generally produce **local** infections (those found in a small area on or in the body). Hospitals have found that this type of infection can spread very easily unless all objects that come in contact with patients are sterilized properly.

Streptococci, on the other hand, usually cause **general infections** (those that are caused by the spread of bacteria through the bloodstream to a large part of the body). Rheumatic fever is an example of a general infection caused by streptococci.

Of course, local and general infections can be caused by many other types of bacteria:

Diplococci (occur in pairs) cause bacterial pneumonia.
Spirilla (spiral) cause cholera and syphilis.
Bacilli (rod-shaped) produce such serious diseases as diphtheria, leprosy, tuberculosis, and typhoid fever.

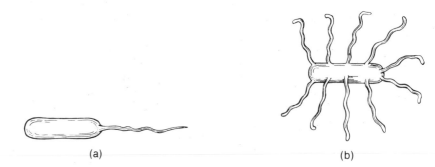

(a)   (b)

Bacilli: (a) with one extension (tail), (b) with many extensions (tails)

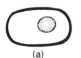

(a)

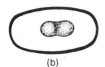

(b)

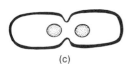

(c)

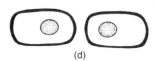

(d)

Cell division: (a) bacteria cell, (b) mature cell, (c) dividing cell, (d) two "new" cells

Both bacilli and spirilla have **flagella** (fleh-JEL-leh) or **cilia** (SIL-ee-ah), which are whiplike extensions (tails) that cause the cell to move in a liquid.

Pathogenic bacteria must have **favorable conditions to grow** and cause disease. Some of the conditions are: **heat, moisture, and the absence of direct sunlight.**

All forms of bacteria multiply (reproduce) by division. As the cell is nourished, it grows larger. When it grows as large as it can, it divides itself into two cells that are the same size. These are called **daughter** cells. This process of cell division is called **mitosis** (migh-TOH-sis). Mitosis can happen as often as once every twenty minutes.

When bacteria are growing and multiplying in favorable conditions, they are in an **active cycle**. When unfavorable conditions exist for bacteria, the cells die or become **inactive**. Some bacteria, including bacilli, can live in an inactive cycle by forming spherical **spores**. These spores, which move through the air easily, are much more **resistant** to heat, chemicals, and sunlight in this inactive state. The bacteria live as spores until their surrounding conditions improve. Then they change back to the original form and return to the active cycle. Although spore formation is not very common among bacteria, it is a factor you should consider when keeping the salon sanitary. Some spores can survive for a long time in extreme heat (water boils at 212 degrees Fahrenheit) and cold (liquid helium freezes at − 507 degrees Fahrenheit).

Viruses are especially important kinds of pathogens. They differ from bacteria in size, characteristics, and activity. They are called **ultramicroscopic** because they cannot be seen unless they are magnified up to one million times by a scan electron microscope.

A virus (VIGH-ruhss) **is essentially a parasite** (an animal or plant that lives in or on another organism without helping it live). Viruses can enter many kinds of cells, reproduce and then destroy the cell. This is called a viral infection. When this happens, thousands of viruses are able to infect other cells.

Viruses probably cause more than half of the diseases affecting humans, animals, and plants. Influenza, chicken pox, the common cold, and certain types of hepatitis are caused by viruses.

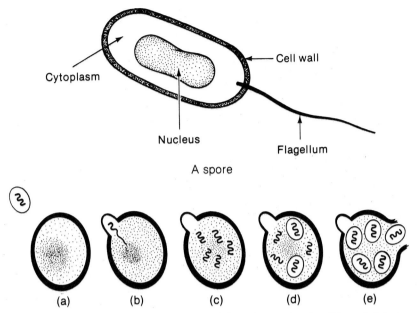

Cytoplasm

Cell wall

Nucleus

Flagellum

A spore

(a)   (b)   (c)   (d)   (e)

Viral infection: (a) virus approaches cell; (b) virus attaches itself to cell; (c) virus multiplies inside cell; (d) virus matures; (e) virus bursts from destroyed cell and spreads to new cells

Safety Tip

Normally, most **illnesses are caused by pathogenic bacteria** that enter the **mouth, nose, ears, or broken skin**, so the cosmetologist must be especially concerned about bacteria that affect the head, arms, and feet. Disease-causing bacteria are often sent into the air by a person who has a disease. These bacteria are also transferred to other people by hands, food, drinking glasses, or other objects touched by a person who has an **infection**. An infection occurs when pathogenic bacteria or viruses have entered a body and multiply to the point of interfering with its normal state. Infections may or may not be **contagious** (kuhn-TAY-juhss). If a disease is contagious, it can be transmitted to another person through touch or through the air. Another term used to describe contagious is **communicable** (koh-MYOO-ni-kah-behl).

A person can carry disease-producing agents and infect others without himself being ill. Such a person is called a **carrier**.

A person who has a contagious disease (such as influenza, ringworm, or head lice) should **isolate** (separate) himself from others. It is very important for cosmetologists who have contagious diseases to isolate themselves since they can infect clients through close contact and handling of implements and equipment. It is just as important for practitioners to refuse service to clients having contagious diseases.

A **susceptible** person is one who is likely to become ill from direct or indirect contact with disease-causing bacteria or viruses. For example, a person in poor health is more likely to become ill from such contact than a healthy person.

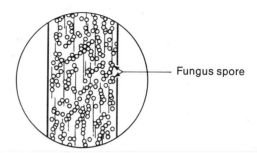

Microscopic view of a hair infected with ringworm

Immunity (ih-MYOO-neh-tee) is the ability of the body's defense mechanisms to fight off disease. The body fights bacterial infections in two basic ways: **active immunity (natural)** and **passive immunity (acquired)**. The body defends itself in the following manner:

1. **Active (natural) immunity** occurs when the body makes **antibodies** (also called white blood cells), which destroy harmful bacteria in the blood. In addition, when certain poisons **(toxins)** develop in the blood, the body produces **antitoxins**, which destroy the poisons.

   The outermost layer of the skin (**epidermis** [ep-eh-DER-mis]) protects the body from bacteria. When this layer of skin is punctured or cut, bacteria can enter, and an infection may develop if the wound is not treated.

   When the active immunity systems are fighting disease, they produce waste products in the same way that a fire produces ashes. These waste products are discarded by the body through the lungs, sudoriferous glands (sweat glands), intestines, and urinary tract.

2. **Passive (acquired) immunity** occurs when antibodies from another person or animal are injected into the body. The most common form of passive immunity is shots, such as polio or flu shots.

KNOWING SUBOBJECTIVE 2

Describe five methods of sanitation.

Now that you have read about the various forms of bacteria, there are two terms that you will want to learn and keep in mind as you clean your working area.

The process of **sterilization** (stehr-il-eh-ZAY-shuhn) is used to kill all bacteria (pathogenic and nonpathogenic) on an implement. The process of **sanitation** destroys pathogenic bacteria. Although sterilizing kills all bacteria and is, really, the ideal way to clean, it is almost impossible to make implements sterile and to **keep** them that way. Bacteria are everywhere, including the air around us. So, even if an implement is sterilized, as soon as it hits the air in the salon, it no longer is sterile. But it will be sanitary—**aseptic** (ay-SEP-tik) (free from pathogenic bacteria)—if the entire school or salon has been cleaned thoroughly. This is why it is very important to keep everything in the salon sanitary. If anything is toxic (unsanitary) so that pathogenic bacteria are in the salon or school, it is called septic (SEP-tik) (from sepsis).

Public health or sanitation describes the set of procedures used to stop the spread of communicable diseases and the development of other infections caused by pathogenic agents. Public health departments and state boards of cosmetology make rules and regulations that require salons and schools to keep their equipment and implements, working areas, and building in a sanitary condition at all times.

The beauty school or salon uses two basic methods of sanitizing implements and equipment: processes involving **chemical** and **physical** agents.

Five kinds of **chemical** sanitizing agents are used: (1) antiseptics, (2) disinfectants, (3) fumigants, (4) bactericides, and (5) germicides.

Antiseptics (an-teh-SEP-tiks) halt or prevent the growth of pathogenic bacteria. They are often used to maintain the sanitary condition of implements already sterilized. A 3–5 **percent hydrogen peroxide** solution is an antiseptic often used by doctors to cleanse the skin.

Disinfectants (dis-in-FEK-tahnts), **fumigants** (FYOO-mi-gahnts), **bactericides** (bak-TIR-eh-sighdz), and **germicides** (JER-meh-sighdz) are chemicals that destroy pathogenic bacteria. You should use these cleaners very carefully. These chemicals are very useful for sterilizing implements, but they are very strong and usually are caustic, which means that they can burn your skin.

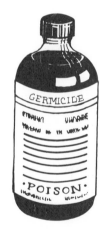

Antiseptics, on the other hand, are not disinfectants. They do not destroy all bacteria. They can be used on the skin. Also, most disinfectants can be diluted with water and used as antiseptics.

You should remember something else when you use any of these cleaners. Sanitizing methods **do not kill bacteria instantly**. Complete destruction of bacteria always requires some time, depending on the agent or method used.

Numerous chemical cleaners are available. Sanitizing chemical agents come in different strengths and forms, including liquid, tablet, capsule, and powder. Many sold by full-service beauty suppliers are ready to use, requiring no mixing or diluting. **In choosing a disinfectant, you should consider the following**:

1. Which chemical agent is recommended by the state board of cosmetology or state health department?
2. Is the chemical agent easy to buy and inexpensive?
3. Is the chemical agent easy and safe to use, or will it cause serious skin irritation?
4. Is it noncorrosive (made so that it does not harm plastic or metal implements) and does it work quickly?

Most sanitizing chemicals are **very poisonous**. If taken internally, they can cause injury or death, so read the directions on the label very carefully.

Safety Tip

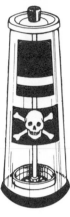

Sanitizer

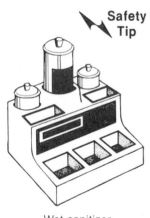

Safety Tip

Wet sanitizer

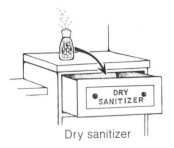

Dry sanitizer

Always follow all safety precautions, directions for diluting, and other procedures recommended by the manufacturer. Chemicals should be poured carefully to avoid waste and damage.

Combing and setting implements are ordinarily sanitized with **quaternary ammonium** (KWOT-er-ner-ee ah-MOHN-ee-um) **("quats")** or **formalin**, which is a **formaldehyde** (for-MAL-deh-highd) solution. **Metal** implements, such as blow-comb attachments, curling irons, manicure implements, scissors, and shapers (razors), are sanitized with **70 percent ethyl alcohol or 99 percent isopropyl alcohol**. Equipment such as shampoo bowls and fixtures in the dispensary and bathroom are sanitized with Lysol or diluted forms of formaldehyde.

Use of quaternary ammonium compounds varies from state to state. To be effective, a quats solution must be as strong as 1 part quats to 200 parts water. For safety, it should not be stronger than 1 part quats to 200 parts water. A ⅔ ounce of quats in one gallon of water will yield a **1:200** sanitizing solution. With this strength formula, it will kill herpes simplex virus, influenza A, New Castle disease, adenovirus type 3, staph bacteria, fungus, and vegetable bacteria. **ALWAYS FOLLOW MANUFACTURER'S DIRECTIONS. WEAR GLOVES WHEN REMOVING IMPLEMENTS** from wet sanitizer with this solution. The ordinary quats usage is 1 part **to 200 parts water**. Formalin is the disinfectant used in some salons. It basically is 37 percent formaldehyde, 6.5 percent methanol, and 56.5 percent water.

The use of quats and formalin brings up an important point you should remember whenever you use any chemical. The kind of disinfectant that is required will vary from state to state (for instance, some states prohibit the use of formaldehyde), so it is very important to **follow the label directions of whatever disinfectant you are using, follow the requirements of your state board of cosmetology or state health department, and consult your instructor or manager before you mix a disinfectant**.

Chemical agents are used in two kinds of sanitizing containers: **wet sanitizers** and **dry sanitizers**.

The **wet sanitizer** is used to sterilize the implements, and the **dry sanitizer** keeps them sanitized until they are used.

The **wet sanitizer** uses water and a chemical agent. The wet sanitizer must be **nonmetal**, large, and deep enough so that combs, brushes, rollers, and other items can be covered by the chemical solution. It also must have a cover to prevent contamination.

The **dry sanitizer** is an airtight cabinet or drawer that has a chemical agent in it. The unit can be made of wood, metal, or plastic. It must be large enough to hold combing, setting, or cutting implements after they have been removed from the wet sanitizer. The germicide called a **fumigant**, which emits bacteria-destroying vapors, is used. The vapors are effective only if the drawer or door of the unit is closed. A solution of formaldehyde is put in a capped salt shaker. This shaker can be placed, standing upright, in the bottom of a dry sanitizer and can be used as an excellent fumigant. The

---

FORMALDEHYDE MIXING CHART

Given 37% formaldehyde (formalin); use the generally accepted conversion of 1000cc (or ml) per quart:

To one quart of water add:

100 cc or 3.2 ounces to obtain a 10% formalin solution
50 cc or 1.6 ounces to obtain a 5% formalin solution
30 cc or .96 ounces to obtain a 3% formalin solution
20 cc or .64 ounces to obtain a 2% formalin solution
10 cc or .32 ounces to obtain a 1% formalin solution

To one gallon of water add:

400cc or 12.8 ounces to obtain a 10% formalin solution
200cc or 6.4 ounces to obtain a 5% formalin solution
120cc or 3.84 ounces to obtain a 3% formalin solution
80cc or 2.56 ounces to obtain a 2% formalin solution
40cc or 1.28 ounces to obtain a 1% formalin solution

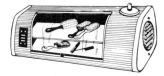

Ultraviolet dry sanitizer

solution should contain one tablespoon of borax and one tablespoon of formaldehyde. Ready-to-use tablets are also available and preferred. Not all states recommend the use of fumigants.

Ultraviolet rays are the salon's most often used sanitation method involving **physical** agents. These rays have a germicidal effect. That is, they kill most bacteria and some viruses. One type of ultraviolet sanitizer has a small blower-heater that dries the combing and setting implements while the rays sterilize them. Although they are expensive, ultraviolet sanitizers are used in some schools and salons.

Two other physical methods for sterilization, **moist heat** and **dry heat**, are **not** ordinarily used in the beauty school or salon. Moist heat, for example, is not used because it takes too long and can damage setting and combing implements.

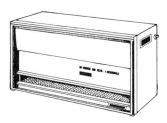

Ultraviolet dry sanitizer

KNOWING SUBOBJECTIVE 3

Sanitary measures must be used for the care of: (1) all implements used in a service, (2) personal habits of the cosmetologist, and (3) the area in which the service is performed.

In this subobjective, you will read about the procedures used to keep the beauty school or salon building in sanitary condition. This will include air purification, plumbing, furnishings, floors, and lighting. The procedures used to sanitize implements will be discussed in the chapters in which the implements are used. Personal habits will be discussed where they apply to the job.

The number of products used daily by the practitioner has increased dramatically. Tiny chemical particles from cold waving solutions, chemical re-

Describe the measures used to sanitize the service area.

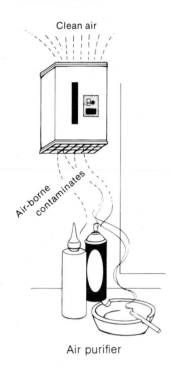

Clean air

Air-borne contaminates

Air purifier

laxers, hair sprays, oxidizing permanent hair colors, bleaches, and other so-lutions are in the air. To a certain extent, this air pollution is an occupational hazard, but the school or salon owner who is aware of this problem can re-duce or eliminate the bad effects of these chemical particles and pathogenic microorganisms.

No single piece of equipment is economically practical to provide proper air purification for the salon or school. A combination of appliances seems to be the best solution.

Electronic air precipitators (air purifier or air cleaner) remove particles and circulate the air. The appliances usually are rated by their CFM (cubic feet per minute). They vary in their capacity to circulate a **cubic foot** of air per **minute**.

Most electronic air precipitators filter the air by drawing air through cel-lulose and/or charcoal filters. Then the air is drawn toward electrodes, and impurities are deposited onto another filter. The cleaned air is then blown back into the salon. Although they are small, they do a good job of remov-ing viruses, bacteria, and chemicals from the air inside the building.

Air conditioners cool, dehumidify (remove moisture), and cleanse pollu-tants from air coming into the building from the outside. Air is ordinarily cleansed through a fiberglass filter and circulated through the building but the air purifier cleans the air better.

Forced-air furnaces heat and, to some degree, cleanse the air. As air in-side the building cools, it returns to the furnace where it is drawn through a fiberglass filter and heated. Then it is blown back into the working area. **Ex-haust fans** (ventilating fans) also can help circulate the air, although they do not clean it. Exhaust fans blow the unhealthy air outside.

The level of humidity in a room is related to the degree of heat needed for comfort. Adjusting the humidity level with a humidifier or dehumidi-fier, with the advice of an appliance dealer, can make the salon more com-fortable. **Humidifiers** add moisture to the air, preventing excessive drying of the skin and reducing static electricity which may be generated during hair combing. **Dehumidifiers** remove excessive moisture from the air.

Schools and salons using a good air-sanitation program generally have fewer lost work days due to illnesses caused by bacteria.

All schools and salons must have **continuous hot and cold water**. Most public health departments also require a **vacuum breaker** for each shampoo bowl. This fixture prevents reverse flow of contaminated water from back-ing up into the fresh water supply system.

Bathroom plumbing fixtures must be sanitized and in good working or-der. Clean, individual hand towels must also be provided.

School and salon furnishings and floors must have surfaces that can be washed and sanitized regularly. Sanitizing chairs and other equipment is covered in the procedures section of this chapter. Curtains should be wash-able and must be kept clean.

Adequate lighting is necessary because of the nature of the services of-fered in the beauty school and salon. Any reputable lighting dealer can pro-vide advice.

Safety Tip

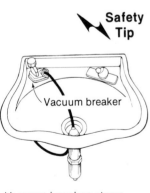

Vacuum breaker

Vacuum breaker stops unclean water from mixing with fresh water

An important part of preparing to be a licensed cosmetologist is recognizing the importance of safety. Knowing how to work in a safe environment is an important part of the licensing requirements. Making the school/salon a safe place to give and receive services is everybody's job—not just the job of the instructor/manager. Everyone has to BE AWARE OF SAFETY and practice hairdressing skills in the most safe manner for everyone in the school/salon. Everyone has to "pitch in."

This subobjective will explain what you can do to make the school/salon a safe place to work and what you should do if a certain kind of accident happens. The information that follows will describe safety considerations when using certain chemicals; how to store chemicals safely, and why; fire safety measures; and first aid for minor cuts and burns.

Describe safety measures for the school/salon— chemical storage, fire safety, first aid.

There are many products used in the school/salon that could be dangerous to you or the client. For example, formaldehyde is a suspected cause of cancer, so many states have prohibited the use of it for sanitizing purposes. Since each state has a different set of laws, you will need to check with your instructor to determine whether formaldehyde (formalin) is used in your state. If it is used, then you should take extra care when using it.

Hazardous Chemicals

Formaldehyde Safety Precautions:

1. Read mixing instructions before use.
2. Mix exactly according to manufacturer's directions.
3. Wear gloves or use forceps when removing combs, brushes or other implements from a wet sanitizer containing formalin.
4. Keep formalin fumes away from your eyes and nose and try not to inhale any fumes, which may irritate the delicate tissues of the eyes and nose.
5. Safely store formaldehyde (formalin) well out of reach of children, who may not know that it is poisonous.
6. Carefully label this and all products if you pour them from their original container into another container, so that anyone picking up a bottle will be able to clearly see what product he/she is about to use.

 Safety Tip

Alcohol, nail polish remover, some instant conditioners, and **hair spray** are other examples of potentially hazardous products, in that they are very **flammable**. Flammable products should always be stored in **metal cabinets** whenever possible, and they should be **kept from** sources of extreme **heat**. For example, the above products should **not** be stored near a water heater, furnace, or other appliances where a spark, heat, or flame may ignite them and cause a fire. A client must not be allowed to smoke cigarettes, pipes, or cigars when these products are in use.

Safety Tip

As a student, you probably wouldn't think that **soiled towels** are very hazardous—but they are—if not stored in a **closed metal or fireproof container**. The problem lies in the fact that the ammonia used to tint hair sticks to a towel and is mixed with a towel used to give a cold wave. The sodium bromate from the cold wave's neutralizer clings to the towel, and mixing towels saturated with ammonia and sodium bromate causes the formation of **bromine gas**. This gas is likely to ignite spontaneously **(spontaneous combustion)**. That is, a fire starts without an outside source of flame such as a match or spark. Storage of these towels in a metal container is very important!

Storage of Chemicals

Light, temperature, moisture, and air are the four most important things to consider when storing products.

Safety Tip

Light   Light, particularly ultraviolet light from the sun changes the chemical makeup of products. Have you ever noticed that some products used in the school, salon, or home are packaged in dark colored, amber bottles? The dark container protects the contents from light. As additional protection, these products should probably be stored in a closed cabinet, rather than displayed in the front window of the salon.

Temperature   Heat in any form also changes the chemical makeup of products. The likely forms of heat found in the school would be as follows: hot sun shining through an undraped window; furnace; hot water heater; hair dryers; wig dryers; towel dryer; and curling irons. It is wise to store all professional products away from any form of heat in a cool, dry area of the salon.

Moisture   Moisture from an extremely damp basement may cause a product to become moldy. Store supplies in a DRY AREA. If beauty supplies are contaminated with water from too much moisture, they may become inactive (won't work).

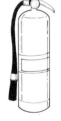
Fire extinguisher

Schools and salons are required by law to have a fire extinguisher. It must be in working order, and you should know how to use it

Air   Air will dilute (water down) most products or allow the active chemicals in a product to escape. Keeping all products tightly capped and in their original box or package will allow you to keep the chemicals in their active state much longer than if you left the products uncapped. Tightly cap all products after use! Clean air makes for a **safe work environment**.

Never store any salon supplies or chemicals in the same area where food is also stored. For example, do not store sanitizing chemicals alongside of breakfast cereal or any other food product.

Fire Safety

Most state, province, county, local, or municipal laws require that any public service business have at least one **fire extinguisher** conveniently located in the school or salon. The fire extinguisher must be regularly inspected and serviced at **least yearly** so that in the event of a fire, it will work. A large business may be required to have several fire extinguishers. In the event of a fire, be sure that your clients leave the school. Call your **local emergency phone number**. Many areas use the "911" emergency phone number, but this may vary from area to area. Check with your instructor to determine the phone number used in your area. Should any client become injured as the result of a fire, or injured elsewhere on the salon/school premises—**seek medical assistance**!

Safety Tip

Minor Cuts   From time to time accidents do happen, so it is important to know what to do if you or the client receives a minor cut from scissors, cuticle nipper, electric clipper, or shaper (razor). The following is a procedure you will find helpful:

First Aid for Minor Cuts and Burns

1. Stop the bleeding using a clean towel/cotton and apply pressure on cut.
2. Sanitize wound with 70% alcohol or another good antiseptic.
3. Apply **Mycitracin Ointment**™ to prevent infection (available over-the-counter in drug stores). Better penetration of the skin is achieved if a bandage is applied at night; however, the bandage should be removed during the day. Mycitracin™ is advised because it has the widest range of antibiotic content to prevent infection.

Safety Tip

If you or your client receives a severe cut, **seek medical assistance** from a physician or hospital. **Take the client to a doctor!**

Chemical Burns   Many of the chemicals used to curl hair, straighten hair, and bleach/color hair could burn your skin or the skin of the client. When using these products **carelessly**, burns often occur in the areas around the client's front hairline, neck, and behind the ears. You will learn how to prevent chemical burns when your instructor assigns those chapters to you. If you should happen to give one of these services to an overly sensitive client and the client develops a chemical burn, you will find the following procedure helpful:

Chemical and Physical Burns

1. Thoroughly flush (rinse) the burned area with cool water. Or, saturate a towel with cool water, wring out, and apply to burned area of skin.
2. Apply a thin layer of Mycitracin™ ointment with clean cotton swab to prevent infection.
3. Cover with a bandage at night for better penetration of ointment, but uncover during the day.

Safety Tip

If the burn is open and seeping fluid, advise the client to go to a physician.

Another effective antibiotic ointment for "over-the-counter" purchase and use is **Neosporin Ointment**™. **Do not use** Gentian Violet Jelly as this is only available with a doctor's prescription, and stains the client's skin and clothes purple. If used on a client, you would actually be practicing medicine, which is against the law.

If any irritating chemicals drip into the client's eye(s), gently flush area with cool water immediately and contact a physician. **Do not apply anything other than cool water to the eye(s).**

Physical Burns   Physical burns are injuries to the skin that result from touching the skin with a mechanical device, such as a curling iron, pressing comb, or other hairstyling implement used carelessly. The following procedure will be helpful if such burns occur:

1. Apply a cold compress (cold water applied to a clean towel, then wrung out) to reduce pain and swelling.
2. Apply Mycitracin™ ointment to prevent infection. Cover with a bandage at night for better penetration. Uncover during the day. For **severe burns, take the client to a physician**.

DOING SUBOBJECTIVE 5

Sanitize the setting, combing, and cutting implements and other equipment in the salon.

Supplies

- ☐ (fumigant) tablets
- ☐ 70 percent alcohol
- ☐ quats (or formalin)
- ☐ comb and brush cleaner
- ☐ paper towels
- ☐ ammonia
- ☐ sponge
- ☐ wet sanitizer
- ☐ laundered towels
- ☐ cotton
- ☐ Lysol (optional)

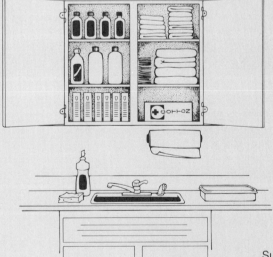

The basic procedure for sanitizing soiled implements:

1. Remove foreign material, such as hair, from combs and brushes.
2. Wash in hot soapy water.
3. Rinse with hot water and place in wet sanitizer.
4. Rinse with hot water, dry, and place in dry sanitizer.

Supply dispensary

PROCEDURE (WHAT TO DO)

1. Remove only the combing and setting implements (clips, combs, brushes, rollers) from your kit.

2. Close the sink drain, add comb and brush cleaner to sink **according to the directions on the label,** and turn on the **hot** water until the desired level is reached.

3. Select a rectangular container with a tight-fitting cover to use for a wet sanitizer; it should be large enough (about gallon-size) to hold clips, combs, brushes, and rollers.

4. Fill this container almost to capacity with **cold** water.

RATIONALE (WHY TO DO IT)

1. Combing and setting implements usually are sanitized with the **same** soaps and chemicals, but cutting implements require a different process.

2. Cleaning excess hair, hair spray, and oil from implements makes it easier to sanitize them. Cleaners dissolve hair spray and oil better in hot water.

3. The cover is necessary to prevent contamination of the sanitizing solution, which will be mixed in it. This container and its solution will be the wet sanitizer.

4. Cold water works better with formalin than hot water does.

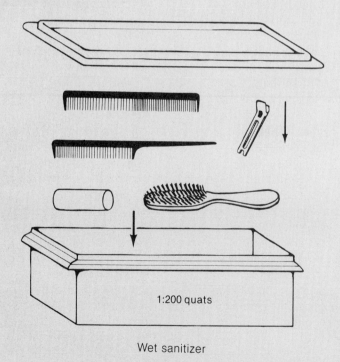

1:200 quats

Wet sanitizer

5. Carefully follow label directions to mix a 10 percent formalin solution with cold water or mix quat solution.

5. Formalin is **poisonous** and can burn your skin. The first time you use it, ask the instructor or manager to be sure that you are using it safely. **Do not smell** any disinfectant because doing so can injure mucous membranes in your nose. Keep formalin away from your eyes! If some does get into your eyes, flush with clean cold water for 15 minutes! **Call a doctor** immediately.

6. Cover the solution in the wet sanitizer and return it to the dispensary cabinet.

6. The chemical should be covered and properly stored when not used.

7. Comb all visible hairs from the brushes before putting them in the solution. The hair should be discarded into a closed refuse container.

7. This helps the sterilizing solution destroy bacteria more easily. To maintain sanitary conditions, the hair must be put into a **closed refuse container**.

8. Immerse combs, clips, and brushes in comb and brush cleaning solution in the sink. Scrub combs and brushes against each other until all have been cleaned.

8. The scrubbing helps the cleaner remove accumulated oil, hair spray, and soil, but bacteria are not destroyed.

9. Rinse all implements with hot water; place them in the sanitizing solution (completed in step 6) and cover.

9. Rinse implements to remove cleaner residue. Covering the container prevents contamination of the solution.

10. Implements should be immersed for 20 minutes.

10. It takes about 20 minutes to destroy bacteria completely. Clips rust easily, so do not leave them immersed for longer than 20 minutes.

11. Fill the sink with hot water and cleaner again.

11. This is the best way to clean hair spray and oil from the rollers and rack.

12. Immerse rollers and rack or tray in the cleaning solution in the sink and stir the solution with your hand. Then drain the sink and rinse the rollers with hot water.

12. This cleaner will dissolve setting lotions and remove temporary hair colors from the rollers. Swishing the solution in the sink speeds cleaning. Rinse the cleaner thoroughly from the rollers.

13. Remove combs, brushes, and clips after they have been in the sanitizer for 20 minutes.

14. Individually dry all combs, brushes, and clips with a clean towel and put the combs and brushes in either an ultraviolet or a dry sanitizer.

15. Place the clips in the implement kit, which contains a fumigant. (Fumigant tablets should be placed in a salt-shaker-type container inside the kit.)

16. Follow the same steps to sanitize the rack and rollers or tray. Thoroughly dry them and put them in a dry sanitizer.

17. Wet a small piece of cotton with 70 percent alcohol and carefully wipe the cutting edges of the scissors and shapers (razors). Then, put them in a dry sanitizer.

18. Remove oils, hair sprays, and setting lotions on curling irons and pressing combs with fine steel wool. Wet a ball of cotton with alcohol, wipe them, and place in a dry sanitizer.

19. Close and return all cleaners to the proper place. Dispose of used cotton in a closed refuse container.

20. Clean all shampoo capes and aprons with an ammonia solution.

13. Use rubber gloves or tongs to remove these implements. The solution could burn or remove a layer of skin.

14. A damp comb or brush used in final styling can straighten the hair and ruin the hairstyle. Also, clips rust easily. So all implements must be dried thoroughly. An ultraviolet or dry sanitizer will keep implements sanitary.

15. This will keep the implements sanitary.

16. Standard procedure. Rollers are dried because bacteria can grow quickly in moist places. Fumigant vapors inside the kit will keep rollers and rack sanitary.

17. This sanitizes metal hairdressing implements. Fumigant will keep them sanitary (see page 26).

18. Remove the buildup from implements before sanitizing them. Electrical implements must not be placed in a wet sanitizer. Electrical shock or damage could result.

19. Exposure to air contaminates and evaporates alcohol. Keep all chemicals well out of a child's reach.

20. This solution works best on plastic and vinyls.

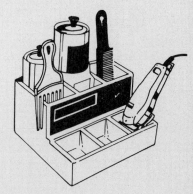

Electric clipper in wet sanitizer

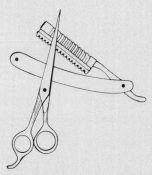

Sanitizing metal implements with 70% alcohol

Safety Tip

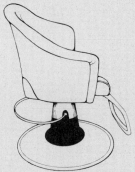

Sanitizing salon equipment with 1:200 quats

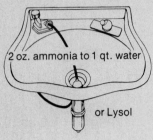

Sanitize neck of shampoo bowl after **each use**

21. Follow label directions to mix a 5 percent formalin solution.

22. Obtain clean paper towels from the dispensary; with solution made in step 21, wipe the back, seat, arms, and hood of each dryer-lounge unit. Also wipe the reception chairs and desk and the hydraulic styling chairs, including their bases.

23. Drain used solution from the sink and place soiled paper towels in a closed refuse container.

24. Mix 2 ounces of ammonia in 1 quart of tepid water to clean soil and hair spray from mirrors, windows, sinks, etc.

21. The strength of this solution usually will not damage upholstery fabrics or counter surfaces as it sanitizes.

22. Since formalin may stain or deteriorate clothing fabrics, each unit should be dried. Although the formalin solution sterilizes the unit, drying with a paper towel to some extent puts bacteria on it again. The units are not sterile, but they are sanitary.

23. This maintains sanitary conditions.

24. Ammonia dissolves soil and hair spray on mirrors, windows, sinks, etc.

When you feel confident that you know the knowing and doing requirements of this task, ask the instructor or manager for the performance checklist and criterion exam. These testing materials should be used with **each chapter** to validate (show) how well you have learned the information in that chapter.

Equivalent Measures

29.573 (approximately 30) milliliters	=	1 ounce		
16 ounces	=	2 cups	=	1 pint
32 ounces	=	2 pints	=	1 quart
64 ounces	=	2 quarts	=	½ gallon
128 ounces	=	4 quarts	=	1 gallon
640 ounces	=	20 quarts	=	5 gallons

GLOSSARY

Antibodies   Substances in the blood that destroy harmful bacteria.

Antiseptics (an-teh-SEP-tiks)   Substances that halt or prevent the growth of pathogenic bacteria.

Aseptic (ay-SEP-tik)   Free from pathogenic bacteria.

Active (natural) immunity   The ability of the body's defense mechanisms to fight off disease by making antibodies (white blood cells) which destroy harmful bacteria in the blood.

Bacilli (bah-SIL-igh)   Rod-shaped pathogenic bacteria that produce such serious diseases as diphtheria, leprosy, tuberculosis, and typhoid fever.

Bacteria (bak-TIR-ee-ah)   One-celled microorganisms, sometimes called microbes.

Bactericides (bac-TIR-eh-sighdz)   Chemicals that destroy pathogenic bacteria.

Bacteriology   The scientific study of bacteria.

Bromine gas   A gas formed when ammonia and sodium bromate combine.

Cells   The basic units of living matter.

Cilia (SIL-ee-ah)   Whiplike extensions that cause the cell to move in a liquid. Also called flagella.

Cocci (KOK-sigh)   Round pathogenic bacteria usually causing pus-forming diseases such as boils, abscesses, and pustules.

Communicable (koh-MYOO-ni-kah-behl)   See **Contagious**.

Contagious (kuhn-TAY-juhss)   Capable of being transmitted to another person through touch or the air.

Dehumidifiers   Devices that remove excessive moisture from the air.

Diplococci (dip-low-KOK-sigh)   Round-shaped bacteria that usually appear in pairs and cause bacterial pneumonia.

Disinfectants (dis-in-FEK-tahnts)   Chemicals that destroy pathogenic bacteria.

Dry sanitizer   An airtight cabinet or drawer containing a chemical agent that is used to keep implements sanitized until they are used.

Electronic air precipitators   Electric air cleaners.

Epidermis (ep-eh-DER-mis)   The outermost layer of the skin.

Flagella (fleh-JEL-leh)   Whiplike extensions that cause the cell to move in a liquid. (Also called cilia.)

Formaldehyde (for-MAL-deh-highd)   A chemical that is in some preparations used to sanitize combing and setting implements.

Formalin   A disinfectant composed of 37 percent formaldehyde, 6.5 percent methanol, and 56.5 percent water.

Fumigants (FYOO-mi-gahnts)   Chemicals that destroy pathogenic bacteria.

Germs   A common name for any pathogenic agent (bacteria or virus) that causes disease.

Germicides (JER-meh-sighdz)   Chemicals that destroy pathogenic bacteria.

Humidifiers   Devices that add moisture to the air, preventing excessive drying of the skin and reducing static electricity.

Immunity (ih-MYOO-neh-tee)   The ability of the body's defense mechanisms to fight off disease.

Inorganic matter   Matter that has never been alive.

Microbes (MIGH-krohbs)   One-celled organisms, sometimes called bacteria.

Microorganisms (migh-kroh-OR-gehn-iz-uhmz)   Organisms that can be seen only by using a microscope.

Mitosis (migh-TOH-sis)   A process of cell division.

Nonpathogenic bacteria   Bacteria that do not cause disease.

Organic (awr-GAN-ik) matter   All things that are living or have been alive in the past.

Passive (acquired) immunity The ability of the body's defense mechanisms to fight disease upon injection of antibodies from another person or animal.

Pathogenic (PATH-ah-jen-ik) bacteria Bacteria that cause disease; commonly called germs.

Public sanitation The set of procedures used to prohibit the spread of communicable diseases and the development of other infections.

Quaternary ammonium (KWOT-er-ner-ee ah-MOHN-ee-um) ("Quats") A chemical used in solution for sterilizing combing and setting implements.

Saprophytes (SAP-roh-fightz) Bacteria that cause dead organic matter to decay and thus help enrich the soil.

Septic (SEP-tik) Toxic, unsanitary.

Spirilla (spigh-RIL-ah) Spiral-shaped pathogenic bacteria that cause cholera and syphilis.

Spontaneous combustion Process by which a fire starts without an outside source of flame such as a match or spark.

Spores (sporz) A spherical state in which some bacteria can survive for long periods of extreme heat and cold.

Staphylococci (staf-eh-low-KOK-sigh) Round, pathogenic bacteria, usually growing in clusters, that generally produce local infections.

Sterilization (stehr-il-eh-ZAY-shuhn) The process of killing all bacteria (pathogenic and nonpathogenic).

Streptococci (strep-tah-KOK-sigh) Round pathogenic bacteria that usually cause general infections.

Susceptible More likely to become ill from direct or indirect contact with disease-causing bacteria or viruses.

Toxins Poisons.

Ultramicroscopic That which can be seen only when magnified up to one million times by a scan electron microscope.

Vacuum breaker A fixture that prevents reverse flow of contaminated water from backing up into the fresh water supply system.

Virus An ultramicroscopic parasitic pathogen.

Wet sanitizer A large, covered, nonmetal container that holds water and a chemical agent to sterilize implements.

QUESTIONS

1. What two words best explain practices that promote and protect good health in the community?
2. Name the term given to anything that takes up space and has weight.
3. Can you name the term given to all basic units of organic matter?
4. What are the small organisms that can't be seen without using a microscope?
5. Can you name the microorganisms cosmetologists study?

6. What is the scientific study of bacteria called?
7. Are pathogenic bacteria harmful to humans?
8. Are nonpathogenic bacteria harmful to humans?
9. Can you list the three types of bacteria and their respective shapes?
10. What conditions must exist for bacteria to grow?
11. Using your own words, explain the difference between sterilization and sanitation.
12. Define the action of antiseptics, fumigants, and disinfectants.
13. If you drank a large amount of a disinfectant, would it be harmful?
14. Can you name two disinfectant chemicals we use?
15. What liquid is used to sanitize metal implements, e.g., scissors?
16. What percentage hydrogen peroxide solution is an effective antiseptic?
17. Is 70% ethyl alcohol the same strength as 70% isopropyl alcohol?
18. What strength quats is needed to kill stubborn viruses such as the herpes simplex virus?
19. Is it necessary to use gloves to remove combs and brushes from a wet sanitizer using quats?
20. Does the filter in an air conditioner clean the air as well as an air purifier?
21. Where should soiled towels be stored?
22. When ammonia fumes and sodium bromate fumes mix together, what hazard will result?
23. Where should flammable beauty products be stored?
24. What over-the-counter medicine will prevent infection from a chemical burn?
25. If the client is burned with a curling iron, should you apply Gentian Violet Jelly?
26. If an irritating chemical drips into the client's eye(s), what should you apply?

ANSWERS

1. Public hygiene. 2. Matter. 3. Cells. 4. Microorganisms. 5. Bacteria. 6. Bacteriology 7. Yes. 8. No. 9. Cocci, spirilla, and bacilli—round, spiral, and rod-shaped. 10. Heat, moisture, absence of sunlight. 11. Sterilization kills all bacteria; sanitation kills only pathogenic bacteria. 12. Antiseptics halt or prevent growth of bacteria. Fumigants (fumes) and disinfectants (generally liquids) kill pathogenic bacteria. 13. Yes, probably fatal. 14. Quaternary ammonium ("quats") and formaldehyde. 15. 70% alcohol. 16. 3–5%. 17. No, ethyl alcohol is stronger. 18. One (1) part quats: 200 parts water; ⅔ ounce quats mixed with 1 gallon of water. 19. Yes. 20. No. 21. A closed metal container. 22. Spontaneous combustion. 23. In a cool, dry place. 24. Mycitracin™ or Neosporin™ ointments. 25. Absolutely not. 26. Only cool water.

Describing the Hair 3

Trichology (tri-KOL-eh-jee) is the scientific study of the hair and its diseases. People who specialize in studying the hair and diseases related to the hair are called **trichologists** (tri-KOL-eh-jists). They are highly educated scientists, and as specialists, they continuously read and study all new information about the hair and diseases related to the hair.

You are studying to become a cosmetologist, not a trichologist. However, most services offered in a beauty school or salon are directly related to the hair. To perform services safely and effectively for your client, you will need to know the composition, structure, function, disorders, diseases, and condition of the hair. While this chapter will give you the knowledge you will need, you should keep in mind that these are only the basics.

The importance of being able to recognize diseases of the hair and scalp has increased greatly in recent years. More and more people use over-the-counter hair products and appliances. As a result, cosmetologists see more complex hair problems today than at any time in history. To cope with these problems, manufacturers have researched and developed many new preparations to help the professional cosmetologist. When should you use which product? The answer to this question is complicated, but it begins in this chapter. Other units will help complete the answer.

Purpose

Provided with the information in the chapter and help from your instructor, define, identify, describe, and analyze the hair, its structure, function, composition, diseases, disorders, and condition.

Major Objective

Score 75 percent or better on a multiple-choice exam on the information in this chapter.

Level of Acceptability

41

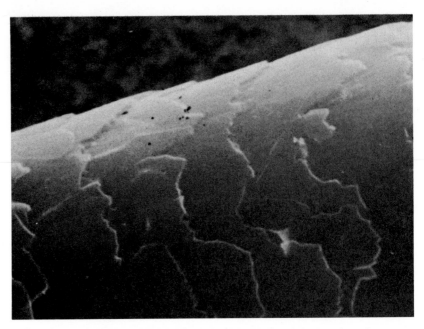

Cuticle layers (imbrications) of a hair seen under the scanning electron microscope (SEM) (Courtesy of 3M Company)

Knowing Subobjectives

1. Define hair and describe the function, location, composition, and types of hair.
2. Describe the basic histology of the hair and surrounding structures.
3. Describe hair growth.
4. Identify factors involved in analyzing hair condition.
5. Describe abnormal conditions, diseases, and disorders of the hair.
6. Describe the removal of superfluous hair.

KNOWING SUBOBJECTIVE 1

Define hair and describe the function, location, composition, and types of hair.

The **two functions** of the hair are **cosmetic** and **protective**. Hair **adorns** the body to improve the appearance of the individual. On certain parts of the body it protects the skin from friction.

Although many animals are protected better and over larger areas of their bodies than humans, we also have hair over most parts of our bodies, except for the palms of the hands, soles of the feet, the lips, and a few other very small areas. But human hair is not easy to see, except on the scalp, face, arms, and legs.

There are two basic types of hair: **lanugo** (lan-OO-goh) **(vellus) hairs** and **terminal hairs**. Lanugo (vellus) hairs are all over the body. They are fine and lightly pigmented (colored). Terminal hairs are **coarser, thicker**, and more pigmented (colored). Terminal hairs are found on the scalp, face, and extremities.

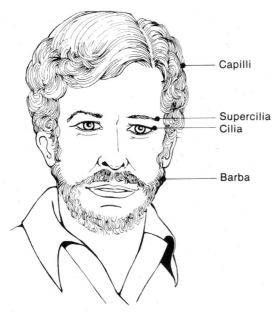

Capilli

Supercilia
Cilia

Barba

Types of facial hair

It is difficult to make general statements about hair because on different parts on the body it varies in length, strength, and rate of growth. Hair is grouped into six types: (1) scalp, (2) eyebrow and eyelash, (3) beard, (4) body, (5) pubic, and (6)underarm (axillary). The technical names for hair involved in salon services are: (1) **capilli** (cah-PIL-igh) (scalp hair); (2) **supercilla** (soo-per-SIL-ee-ah) (eyebrows) and **cilia** (eyelashes); and (3) **barba** (beard).

Scalp hair provides a cushion that helps the skull protect the brain. The eyebrows and eyelashes shield the delicate tissues of the eyes (for instance, from a speck of dirt or dust). Beard hair protects the face. Both men and women have beard hair, but male hormones make men's beard hair much coarser than women's. Pubic hair protects the genital region, and axillary hair shields the soft underarm skin.

Hair is a slender, threadlike **appendage** (ah-PEN-dij), or extension of the skin. It is made of hard, keratinized protein. **Keratin** (KER-eh-tin) is a protein found in the human skin. It is located in the **epidermis** (the outer layer of skin made of soft keratin that protects the body—you will hear more about the layers of the skin in chapter 22). There are two kinds of keratin: soft and hard. The chemical basis of hair is hard keratin. Hair is made up of approximately 51 percent carbon, 7 percent hydrogen, 18 percent nitrogen, 5 percent sulfur, and 19 percent oxygen. Hair is nourished (fed) by protein that comes from food. Protein is carried to the hair by blood vessels.

A **molecule** (MOL-eh-kyool) is the smallest possible unit of any compound. It is made up of two or more atoms chemically combined. These atoms are joined, or connected, by bonds. The building blocks of the protein molecule are organic substances called **amino acids**. Healthy hair has eighteen or more of these amino acids. (See chapter 32, Chemistry.)

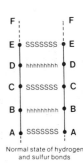

Normal state of hydrogen and sulfur bonds

Amino acids form proteins, and peptide linkages strengthened by cross bonds

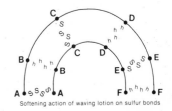

Softening action of waving lotion on sulfur bonds

Cross bonds are broken when hair is stretched on rollers

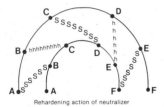

Rehardening action of neutralizer

The bonds are re-formed as hair dries on rollers

As a cosmetologist, you will be especially interested in two amino acids: **cystine** (SIS-teen) and **tyrosine** (TIGH-rah-seen). Cystine is important for cold waving and chemical relaxing, while tyrosine is involved in hair coloring.

Hair is made beneath the scalp. Amino acids form proteins. As this happens, chemical reactions that produce **peptide** (PEP-tighd) **linkages** take place. These peptide linkages are held together by cross-bonds. The types of cross-bonds in the hair are cystine, hydrogen, and salt (the salt bonds are less important). When joined together in the hair, these cross-bonds are called **poly** (many) **peptide bonds**. During hair-care services the polypeptide bonds are broken and re-formed by both physical and chemical actions.

Hydrogen bonds are broken physically when the hair is stretched, while it is still wet and wound around a roller. The bonds re-form as the hair dries in a curled position or shape.

Cystine bonds (also called disulfide bonds) are broken chemically by applying reducing agents to the hair. Then the bonds are re-formed by oxidation. In cold waving, for example, the bonds are broken by ammonium thioglycolate (waving lotion) and are re-formed by hydrogen peroxide (the neutralizer).

KNOWING SUBOBJECTIVE 2

Describe the basic histology of the hair and surrounding structures.

Hair histology (his-TAHL-eh-jee) involves the study of the microscopic structures of the hair. As was mentioned in Subobjective 1, hair is like a thread. This thread is called the hair shaft.

The **hair shaft** is the dead portion of a hair that is above the skin. The basic layers of the hair shaft from the inside outward are: the medulla, the cortex, and the cuticle. The part of the hair below the skin is called the **hair root**.

The **medulla** (med-DUHL-ah) is the innermost layer of the hair. It may contain soft keratin. The medulla is the least important layer of the hair. Some hair, such as lanugo hair (the short, soft hair found on some parts of the body, such as the arms), does not have a medulla (see photos, p. 45).

The **cortex** (KOR-teks), or middle layer, is the largest layer of the hair. It makes up about 75 percent of a single hair. It contains the coloring pigment (melanin). Natural hair colors have one or a combination of the following pigments: Yellow, red, brown, and black.

The **cuticle** (KYOO-ti-kehl) is the outside layer of clear, horny cells that overlap (imbricate) each other to form the outer layer of the hair shaft. The density of the cuticle varies from 5 to 15 layers of cells, depending on a person's race. Caucasians usually have fewer than 7 layers; Orientals usually have from 7 to 10 layers; and Blacks may have as many as 15 cuticle layers.

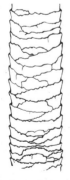

Hair shaft (note imbrications)

The hair grows through the **follicle** (FAHL-i-kehl), which encases the root. The follicle is a long, slender, pocketlike depression in the skin. Two glands and one muscle are near the follicle. The two glands are an apocrine sweat gland and a sebaceous gland. (A **gland** is a cell or group of cells that removes material from the blood, changes that material in some way, and secretes it either to another part of the body for further use or eliminates it from the body.) These glands empty into the follicle through ducts.

The **arrector pili** (ah-REK-tehr PIGH-ligh) **muscle** is attached to the follicle below these two glands. Changes in skin temperature cause this muscle to contract (become shorter), resulting in "goose bumps." Sudden fright also causes contraction. During this contraction, the hair stands straight up. The contraction of this muscle also forces sebum into the follicle, where it lubricates the hair and skin.

At this point, you have traced the hair backwards, in a sense, from the hair shaft to the follicle. The glands and the muscle are at the top of the follicle. Hair is made at the other end of the follicle, farther down.

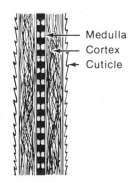

Cross-section of the hair shaft

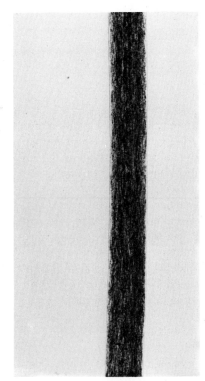

Microscopic photo of a hair without medulla (Courtesy of 3M Company)

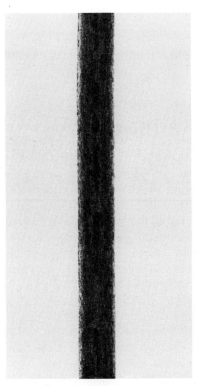

Microscopic photo of a hair with intermittent medulla (Courtesy of 3M Company)

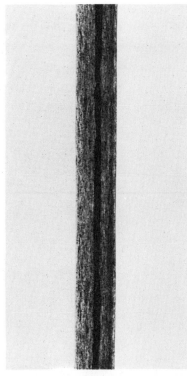

Microscopic photo of a hair with continuous medulla (Courtesy of 3M Company)

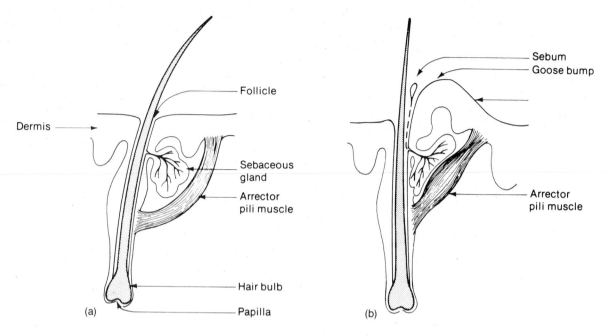

(a) Arrector pili muscle relaxed (b) Arrector pili muscle contracted

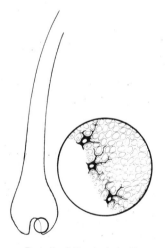

Detail of the hair bulb showing melanocytes forming pigment

The **hair bulb** is the bottom part of the follicle. The hair bulb almost completely surrounds a small, nipplelike projection called the **papilla** (pap-PIL-ah), which grows from the dermis (the layer of skin just below the epidermis). The papilla contains a nerve and the blood supply (one capillary—a very small vessel) needed to form hair and keep it growing.

In the middle and upper parts of the hair bulbs are **melanocytes** (MEL-an-oh-sights) that make melanin and cells for making hard keratin. **Melanin** (MEL-eh-nehn) gives hair its color. When the melanocytes cannot make melanin, a person's hair turns gray. Cosmetologists call gray hair **canities**.

Have you ever seen a child with gray hair? His (or her) gray hair is probably **congenital** (since birth). This is one classification of gray hair. The other category, acquired gray hair (canities), often occurs by the early forties, though it can occur at almost any age. If and when your hair will turn gray is usually determined by **heredity**.

The keratin that is made in the hair bulb is actually turned into keratinized protein just above the hair bulb in two layers of the follicle called Henle's layer and Huxley's layer.

The process of keratinization (changing keratin into hard protein) is slow. It occurs in stages, but as the hair comes out of the follicle, it has been completely changed into hard protein.

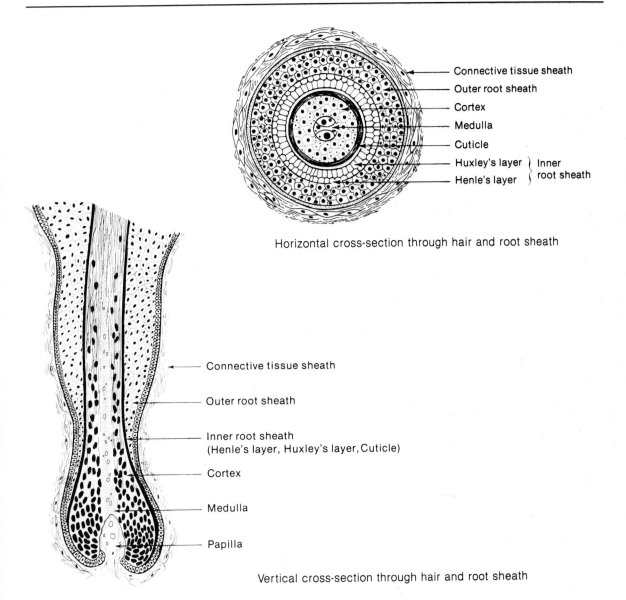

Horizontal cross-section through hair and root sheath

Vertical cross-section through hair and root sheath

What can happen at the mouth of the follicle (right next to the skin, where the hair emerges) is a good reason for good personal hygiene. There is a depression in the skin at the mouth of the follicle. This depression is a perfect place for bacteria, sebum, and soil to collect. If this happens, it can cause either a minor infection or serious disease.

As you know, hair can have different shapes and degrees of curliness. You often can see the four different categories by looking at cross-sections of hair shafts under a microscope. A **flat** hair shaft is super-curly. A **semi-oval** one is curly. An **oval** one is wavy. A **round** one is straight (see p. 50).

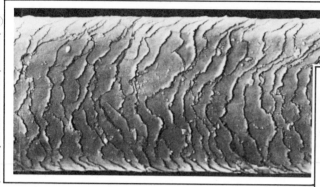

(Courtesy of the Wella Corporation.)

Magnified 1,000 times, the hair cuticle is composed of overlapping layers that extend over a large portion of the circumference of the hair

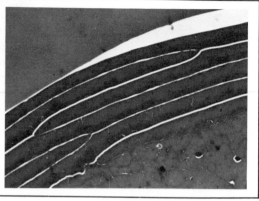

(Scanning electron micrograph supplied by Scruples.)

Using a magnification of 15,000X, this micrograph indicates that the cuticle layers are held together with a glue-like substance, appearing as a white membrane between cuticle layers. When this substance is damaged, for instance by chemicals, environmental causes, and excessive heat from curling irons and blow dryers, it deteriorates, allowing the layers to separate. This causes the hair to lose luster and sheen

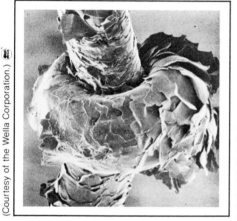

(Courtesy of the Wella Corporation.)

A knotted hair shows severe damage with cuticle layers separating, particularly where knot is. The loose cuticle causes the hair to feel rough and become tangled during styling. 400X magnification

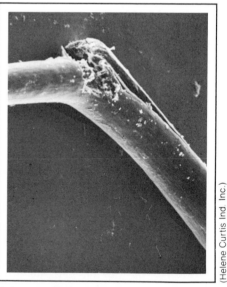

(Helene Curtis Ind. Inc.)

Hair magnified 1,000X shows break (split) from using brush rollers

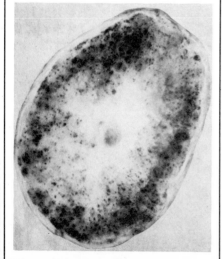

(Helene Curtis Ind. Inc.)

This cross section of the hair shows the medulla at the center, the color pigmented cells of the cortex, and the cuticle as one layer. 2000X

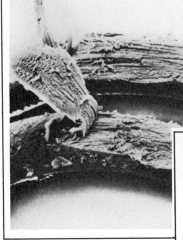

By nicking hair wound around a pin with a razor blade, a split is clearly visible at a magnification of 200X. When the split section is torn, the longitudinal fibers of the cortex are revealed

(Courtesy of the Wella Corporation.)

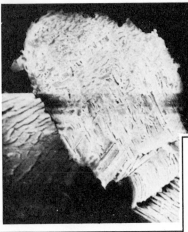

At 400X, the flap shows that where cut, the details of the fibers of the cortex are obscured by a plastic-like or adhesive coating. Where torn, the structural details of the fibers are visible

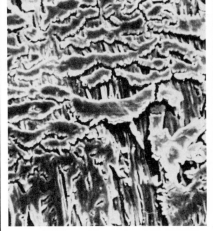

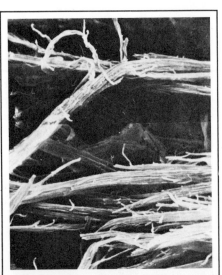

(*right*) At 2,000X, the coating now believed to be a micropolysaccharide (carbohydrates bound to protein and mucoproteins which forms a cement substance) is apparent where the long fibers have been cut

(*left*) With 2,000X magnification, the boxed portion shows greater detail of the fiber development into the cable

(*bottom*) This 200X SEM shows the fibers from the cortex which have been pulled from the split hair by adhesive tape. The fibers do not lie parallel but are twisted and often cross each other. They also form a cable, similar to spun sewing thread. The entanglement of the individual fibers gives the hair its strength and elasticity

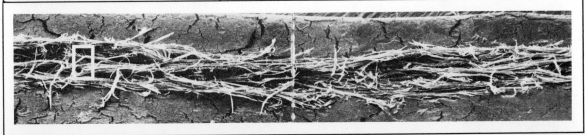

(Courtesy of the Wella Corporation.)

(Courtesy of the Wella Corporation.)

(Courtesy of the Wella Corporation.)

(Courtesy of the Wella Corporation.)

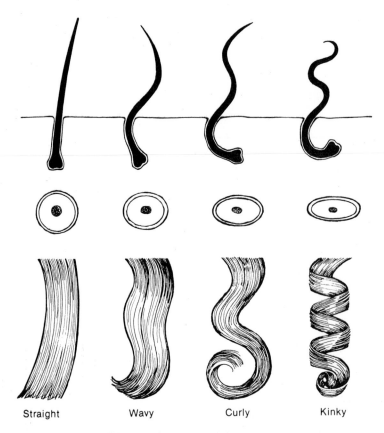

| Straight | Wavy | Curly | Kinky |

Effect of the angle of the follicle

The **angle** at which the **follicle** approaches the surface of the skin can affect the shape of the hair. A follicle that is curved and parallel to the skin produces a super-curly hair shaft. A follicle that approaches the skin at a slight angle forms a wavy shaft. The angle of the follicle for a curly shaft is in between that for a kinky and wavy shaft. A follicle that is perpendicular to the surface of the skin produces a straight hair.

KNOWING SUBOBJECTIVE 3

Describe hair growth.

Hair appears very early on the human body. In fact, it appears on the human embryo near the eyebrows by the sixth or seventh week after conception (in other words, even before birth). Other hairs appear after the twelfth week.

All human hair grows in cyclical periods that differ from one region of the body to another. Scalp hair, for example, grows for 2 to 5 years before it goes into a resting phase. Hair growth on the trunk, limbs, and other areas occurs in periods of 4 to 6 months.

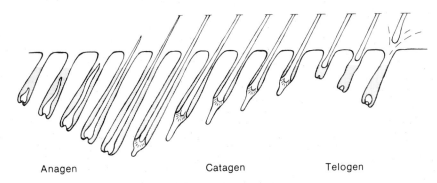

Anagen   Catagen   Telogen

The three stages of hair growth

There are 3 recognized cycles of growth. They are **anagen, catagen,** and **telogen.**

The **anagen** (AN-ah-jen) **stage** is the **growth period**. The length of the anagen stage determines the length of the hair shaft. The anagen stage has 2 phases. The first period is when the hair bulb stretches itself out into the follicle. The second period is when hard keratin is being synthesized in the follicle. Although the anagen stage normally lasts from 2 to 5 years, periods of 25 years have been recorded. In the anagen stage, scalp hair grows at a rate of about one-half inch per month.

During the **catagen** (KET-eh-jen) **stage** hair growth slows and club hairs form. Keratinization does not take place during this stage.

The **telogen** (TEL-oh-jen) **stage** is a resting period which continues until the next anagen stage begins. Although scientists do not know exactly how long the telogen stage lasts, they think it is short—3 or 4 months.

The number of hairs on normal scalps varies according to hair color as follows: **90,000—red; 105,000—black; 110,000—brown, and 140,000—blonde.**

During the telogen stage, the hairs are removed easily by vigorous brushing. Under normal conditions, 85 to 95 percent of the terminal (coarse) scalp hairs are in the anagen stage; 1 percent in the catagen; and from 4 to 14 percent in the telogen stage. So, hair grows almost continuously. However, nearly all of the tiny vellus hairs on the scalp are in the telogen stage. On an average, humans lose between 50 and 75 hairs per day.

Affecting Hair Growth

Hair is affected mainly by **climate** and **seasons** of the year. Hair grows faster in warmer climates than in colder ones and faster in summer than in winter.

Hormones increase hair growth on the scalp. Since women generally have proportionately more female hormones than men have male hormones, women rarely become bald. On the other hand, many men gradually lose their hair. During menopause, women may find that their vellus hairs have a coarser texture.

Nutrition affects general body health, which in turn influences hair growth.

Stimulation may affect hair growth, although this has not been proved. For instance, if trauma (shock) to nails, also appendages of the skin—such as nail biting, causes the nails to grow faster, hair growth similarly might be stimulated by frequent (more than once a week) scalp massages. However, the hair shaft is a **dead** structure, and the papilla, where growth begins, is at the base of the follicle; so close shaving, trimming, plucking, cutting, or singeing (burning the ends of the hair), and cremes, gels, or ointments will not make hair grow faster.

Hair seems to grow faster when it is cut short because any growth is noticeable, but it doesn't grow faster.

KNOWING SUBOBJECTIVE 4

Identify factors involved in analyzing hair condition.

As a student and later as a practicing cosmetologist, you will learn to watch for certain signals or signs when you prepare treatments for a client. The condition of a client's hair shaft—determined by its texture, porosity, elasticity, appearance, and feel—will rank high on your list of concerns.

Hair texture is related to its **diameter. Fine** hair has a smaller (thinner) diameter than **medium** hair, and **coarse** hair has a larger diameter than medium hair. At least two structures can influence the diameter of the hair: the medulla and the cuticle.

As was stated previously in this chapter, some hair does not have a medulla. You can see whether a hair has a medulla or not by looking under a microscope. (The medulla also can be distributed unevenly through a hair.) Overall, this is not particularly important. This type of hair may have a smaller diameter than hair that has a medulla.

For many years, scientists thought that the cuticle protecting the cortex was made up of only one layer. However, in recent years, scientists, aided by the scan electron microscope, have learned that hair has from 5 to 15 imbricated (overlapping) cuticle layers.

You must consider hair texture when selecting products. Products are made in strengths that are best for various conditions of the hair. Fine hair ordinarily does not have as much tensile strength (the ability to stretch without breaking) as medium hair, and coarse hair has greater tensile strength than medium hair.

Hair **porosity** (poh-RAHSS-eh-tee) refers to the amount of moisture that can be absorbed by the cuticle layers. There is a direct relationship between porosity and the number of cuticle layers in the hair. Porosity is also affected by the acidity or alkalinity of products used. **Alkaline** (AL-kah-lin) preparations cause the overlapping cuticle scales to "open," or stand away from the cortex, to a certain extent. **Acid** preparations have a tendency to "close" or lay the overlapping cuticle layers tightly against the cortex.

You can test the porosity of hair by the following procedure. Hold a one-square-inch strand of dry hair straight away from the scalp between the mid-

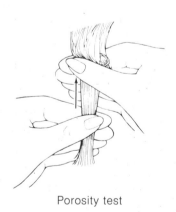

Porosity test

dle and index fingers of your left hand. Slide the middle and index fingers of your right hand along the strand toward the scalp. The more that the strands pile up or slide toward the scalp, the more porous the hair is. This is true because the fingers of the right hand will "catch" the cuticle scales of the hair that are *not* closed. If the cuticle scales are tightly packed against the cortex, the hair is **not porous**. For certain services, this nonporous hair is considered resistant because its cuticle is difficult to penetrate.

The **elasticity** of the hair refers to its ability to stretch without breaking and to return to its original form. **Dry hair** with good elasticity can normally be stretched one-fifth, or **20 percent**, of its length, while **wet hair** can be stretched two-fifths or **40 percent (sometimes 50 percent)**, of its length without breaking. Some companies make instruments that measure the tensile strength of hair. Your instructor may wish to demonstrate one of these instruments in class.

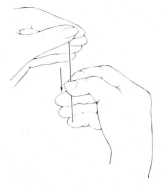

Elasticity test

Although small machines are sold to determine the exact **tensile strength**, or elasticity of the hair, you can perform a simple manual test that is quick and very accurate. Pluck one hair from your client's head. Holding the hair between the middle and index fingers of your left hand, slide the hair between the thumbnail and index finger of your right hand *with* the direction of the cuticle scales. This action produces a "ribboning" effect; the hair will spiral like a piece of wrapping ribbon. The number of spirals the hair makes indicates the elasticity of the hair. The *more* the hair spirals, the stronger it is. Few spirals indicate that the hair is weak or fragile. Hold the hair at each end in a straight position for three seconds; then release one end and watch how closely it returns to its original spiraled position. If the hair hangs straight with very little or no curl, its elasticity is not very good.

The **appearance** of the hair should be lustrous and shiny. The sebaceous gland secretes oil (sebum) into the hair follicle. The sebum works its way to the scalp, where brushing transfers the sebum onto the hair shaft and gives the hair sheen and luster. The sebum seals moisture in the hair and protects it from the sun, wind, and weather. Without sebum, the hair appears dry and lusterless.

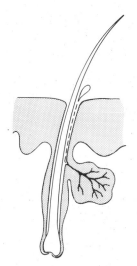

Sebaceous gland secreting sebum

The **feel** of the hair is another indicator of its condition. In some cases, touching the hair is the only, or best, way to check hair texture and to detect some condition, such as color buildup. There is no "magic formula" for learning how hair should "feel." This is a sense that you can develop only through experience and help from your instructor or manager.

KNOWING SUBOBJECTIVE 5

As a student and later as a cosmetologist, you will probably see abnormal conditions (maybe even very serious disorders and diseases) of the hair. Although you do not—in fact cannot—treat these diseases, you should be able to recognize them. **Trichosis** (tri-KOH-siss) is any diseased condition of the hair.

Describe abnormal conditions, diseases, and disorders of the hair.

Conditions of Overgrowth

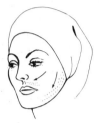

Superfluous hair

Hypertrichosis (high-per-tri-KOH-siss)—excessive growth of unwanted hair—is also called **superfluous** hair or **hirsutism** (HIR-soot-iz-uhm). **Congenital** hypertrichosis is considered hereditary.

Localized hypertrichosis may be seen in two forms. Sometimes it appears as two or three hairs growing in a mole or as considerable growth over large areas of the body. Refer persons with hypertrichosis to a dermatologist. Electrolysis may be necessary to treat this condition, but only on a doctor's recommendation. If moles are not involved, it is all right to bleach or pluck a few hairs on a small area of skin. Removal of excess hair will be treated in the next subobjective (see p. 57).

Classification of Hair Loss

Alopecia (al-ah-PEE-shee-ah) means hair loss. There are many kinds of alopecia and many reasons for it. The kind that you probably think of first is alopecia occurring on the scalp. It is particularly important in beauty-care services because it is so noticeable, but there are many other forms.

There are two categories of alopecia of the scalp: (1) diffuse (scattered) and (2) patchy. There are two varieties of patchy alopecia. One causes scars; the other does not. In the scarring variety, hair cannot grow because the papilla of the follicle has been destroyed.

Types of **diffuse hair loss** are:

1. Male pattern hair loss.
2. Female pattern hair loss.
3. Temporary hair loss in females.
4. Hair loss due to trauma caused by physical or chemical interference with natural growth.
5. Hair loss due to disorders of the body.

1. **Male pattern hair loss** is a receding hairline caused by heredity, aging, or a decrease in hormones. Young clients should consult a dermatologist for preparations that may at least slow the hair loss.

2. **Female pattern hair loss** occurs in women over fifty as a result of a relative increase in the male hormone. There is no effective treatment, but maintenance of a healthy scalp is important.

3. **Temporary hair loss in females** can follow childbirth, nervous upset, the use of anesthetics, or for no apparent reason. During pregnancy, hair growth increases, but after delivery, hair loss occurs until the body returns to its normal state. Baldness seldom results from childbirth.

4. **Different kinds of trauma,** both physical and chemical, can cause hair loss. Accident, injury, or infection (such as pneumonia) can cause hair loss because of the shock to the nervous system. Some chemicals used to treat certain diseases and conditions also can cause hair loss.

5. Some **disorders of the body** also can cause loss of hair. Diseases of the endocrine system of the body, such as an underactive thyroid or pituitary gland, can lead to loss of hair. Some congenital (birth) defects can cause loss of nails as well as hair.

Types of **patchy nonscarring hair loss** are:

1. Alopecia areata.
2. Tinea of the scalp (ringworm).

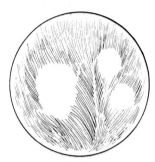

1. **Alopecia areata** (ay-reh-AT-ah) refers to an **oval bald patch** usually caused by bodily disorders. There may be one or several patches, but there is no scaling or infection. This usually affects the scalp, eyebrows, eyelashes, and beard, but it can occur in any area. In 6 to 12 months the hair is usually (though not always) restored.

Alopecia areata (oval bald patches)

2. **Tinea** (TIN-ee-ah) of the scalp is characterized by broken-off hairs, scaliness, and occasionally infection. This is a ringworm infection. The scales on the surface of the scalp are silvery white or gray. Do not serve a client with tinea of the scalp; advise the client to see a doctor.

Although they do not fall into the category of patchy nonscarring hair loss, there are four other types of alopecia. Total loss of scalp or body hair is called **alopecia totalis** (toh-TAL-iss); it is usually permanent. Its cause is unknown, but it may be linked to infections (teeth, prostate, sinuses, gall bladder, etc.) and emotional problems. Heredity is involved. **Alopecia universal** is a loss of hair all over the body. **Alopecia senilis** (seh-NIL-iss) refers to loss of hair occurring in old age, and **alopecia prematura** refers to hair loss early in life.

Three types of patchy hair loss that cause **scars** are:

1. Rare tinea of the scalp.
2. Bacterial infection of the scalp.
3. Damage to skin from third-degree burns, overdose of X-rays, trauma, caustics, and other severe skin injuries.

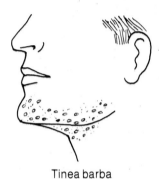

Tinea barba

Diseases and Disorders of Hair Other Than Loss

In many cases you will be able to recognize hair diseases or disorders quickly and simply because you will notice that the client has lost a considerable amount of hair.

Trichorrhexis nodosa (tri-koh-REK-siss no-DOH-sah), knotted hair, is an uncommon disease of the beard and pubic hair of adults; it is characterized by nodular swellings along the hair shaft. If you look at hair having this disease under a microscope, you will see a definite pattern of breaks across the hair.

Monilethrix (mon-i-LETH-riks) **(beaded hair)** involves rhythmic, alternating constrictions that look like nodes or beads along the hair shaft. Hairs having this disease are usually coarse, dry, and dull. They eventually break off at the constrictions, leaving a stubble either over the entire scalp or in localized areas. Alopecia does not result from this condition. Its cause is unknown, but both the hair shaft and the follicle are involved, and the keratinization process obviously is affected.

Pili (PIGH-ligh) is a general term that means pertaining to the hair. It appears in the names of many hair disorders.

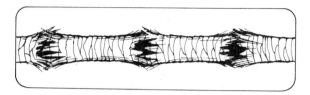

Knotted

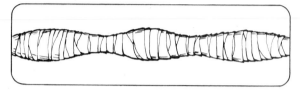

Beaded

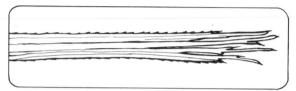

Split ends

Pili annulati (PIGH-ligh an-nyoo-LAY-tigh) **(ringed hair)** is characterized by dark and white bands in some or all of the scalp hair. If a client has this condition, you will be able to spot it easily—in ordinary light. This hair may appear to lack pigment, but it doesn't. Heredity seems to be a factor. There is no treatment.

Pili incarnati (PIGH-ligh in-CAR-nay-tigh) **(ingrown hair)** occurs in individuals who have short, bristly, recurved hairs. This disorder affects facial areas that are shaved every day. The hair simply reenters the skin, irritates it, and causes a pimple. This irritation can be complicated further if the disease does not stop when the hair is allowed to grow.

Trichoptilosis (tri-kop-ti-LOH-siss) **(split ends)** or **fragilitas crinium (fragile hair shaft)** is characterized by splitting along the length of hair shafts. This is not a disease, and its cause is not known. Professional conditioning treatments should improve this disorder.

KNOWING SUBOBJECTIVE 6

Describe the removal of superfluous hair.

Many of your clients will want superfluous hair removed. There are two basic processes used to remove unwanted hair temporarily: **epilation** (pulling the hair shaft from the follicle) and **depilation** (removing part of the hair shaft at skin level).

1. **Tweezing** (plucking or epilation), involves pulling the hairs from the follicle in the areas of the eyebrows, upper lip, chin, and neck.
2. Cutting (depilation) involves applying shaving cream and cutting the hair with a safety razor. Some people, feeling that shaving cream is unnecessarily messy, use an electric razor instead.

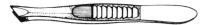

Tweezers for removing hair (epilation).

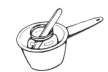

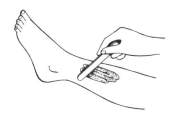

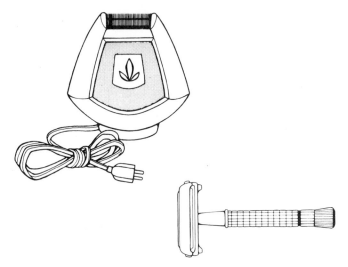

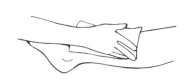

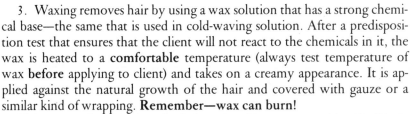

Razor for cutting hair (depilation)

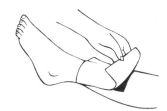

Removal of superfluous hair by hot waxing method

 Safety Tip

3. Waxing removes hair by using a wax solution that has a strong chemical base—the same that is used in cold-waving solution. After a predisposition test that ensures that the client will not react to the chemicals in it, the wax is heated to a **comfortable** temperature (always test temperature of wax **before** applying to client) and takes on a creamy appearance. It is applied against the natural growth of the hair and covered with gauze or a similar kind of wrapping. **Remember—wax can burn!**

This preparation dissolves the hair and enables you to peel it off safely in about ten minutes. If you follow the label directions, you will find that this type of depilatory is simple to use, painless, and leaves the skin soft and pliable.

4. A variety of over-the-counter foam and liquid depilatories (depilation) is available. However, **always give a skin test** (allergy test) on a hairless part of a client's arm **before using a depilatory**. Use them very carefully because they are very strong and may irritate the skin (do not use on client's arms). Their basic ingredient, thioglycolate, dissolves hair. All temporary measures are just that; the hair will soon grow out again, and the procedure will have to be repeated.

The only permanent way to remove hair is through **electrolysis** (eh-lek-TRAHL-eh-siss). The licensed or registered person who performs electroly-

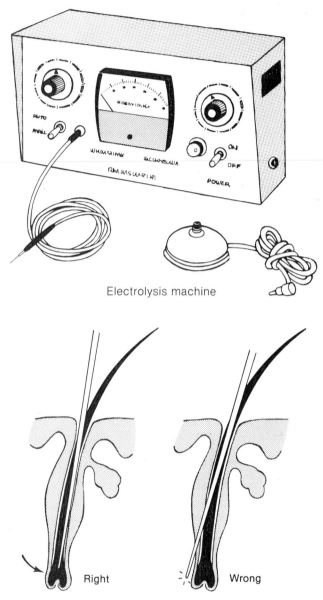

Electrolysis machine

Inserting electric needle to destroy the papilla of the
hair follicle

sis is called an **electrologist**. In some states any licensed cosmetologist may
remove hair by electrolysis; in others, a separate license is needed.

The electrologist uses a **short-wave machine**, approved by the Federal
Communications Commission, to remove hairs **only** in the hairline, eyebrows, cheeks, lips, chin, underarms, arms, and legs.

The electrologist follows several steps to remove the hair. He or she inserts a short-wave needle ⅛ to ¼ inch into the hair follicle along the angle

of its growth in respect to the scalp. The operator inserts the needle manually and steps on a foot pedal that starts the machine, but once started, the machine works automatically. The current stops and starts according to the selection set on the time and intensity controls. The current destroys the papilla of the hair follicle. The hair then slides easily from the skin. The strength of the current and the length of time it runs are determined by the texture of the hair, e.g., fine, medium, or coarse (coarser hair may require more current and time); the machine used; and the electrologist.

An electrologist **never** removes hair from eyelids, ears, inside the nose, from moles or warts, or from inflamed or diseased skin. Clients who have diabetes cannot be treated. If the electrologist is unsure of the client's health, he or she should receive written permission from the person's doctor prior to giving the service. The electrologist always maintains a sanitary work area and implements. Additional information about electrology will be covered in the electricity chapter.

Superfluous hair can be bleached instead of removed. Lightly pigmented hair on the arms, legs, and face can be bleached, but hair growing from moles or warts must not be lightened. Handle bleaches carefully to protect the skin and eyes.

Safety Tip

GLOSSARY

Acid preparations   Products that cause the cuticle layers of the hair to "close" or lie tightly against the cortex.

Alkaline (AL-kah-lin) preparations   Products that cause the cuticle layers of the hair to "open" or stand away from the cortex to a certain extent.

Alopecia (al-ah-PEE-shee-ah)   A hair loss or baldness of a temporary or permanent nature. Some of its forms are **alopecia areata** (ay-reh-AT-ah), an oval bald patch; **alopecia prematura**, hair loss occurring before middle age; **alopecia senilis** (seh-NIL-iss), hair loss due to age; **alopecia totalis** (toh-TAL-iss), a permanent total hair loss; and **alopecia universal**, hair loss all over the body.

Amino acids   Organic substances that are the building blocks of the protein molecule.

Anagen (AN-ah-jen) stage   The growth period of hair.

Appendage (ah-PEN-dij)   An extension of something; used in this chapter to refer to hair as an appendage of the skin.

Arrector pili (ah-REK-tehr PIGH-ligh)   A muscle attached to the follicle that contracts with changes in skin temperature.

Barba   Beard hair.

Canities   Gray hair.

Capilli (cah-PIL-igh)   Scalp hair.

Catagen (KAT-en-jen) stage   The period in which hair growth slows and club hairs form.

Cilia (SIL-ee-ah)   Eyelashes.

Congenital   Existing since birth.

Cortex (KOR-teks)   The middle and largest layer of the hair; contains the coloring pigment.

Cuticle (KYOO-ti-kehl)   The outside layer of clear horny cells that overlap each other to form the outer layer of the hair shaft.

Cystine (SIS-teen)   An amino acid found in hair important in cold waving and chemical relaxing.

Cystine bonds   Chemical bonds in the hair that are broken by applying strong alkalines and acids to the hair. They are re-formed during oxidation or by applying a chemical neutralizer. Also called disulfide bonds.

Elasticity   The ability of the hair to stretch without breaking and return to its original form.

Electrologist   A person trained to remove hair by destroying the hair root by electrolysis.

Electrolysis (eh-lek-TRAHL-eh-siss)   Permanently removing the hair by destroying the hair root with an electric needle.

Follicle (FAHL-i-kehl)   A long, slender, pocketlike depression of the skin from which the hair grows.

Gland   A cell or group of cells that removes material from the blood, changes that material, and secretes it to another part of the body or eliminates it.

Hair bulb   The bottom part of the follicle surrounding the papilla.

Hair histology   The study of microscopic structures of the hair.

Hirsutism (HIR-suh-tiz-uhm)   An excessive growth of hair in unwanted places.

Hypertrichosis (high-per-trik-OH-siss)   Excessive unwanted growth of the hair; also called superfluous hair or, in extreme cases, hirsutism.

Keratin (KER-eh-tin)   A protein found in the human skin and its appendages: hair and nails.

Lanugo (lan-OO-goh) hairs   Fine, lightly pigmented hairs occurring all over the body; also called vellus hairs.

Medulla (Meh-DUHL-ah)   The innermost layer of the hair. Not all hairs have a medulla.

Melanin (MEL-eh-nehn)   A kind of pigment that gives hair its color.

Melanocytes (MEL-an-oh-sights)   Cells that make melanin.

Molecule (MOL-eh-kyool)   The smallest possible unit of any compound, made up of two or more atoms chemically combined.

Monilethrix (mon-i-LETH-riks)   A condition in which hair appears to have nodes or beads along the shafts.

Papilla (pap-PIL-ah)   A small, nipplelike projection growing from the dermis that contains a nerve and the blood supply needed to form hair and keep it growing.

Peptide (PEP-tighd) linkages   Amino acid combinations held together by cross-bonds that form the hair. These bonds are broken and re-formed by physical and chemical actions during hair-care services.

Pigment   A substance that gives hair its color.

Pili (PIGH-ligh)   A prefix that means pertaining to the hair.

Pili annulati (PIGH-ligh an-nyoo-LAY-tigh)   A condition characterized by dark and white bands in some or all the scalp; also called ringed hair.

Pili incarnati (PIGH-ligh in-CAR-nay-tigh)   Ingrown hairs.

Porosity (poh-RAHSS-eh-tee)   The amount of moisture that can be absorbed by the cuticle layers of the hair.

Porous   Capable of absorbing moisture.

Short-wave machine   A machine used by an electrologist to remove superfluous hair.

Supercilia (soo-per-SIL-ee-ah)   Eyebrows.

Superfluous (soo-PER-fluh-wuhs) hair   Unwanted hair.

Telogen (TEL-oh-jen) stage   The resting period of hair growth.

Tensile strength   Elasticity.

Tinea (TIN-ee-ah) of the scalp   A condition of broken hairs, scaliness, and, occasionally, infection caused by bacteria. Ringworm.

Terminal hair   Coarse, thick, pigmented hair found on the scalp, face, and extremities.

Trichology (tri-KOL-eh-jee)   The scientific study of the hair and its diseases.

Trichologists (tri-KOL-eh-jists)   People who specialize in studying the hair and diseases related to the hair.

Trichoptilosis (tri-kop-ti-LOH-siss)   Hair that splits along the length of the hair; commonly called split ends.

Trichorrhexis nodosa (tri-koh-REK-siss no-DOH-sah)   An uncommon disease of beard and pubic hair characterized by nodular swellings along the hair shaft.

Trichosis (tri-KOH-siss)   Any diseased condition of the hair.

Tyrosine (TIGH-rah-seen)   An amino acid found in the hair involved in hair coloring services.

QUESTIONS

1. What is the technical term for the scientific study of the hair and its diseases?
2. Aside from protection, what is the other function of hair?
3. Briefly define lanugo hair.
4. What is a threadlike appendage of the skin called?
5. Can you name the outer layer of the skin?
6. What is the smallest unit of a compound?
7. The basic building block of the protein molecule has a two part name. What is that name?
8. What is the other name for cystine bonds?
9. Using your own words, write a definition for hair histology.
10. Using the text, write definitions for the following terms: hair shaft, medulla, cortex, cuticle.
11. What is the hair follicle?
12. What muscle causes "goose bumps" on the skin?
13. Where is the papilla located, and what does it do?
14. What is melanin?
15. What is a simple two-part word for canities?
16. What is the technical term for the process that changes soft keratin to hard protein (keratin)?
17. Can you name the three growing cycles of the hair?

18. What are the four types of hair on the head?
19. Does hair grow faster in summer or winter?
20. What is the technical name given to an oval, bald patch on the head?
21. What is another name for ringworm of the scalp?
22. Before giving a service to a client using a depilatory, what should you do first?
23. Why do you have to be extremely careful when using hot wax on the client?

ANSWERS

1. Trichology 2. Adornment—it improves our individual appearances 3. Lanugo is fine, lightly pigmented hair found almost all over the body 4. A hair 5. Epidermis 6. Molecule 7. Amino acid 8. Disulfide bonds 9. (Check text for correct answer) 10. (See text) 11. The pocket-like depression in the skin through which the hair grows 12. Arrector pili muscle 13. Base of the follicle/supplies blood and nerves to the hair bulb so hair will form and grow 14. Cells that give hair its color 15. Gray hair 16. Keratinization 17. Anagen, catagen, and telogen 18. Capilli—scalp; supercilia—eyebrows; cilia—eyelashes; barba—beard 19. Summer 20. Alopecia areata 21. Tinea of the scalp 22. Allergy test 23. To prevent a severe skin burn

Shampooing the Hair 4

Shampooing cleanses the scalp and hair of dust, dirt, hair spray, sebum (oil), and other residue. Ordinarily, the hair should be shampooed once a week; however, persons who have very oily hair may need a shampoo daily or several times a week.

Because shampooing is a vital preliminary step for many services, it is performed frequently in the school or salon. The clients enjoy this service since effective shampooing manipulations relax the body and are good for the hair and scalp. Therefore, you must master this task early in the training program.

Use shampoo supplies to cleanse the scalp and hair using the proper steps given in this chapter.

Perform the service within 10 to 15 minutes. Score 75 percent or better on a multiple-choice exam on the information in this chapter.

1. Describe the physical and chemical actions of shampooing, the effects of alkaline shampoos and acid rinses, and the effects of cationic, anionic, and nonionic agents.
2. Describe the characteristics and contents of specific kinds of shampoos. Identify appropriate products for conditioning the client's scalp and hair.
3. Recognize scalp and hair irregularities and suggest corrective measures.

4. Cleanse the scalp and hair.

KNOWING SUBOBJECTIVE 1

Describe the physical and chemical actions of shampooing, the effects of alkaline shampoos and acid rinses, and the effects of cationic, anionic and nonionic agents.

Physical and Chemical Actions of Shampooing

Shampooing involves both **physical** and **chemical** actions. The cosmetologist physically spreads the shampoo and exposes all surface areas of the hair for cleansing. Particles of oil, dirt, and other foreign substances are chemically attracted to shampoo molecules. These particles then are attracted to molecules of rinse water flowing along the hair shaft and are washed away. The rinse water provides both chemical action (attraction) and physical action (washing away) to complete cleansing.

pH Ratings of Shampoos

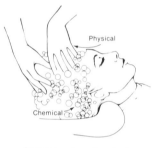

Shampooing the hair

It is important to understand the pH factor of shampoos so that you will know a product's chemical effects and its proper use. (See color plate 4.) The term **pH (potential hydrogen)** indicates the concentration of hydrogen in a solution. This concentration determines a shampoo's pH rating, that is, whether a shampoo is **acid** or **alkaline** (AL-kah-lin). There are various degrees of acidity and alkalinity. The pH scale shows those degrees. The middle of the scale, 7, is the **neutral point**. At 7, the acidity and alkalinity balance each other off so that the solution is neutral. Distilled water has a neutral pH, 7. The numbers 0 to 6.9 indicate acidity; 7.1 to 14 represent alkalinity.

Skin and hair are acid. They have a pH of **4.5–5.5**. Salon products that have the same pH as skin and hair are **acid-balanced**. This means that they do not change the natural pH of the skin or hair.

Shampoos are either alkaline (pH of 7.1–14) or acid-balanced (4.5–5.5). If a client has many hair services using alkaline products, you should recommend an acid-balanced shampoo, especially since many setting lotions have a pH higher than 5.5. Alkaline shampoos are powerful cleansers, but they should be neutralized by an acid rinse, which brings the hair back to its natural pH.

The Effects of Alkaline Shampoos and Acid Rinses

To understand the importance of neutralizing an alkaline shampoo, you must identify the shampoo's chemical effects on the hair. Alkaline products and water with a high alkaline content cause the cuticle of the hair to swell and the hydrogen bonds to **soften**. In this process, the overlapping layers of cuticle scales, called **imbrications** (im-breh-KAY-shunz), open. Thus the hair becomes more porous and its tensile strength, or elasticity, is reduced. Natural oils are removed and moisture evaporates from the cortex.

Acid products shrink and harden the swollen cuticle. The imbrications close, which reduces the hair's porosity and enhances its luster. In addition to neutralizing the alkalinity of shampoos and some water, an acid rinse also eliminates soap curds produced by the interaction of hard water with fatty acids in soaps contained in some shampoos.

When you use an alkaline shampoo, you should explain to the client why an acid rinse is needed; otherwise, the client might think you are insisting on unnecessary products and expense.

Both natural acids and formulated products may be used as neutralizing rinses after you have used alkaline shampoos or other alkaline products. Effective natural acids are apple cider vinegar **(acetic acid)**, white vinegar **(acetic acid)**, and lemon juice **(citric acid)**. Neutralizing products are also made by cosmetics manufacturers. Many names are used to describe them, such as normalizing cremes, creme rinses, stabilizing conditioners, and instant conditioners.

To understand the effects of shampoos, you should also be aware of these three categories of agents: cationic, anionic, and nonionic.

Cationic (KAT-igh-ahn-ik) **agents**, which have positively charged ions, are less damaging to hair than anionic agents and are less likely to leave hair unmanageable.

Anionic (AN-igh-ahn-ik) **agents** are in many shampoos, soaps, and detergents that lather. They can damage hair.

Nonionic (NAHN-igh-ahn-ik) **agents** in shampoo formulas usually are the cleansers. The cationic portion is attracted to the hair's surface and helps increase manageability.

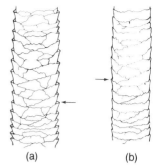

Imbrications of the hair shaft: (a) open, (b) closed

The Characteristics and Contents of Shampoos

Three kinds of shampoos used in salons are liquids, semi-liquids, and solids. These shampoos come in several forms: thin liquids, gels, cremes, foams, pastes, and powders. They come in a variety of containers.

Some shampoos are ready to use; others are concentrates that must be mixed with water. For example, 1 pint of concentrate might make 1 gallon of shampoo. Some superconcentrates make as much as 5 gallons from 1 pint of base. **Always read** and **follow manufacturer's directions** before mixing and using shampoos.

The fragrances added to shampoos serve two purposes. They mask unpleasant chemical odors and provide pleasant ones of their own that complement perfume or cologne. Although fragrances may be pleasant, they may also be a problem. Some persons are allergic to substances that create these fragrances. **Orrisroot**, which is in many products, is one example. Orrisroot may cause skin and scalp irritation and/or sneezing and coughing. Because of the possibility of allergic reactions, you should be particularly careful to dilute superconcentrates according to the directions on the label.

Some shampoos produce more lather than others. Many cosmetologists prefer to use a shampoo that lathers or foams heavily. Many people think that lather is a sign of cleansing power. This is **not necessarily** true. Some shampoos that produce little lather **cleanse the scalp and hair very well.**

Describe the characteristics and contents of specific kinds of shampoos and identify the appropriate products for conditioning the client's scalp and hair.

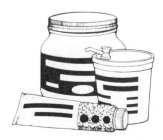

Most shampoos used in salons contain surface-active, complex detergents that have better cleansing power than plain bar soaps or soap-based shampoos. These detergents are more effective than soaps in emulsifying (or breaking up) soil and other unwanted substances. They also have the **advantage** of cleansing with little or no residue (film) like the kind left by the interaction of soaps and hard water. The final test for any shampoo is its effect on the hair and how well you like to use it.

Classifying Shampoos According to Their Uses

Shampoos can be classified according to their special uses. These categories include: nonstripping, medicated, all-purpose, conditioning, herbal, acid-balanced, powder-dry, and liquid-dry shampoos.

Nonstripping shampoos (non-strip shampoo) are made to cleanse without removing permanent hair coloring or toning colors used on prelightened hair. Always use a non-strip shampoo on bleached hair.

Medicated shampoos contain ingredients for treating scalp and hair problems or disorders. Some are available from your beauty supply dealer; others are obtained only by prescription from the client's doctor.

All-purpose shampoos are available from most shampoo manufacturers. They do not strip color, and they have a lower alkaline content than some specialty products. Some even include antifungus and antidandruff agents, besides ingredients that are very mild for hands. If this type of product meets the needs of the client, it can save both clients and salons many dollars in avoiding **product duplication.**

Conditioning shampoos have small amounts of animal, vegetable, or mineral additives that improve the tensile strength and porosity of hair. Some of these additives are proteins, which may go into the cortex or attach themselves to the cuticle of the hair shaft. Proteins in the better conditioning shampoos usually remain in the hair for more than two or three salon visits.

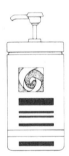

Herbal shampoos contain natural ingredients. Their appeal is based on the "back-to-nature" trend. Although these natural ingredients may be helpful, the products often are expensive. Their value should be judged carefully and compared with less expensive products.

Acid-balanced shampoos, as already mentioned, have about the same pH (4.5–5.5) as hair, so they do not change the hair's natural pH.

Powder-dry shampoos are designed for clients who cannot wet their hair. They are particularly helpful to bedridden persons. They are granules that absorb soil and oil as they are brushed through the scalp and hair.

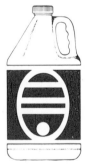

Liquid-dry shampoos also are used on clients who cannot wet their hair in a regular shampooing service. The solution is applied on cotton to small strands of hair. It loosens soil and residue that can be removed by towel-blotting immediately after the shampoo has been applied. The remaining solution evaporates. Liquid-dry shampoos are used mainly on hand-tied hairpieces, such as wigs and wiglets, because ordinary shampoos deteriorate the wefting (base material to which the hair is sewn) of hairpieces.

Because liquid-dry shampoos may be very **flammable** or **combustible**, the following precautions must be taken:

 Safety Tip

1. **Never** use liquid-dry shampoo near an open flame or gas or electric appliances.
2. **Never** smoke cigarettes or allow clients to smoke when liquid-dry shampoo is being used on them.
3. **Always** use liquid-dry shampoos in an open, well-ventilated area. Fumes from these products can burn your lungs.

KNOWING SUBOBJECTIVE 3

Prior to shampooing (or any other service), you must examine the scalp and hair to: (1) check for disease and (2) analyze the condition of the scalp and hair to select appropriate products. If a **communicable disease** (one that can be transmitted from one person to another) is present, **do not serve the client. Don't shampoo the hair before giving a permanent wave, chemical relaxer, frosting, or other chemical service.** If you are not sure, ask your instructor.

Although when you are a cosmetologist you will be concerned about recognizing communicable diseases, you also will need to recognize the differences between congenital, chronic, and acute diseases. A **congenital disease** is a disorder that has existed from birth. (A person born with a heart condition has a congenital disease.) A **chronic** (KRON-ik) **disease**, such as emphysema, is a **long-term** or recurring disorder. A **short-term** condition, such as the common cold, is called an **acute disease**.

In examining the scalp and hair, you should watch for **skin diseases** (infections of the skin). Probably the most common skin disorder observed in the beauty salon is **dandruff**. It is characterized by an excessive number of small or large white flat scales or flakes shed from the outermost layer of the skin of the scalp. This layer of skin is the **epidermis**.

The medical term for dandruff is **pityriasis** (pit-i-RIGH-ah-siss). There are two forms of pityriasis. **Pityriasis capitis simplex** (KAP-eh-tis SIM-pleks) is characterized by dry flaky, white scales on the scalp, hair, and shoulders. A cosmetologist can lessen it by using **nonprescription** medicated shampoos.

Pityriasis steatoides (pit-i-RIGH-ah-siss stee-ah-TOI-deez) is characterized by yellow, oily or waxy scales located close to the scalp. Sebaceous (si-BAY-shuhs) glands in the scalp produce a lubricating substance called sebum. If the sebaceous glands become overactive when dandruff is on a person's scalp, the scales become stuck together and attached to the scalp and hair. Ordinary shampoos will not remove these scales, flakes, and oil deposits. This condition may require a medicated shampoo prescribed by a doctor.

About two out of three persons in the United States have dandruff. Although its cause has not been determined, scientists have had several theor-

Recognize scalp and hair irregularities and suggest corrective measures.

 Safety Tip

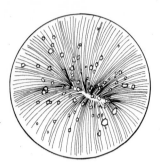

Dandruff

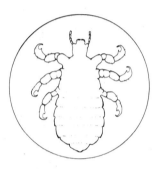

Head louse (pediculosis)

Safety Tip

ies. One theory is that dandruff is caused by nervous disorders related to high blood pressure (hypertension) and emotional stress. People living in cities get dandruff more often than people who live in small towns and on farms. This fact might be due to the difference in their lifestyles.

Psoriasis (sah-RIGH-eh-siss) is a skin disease that can be chronic or acute. It is characterized by inflamed (red) patches and overlapping yellow or white scales. It is **not** contagious, and though the crust will bleed if disturbed, clients having it may receive cold waves and use hair colors. You should ask the client to give you a letter from a doctor stating that hair treatments are permissible.

Herpes simplex (HEHR-peez SIM-pleks) is a viral infection (from a virus) characterized by inflammation of skin and mucous membranes, especially those of the face and lips. Such inflammations are called **cold sores**. Exactly how this condition develops is not known, but it usually clears up in six to ten days.

Pediculosis (pi-dik-yah-LOH-siss) is an animal parasitic condition. (A parasite is an organism or microorganism that lives on another organism.) Pediculosis involves **head lice** that lay their eggs on the scalp and hair. Because of improved personal hygiene in the United States, head lice was not a common disease during recent decades. However, there has been some increase in the occurrence of head lice since more people began to grow their hair long and because some people probably do not shampoo their hair as often as they should. Since **pediculosis is contagious**, a client having it **cannot be served** in the school or salon. Effective treatment, including a medicated shampoo prescribed by a doctor, can eliminate the condition in three or four days.

Scabies is another animal parasitic condition. It is an infestation of the **itch mite**, which burrows into the scalp and causes irritation leading to scratching of the scalp. **Refuse service** to a person having scabies and refer her or him to a doctor.

Tinea (TIN-ee-ah), a skin infection caused by a fungus (vegetable parasite), is **very contagious**. This condition, commonly called **ringworm**, appears as circular inflamed areas of little blisters. A person having it **cannot be served** and should be advised to see a doctor.

Seborrhea (seb-ah-REE-ah) is a disorder of the sebaceous glands causing **excessively oily scalp and hair. Hyper**activity (**over**activity) of the sebaceous (si-BAY-shuhs) **glands** causes this excessive secretion of **sebum**, which is transferred from the scalp to the hair. Seborrhea can be controlled by using a medicated shampoo for oily hair or by using frosting or streaking the hair. One or both methods may be used. Daily shampoos also may be needed.

Asteatosis (as-tee-ah-TOH-siss) is caused by **hypo**activity (**under**activity) of the sebaceous glands. Too little sebum is produced, resulting in dry, scaly skin and/or hair that lacks luster. This unusual condition seldom is seen in the salon.

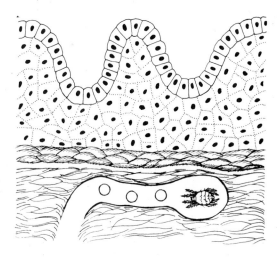

Itch mite

A **steatoma** (stee-ah-TOH-mah), or **wen**, is a subcutaneous (beneath the skin) cyst occurring when the duct from the sebaceous gland to a hair follicle becomes clogged or blocked. Sebum accumulates and hardens beneath the skin until the duct is open again.

Acne (AK-nee) is an eruptive skin disease caused by inflammation (irritation) of the sebaceous glands. It usually appears on the face, chest, and back. The condition can be controlled by a dermatologist. Clients having acne can be served in the salon and school.

Comedones (kahm-eh-DOH-neez), also called **blackheads**, occur when the skin is not cleansed properly and regularly. Sebum hardens around a speck of dirt or dust, clogging a pore and creating a slightly raised area.

Milia (MIL-ee-ah), also called **whiteheads**, are cysts that contain sebum trapped in a sebaceous duct.

Miliaria rubra (mil-ee-AR-ee-ah ROOB-rah) is an acute irritation below the top layer of skin. It is an inflammation of the sudoriferous (sweat) glands. Commonly called **prickly heat**, this noncommunicable disorder usually occurs during hot weather.

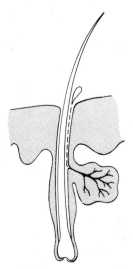

Sebaceous gland
secreting sebum

DOING SUBOBJECTIVE 4

Supplies
- ☐ client release form*
- ☐ laundered towel
- ☐ sanitized comb and brush
- ☐ neck strip
- ☐ shampoo cape
- ☐ shampoo
- ☐ neutralizing rinse, if necessary

Cleanse the scalp and hair.

*To avoid excessive repetition, the release form will not be listed for all procedures. It is included, however, in all chemical services and in a few others as a reminder of its importance. You must follow the policy of your school or salon.

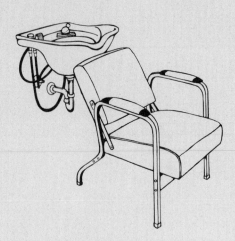

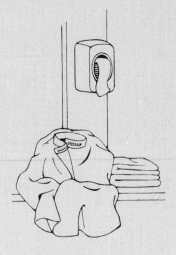

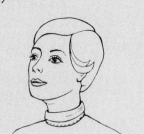

PROCEDURE

1. Ask client to sign release form. Take off any jewelry you are wearing. Greet the client and politely ask for his or her jewelry. Put it in a safe place, such as a drawer.

2. Wash your hands with soap and hot water before beginning this and every other service.

3. Place a neck strip or towel around the client's neck before securing the shampoo cape.

Safety Tip

RATIONALE

1. Since services are performed by students, clients need to sign form. Removing jewelry protects it from chemicals and from getting lost. Always treat the client courteously.

2. **Preventing the spread of disease causing bacteria is the** responsibility of everyone.

3. Since a cape is used on more than one person, a laundered towel or new neck strip is placed around client's neck as a sanitary precaution before cape is used.

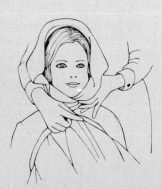

Secure towel around neck

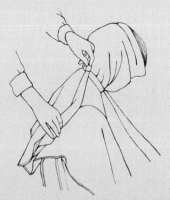

Hook cape lock around neck

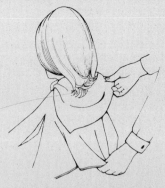

Place bottom of cape over back of shampoo chair

4. Observe the client's hairstyle before wetting the hair.

5. Ask the client what services are scheduled.

6. Determine step-by-step procedures to be followed.

7. Remove hairpins, bobby pins, and hair ornaments.

8. Examine the scalp for cuts, scratches, abrasions, irritation, and other abnormal conditions. Consult your instructor or manager if abnormalities are visible.

9. Begin brushing on left front of head using horizontal ½- to ¾-inch partings.

10. Rotate the brush 180 degrees in your right hand while holding the section of hair in your left hand.

11. Be certain to rotate the brush on the scalp and then into the hair.

4. If the client requests a similar hairstyle, you will have a clear mental picture of it.

5. Shampooing procedures vary according to services that follow.

6. The hair usually is **not brushed or shampooed before applying a lightener, permanent color retouch, permanent color for virgin hair, or chemical relaxer.** The hair is brushed before a shampoo and set unless the scalp is irritated. It is also brushed before a frosting. Also, some clients will ask you to remove back-combing. If the client has an extraordinary accumulation of hair spray or soil, plan to shampoo twice or even three times.

7. If the brush catches on something in hair, the client will be uncomfortable.

8. **Examination is necessary because you must refuse service to anyone who has a contagious scalp disease.**

9. **This sectioning insures** that all the scalp and **hair** will **be** brushed and **examined for scratches, abrasions, and diseases.**

10. Brushing increases the blood supply to the scalp and normalizes the activity of the sebaceous glands.

11. Brushing the scalp loosens soil and flaking skin so that the shampoo will cleanse more thoroughly.

Safety Tip

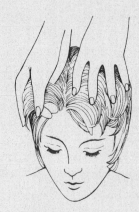

Examine the scalp

Safety Tip

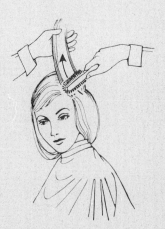

Scientific brushing

12. Each section should be brushed thoroughly 3 times.

12. This insures that the entire scalp and hair are brushed thoroughly.

13. Lay the first section over on the right front area, then bring your hand down and part off another ½- to ¾-inch horizontal section.

13. Brush from the top to the bottom of the left side of the head so that the section just brushed will not be in the way when you brush the next section down.

14. Repeat steps 10, 11, and 12 until all hair in that section has been brushed.

14. Again, immediately report any abnormal conditions to your instructor or manager.

15. Go on to the crown section on the left side of the head and begin brushing. Use ½-inch horizontal partings. Work from the top of the section until all scalp and hair have been brushed. Repeat step 12.

15. This procedure will save time because the brushing proceeds around the head—from left side of head to both the crown and nape sections and on to the right front section.

16. Using the information presented in this unit, analyze the condition of the client's scalp and hair and select the appropriate shampoo.

16. In performing the first 7 shampoos on clients, consult your instructor or manager on the choice of shampoo. Depending on the condition of scalp and hair, plain, non-stripping, medicated, and conditioning shampoos may be needed.

17. Check to make sure that the cape is secure but comfortable and that it drapes over the back of the chair.

17. **A loose or poorly secured cape can cause water damage to the client's clothing. Draping it over the chair will cause water to run onto the floor.**

Shampoo the Hair

Safety Tip

PROCEDURE

1. Standing by the client's left side, place your left hand behind the **client's head and** carefully lower it to the shampoo bowl. Make any necessary adjustments.

RATIONALE

1. Shampoo bowls are made of porcelain-covered iron. If unassisted, **a client could be injured by lowering his or her head too quickly.**

2. Pick up the nozzle of the spray hose and point it toward the drain. Then turn on cold water.

3. Hold the nozzle between your thumb and index and middle fingers. Slide the little finger of your right hand into the water's spray.

4. Any time that water is directed at client's head, the little finger should be in the water's spray.

5. Gradually saturate the hair in the crown. **Use back of your hand to shield the client's face from the water spray**. Cup your left hand around the client's left ear as you move the spray around the head.

2. If water is turned on before nozzle is pointed downward, someone may be sprayed. Always turn on cold water first, adding hot water as necessary.

3. In this position the little finger can monitor water temperature. A good, comfortable temperature for the average client is 90° to 110°F. (The following terms indicate water temperatures: cool, 65°–70°F.; tepid, 85°–90°F.; warm, 95°–100°F.; hot, 105°–110°F.)

4. **Water pressures and temperatures can change quickly. The little finger will detect changes so that water can be directed away from client's head when necessary**.

5. This allows the client to react if water temperature is uncomfortable. Always protect the client from the spray.

◣ **Safety
   Tip**

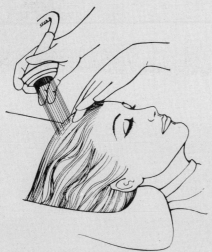

Use one hand to protect the eyes and face from the water

6. Gently move the side of the client's right ear forward with your left hand as you saturate the hair on that part of the head.

6. Same as step 5.

7. Use your left hand to protect the client's nape area as you saturate it.

7. This will protect the client's clothing.

8. After all the hair is saturated, turn off **hot water first** then cold. Check the shampoo you have selected.

8. If cold water were turned off first, client might be burned. Checking shampoo for correct viscosity, color, and fragrance is a good safety measure.

9. Apply shampoo sparingly about 2 inches from the hairline in small, even sections across the crown.

9. Since soiled hair doesn't lather well during a first application, using a large amount is wasteful and unnecessary. If shampoo were applied at the hairline, some might drip on the client's forehead and in the client's eyes. **If the shampoo does get in the client's eyes, use the corner of a clean towel saturated with cold water to blot the eyes immediately.** Consult your instructor or manager for help.

Safety Tip

10. Using both of your hands on both sides of the client's head, manipulate your fingertips firmly in a zigzag pattern from the hairline toward the back of the head.

10. This lathers and evenly distributes the shampoo so that it can clean all the scalp and hair. Use the cushions of your fingertips to avoid scratching the scalp.

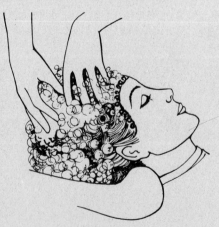

Cosmetic hairline is the place where makeup can collect around the client's face

11. Repeat this procedure 3 times.

11. This insures thorough cleansing.

12. Lift the client's head with your left hand while the client braces his or her neck against the shampoo bowl.

12. This procedure gives the client's head the proper support. The client braces his or her head against the bowl to keep shampoo from dripping onto his or her clothing.

13. Begin manipulations with your right hand behind the client's right ear and zigzag firmly across the back of the crown to the left ear.

13. This procedure cleanses the crown evenly.

14. Repeat preceding step 3 times.

14. This insures thorough cleansing.

15. Repeat these manipulations in the nape area, working across from the right ear to the left ear.

15. Same as step 14.

16. Use your thumbs to shampoo the "**cosmetic hairline**."

16. The **cosmetic hairline** is that area in which makeup has accumulated because of attempts to clean the face without disturbing the hairstyle.

17. Carefully lower the client's head into shampoo bowl.

17. This protects the client.

18. **Rinse the hair thoroughly** by saturating it with water.

18. Rinsing removes soil, sprays, and other unwanted substances.

19. Repeat the steps for cleansing and rinsing the hair. No visible traces of shampoo should remain in the hair, particularly in the **nape** area.

19. **Shampoo left in hair will interfere with other services**.

20. Raise the client upright and towel-dry hair.

20. This removes excess moisture that could interfere with the next service.

21. Select and mix the creme rinse conditioner.

21. The rinse neutralizes the alkalinity of shampoo. Most creme rinses have a low pH so that they, too, can neutralize.

22. Lower the client's head to shampoo bowl and apply the rinse according to manufacturer's directions.

22. Products vary widely. Always read and follow directions.

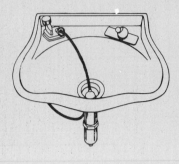

23. Thoroughly rinse again.

23. A product left in the hair could interfere with the next service.

24. Raise the client to a sitting position and towel-dry the hair.

24. The client is more comfortable.

25. Sterilize the shampoo bowl. Give special attention to the neck rest after each client.

25. This protects other clients.

26. Return hose nozzle to drain position.

26. Leaving the nozzle as shown here allows any dripping water to drain in the sink, rather than onto the floor.

GLOSSARY

Acetic acid   A natural acid; vinegar.

Acid   A product that has a pH rating of under 7.

Acid-balanced products   Products that have the same pH rating as skin and hair (4.5–5.5).

Acid-balanced shampoos   Shampoos that do not change the hair's natural pH.

Acne (AK-nee)   An eruption of the skin caused by irritation of the sebaceous glands. It usually appears on the face, chest, and back.

Acute disease   A short-term disease (such as the common cold).

Alkaline (AL-kah-lin)   A product having a pH rating of over 7.

All-purpose shampoos   Shampoos that have a lower alkaline content than some specialty shampoos and will not strip color.

Anionic (an-igh-AHN-ik) agents   Substances having negatively charged ions.

Asteatosis (as-tee-ah-TOH-siss)   Dry, scaly skin and/or hair that lacks luster resulting from underactivity of the sebaceous glands.

Blackheads   See **Comedones.**

Cationic (Kat-igh-AHN-ik) agents   Substances that have positively charged ions.

Chronic (KRON-ik) disease   A long-term or recurring disorder (such as emphysema).

Citric acid   A natural acid found in lemon juice.

Comedones (kahm-eh-DOH-neez)   Raised, clogged pores caused by sebum hardening around a speck of dirt or dust; commonly called blackheads.

Conditioning shampoos   Shampoos that have small amounts of animal, vegetable, or mineral additives that improve the tensile strength and porosity of hair.

Congenital disease   A disorder that has existed from birth (such as a heart condition).

Dandruff   See **Pityriasis.**

Epidermis (ep-eh-DER-mis)   The thinnest, outermost layer of the skin.

Herpes simplex (HEHR-pees SIM-pleks)   An inflammation of the skin and mucous membranes, especially those of the face and lips, caused by a virus. Often called cold sores.

Imbrications (im-breh-KAY-shunz)   Overlapping layers of cuticle scales of the hair.

Liquid-dry shampoo   A solution that loosens soil so that it can be removed by towel-blotting the hair. It then evaporates. Used mostly on wigs and hairpieces.

Medicated shampoos   Shampoos containing ingredients for treating scalp and hair problems.

Milia (MIL-ee-ah)   Cysts that contain sebum trapped in a sebaceous duct, commonly called whiteheads.

Miliaria rubra (mil-ee-AR-ee-ah ROOB-rah)   An acute, noncontagious inflammation of the sweat glands, usually occurring in hot weather; commonly called prickly heat.

Neutral point   A point (7) on the pH scale where a product is neither acid nor alkaline.

Nonionic (NAHN-igh-ahn-ik) agents   Substances composed of molecules which are neither positively nor negatively charged.

Nonstripping shampoos   Shampoos that cleanse without removing permanent hair coloring or toning colors used on prelightened hair.

Orrisroot   An ingredient found in many fragrances known to cause an allergic reaction.

Pediculosis (pi-dik-yah-LOH-siss)   A parasitic condition of the scalp caused by head lice that lay their eggs on the scalp and hair.

pH (potential hydrogen)   Indicates the concentration of hydrogen in a solution. This concentration determines whether a product is acid or alkaline.

Pityriasis (pit-i-RIGH-ah-siss)   An excessive number of flat scales or flakes shed from the outermost layer of the skin of the scalp, commonly called dandruff. The two types are pityriasis capitis simplex (KAP-eh-tis SIM-pleks), which are dry, flaky, white scales; and pityriasis steatoides (stee-ah-TOI-deez), which are yellow, oily, or waxy scales close to the scalp.

Powder-dry shampoos   Shampoos consisting of granules that absorb soil and oil as they are brushed through the scalp and hair.

Psoriasis (sah-RIGH-eh-siss)   Noncontagious inflamed (red) patches and overlapping yellow or white scales on the skin; can be chronic or acute.

Scabies   A parasitic condition of the scalp caused by itch mites that burrow into the scalp.

Sebaceous (se-BAY-shuhs) glands   The glands that supply sebum (oil) to the hair.

Seborrhea (seb-ah-REE-ah)   A disorder of the sebaceous glands causing excessively oily scalp and hair.

Steatoma (stee-ah-TOH-mah)   A cyst beneath the skin occurring when the duct from the sebaceous gland to a hair follicle becomes clogged or blocked; commonly called a wen.

Tinea (TIN-ee-ah)   A very contagious skin infection caused by a fungus, which appears as circular inflamed areas of little blisters; commonly called ringworm.

Whiteheads   See **Milia**.

QUESTIONS

1. What is a shampoo?
2. The letters pH are an abbreviation for what two words?
3. When a product is acid-balanced, what range of numbers would indicate that?
4. Can you name at least six different classes of shampoos?
5. What is herpes simplex?
6. What is another name for whiteheads?
7. Does a shampoo have to lather heavily in order to clean the hair?
8. What type of shampoo would you recommend for lightened (bleached) hair?
9. Why would you refuse to allow a client to smoke a cigarette while you applied a liquid-dry shampoo?
10. What is the name given to small white flakes on the scalp?
11. What is the medical name for dandruff?
12. Would you serve a client with pediculosis?
13. Tinea of the scalp is another name for what condition?
14. Would you serve a client who has psoriasis?
15. What is the technical term for an oily scalp?
16. What is the cosmetic hairline?
17. After finishing with the shampoo bowl, where should you leave the nozzle of the hose?

ANSWERS

1. The cleansing of the hair and scalp 2. Potential hydrogen 3. 4.5–5.5 4. Non-stripping, medicated, conditioning, herbal, powder-dry and liquid-dry 5. A viral infection which causes cold sores 6. Milia 7. No 8. Nonstripping shampoo 9. It is flammable 10. Dandruff 11. Pityriasis 12. Absolutely not 13. Ringworm of the scalp 14. Yes 15. Seborrhea 16. The area around the face where makeup collects 17. In drain position

Conditioning the Hair 5

You may have already seen a few of the available products that have been designed to improve the condition of the hair. At this point you may even feel that you have "seen them all," but in fact, you probably have only scratched the surface. When you become a practicing cosmetologist, you will be exposed to hundreds, if not thousands, of hair conditioners. How can you know which one to use? This chapter is designed to answer a few basic questions:

1. **Why** is the hair conditioned?
2. **What** is used to condition it?
3. **When** should it be conditioned?
4. **How much** conditioning should be done?
5. **How** should the conditioning be sold to the client?

Because so many different conditioners are available both professionally and over the counter, it would be impossible to include all types and their effects. Hair conditioning is one of the most frequently requested services, so it is very important that you learn as much as possible about it. As in all other cases, ask your **instructor or manager** about the use of a particular conditioner to solve a specific hair-conditioning problem.

This chapter will discuss the composition, use, and application of the **general types** of conditioners.

Select a specific conditioner that will improve the condition of a client's damaged hair.

Major Objective

Level of Acceptability

Perform the major objective according to the principles discussed in this chapter.

Knowing Subobjectives

1. List the physical and chemical actions that damage hair, and define 5 terms that describe hair condition.
2. Describe the use of proteins in conditioning the hair.
3. Classify and describe the different types of conditioners.

Doing Subobjective

4. Assess hair damage and select and apply the appropriate conditioner.

KNOWING SUBOBJECTIVE 1

List the physical and chemical actions that damage hair, and define 5 terms that describe hair condition.

To use any conditioner effectively, you must understand why conditioners are needed at all! Conditioners are needed to correct physical or chemical damage to the hair.

Physical damage to the hair may be caused in a natural way due to: sunlight (ultraviolet rays), drying winds, air oxidation, hard (high mineral content) water, or chlorinated water.

Physical damage may also occur unnaturally from:

1. **Brush rollers** (used at home), which split and break hair.
2. **Heated rollers,** which have points that can split and break the hair and damage the scalp.
3. **Thermal curling irons** (used at home), which burn and singe the hair.
4. **Incorrect teasing** (back-combing), which causes the hair to break.
5. **Incorrect brushing** using a nylon brush without rounded bristles. A natural boar-bristle brush is better for use at home. Sharp-pointed nylon-bristle brushes tend to cut the hair shaft and scrape the scalp.

The scalp and hair can be damaged chemically by the improper use of chemical relaxers, cold waves, hair lighteners (bleaches), tints, setting lotions, and conditioners.

Physical and chemical damage to the hair affects its porosity, elasticity, texture, appearance, and manageability.

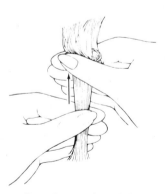

Porosity test by a left-handed person

1. **Porosity** of the hair refers to the amount of liquid the hair strand can **absorb**. Damaged hair is said to be overporous if the imbricated outer layers of the cuticle are in an open position.

2. **Elasticity** refers to the degree to which a hair can be stretched without breaking. The amount of "stretch" or elasticity hair has relates to its **tensile strength.** A hair can be stretched almost 50 percent when wet, but only 10 to 20 percent when dry. If the hair has been physically and/or chemically damaged, it may be very weak and break **easily** when stretched.

3. **Texture** refers to the feel and diameter of the hair shaft. If the hair shaft feels smooth, hard, and "glassy," the imbricated layers of the outer cuticle are lying flat against the hair shaft. When the imbrications are open, the hair shaft feels rough. If the hair "feels" soft, fluffy, and has a small diameter, it is called **fine hair.** Hair that has a larger diameter is **coarse hair.** Hair diameters in between are referred to as average or **medium hair.**

4. **Appearance** refers to the luster, sheen, or shininess of the hair. Damaged hair is lackluster. It does not shine. This is caused by the loss of natural scalp oil through physical or chemical abuse. This natural lubricant from the scalp that gives hair its beautiful shine is called **sebum.**

5. **Manageability** of hair refers to the ease or difficulty with which the comb passes through the hair, both when the hair is wet and when it is dry. For example, if it is very **difficult to comb through** the hair when it is wet, the hair is said to be "unmanageable," and it needs conditioning. Dry, "flyaway" hair can be caused by static electricity created by low humidity. The humidity inside buildings, especially in colder climates, often is too low.

Dry hair also may be unmanageable and difficult to comb. Manageability is affected by the overall condition of the hair, which takes into account porosity, elasticity, texture, and appearance. Therefore, whenever one of these natural hair qualities is lost or weakened, the hair is said to be "damaged."

Whenever you see that the scalp is red and irritated or has cuts and abrasions, you should advise the client to visit the family doctor or a dermatologist. Only a medical doctor can treat diseases or injuries of the skin. You **cannot** legally **treat** such conditions and must **refuse** service to clients who have them.

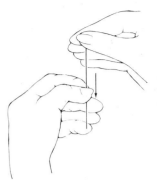

Elasticity test by a left-handed person

KNOWING SUBOBJECTIVE 2

As was stated earlier in the text, **keratin (KER-eh-tin)** is the basic protein that forms the structure of the hair shaft. All preparations that are labeled or called protein conditioners do contain protein. The differences in proteins used on the hair are mainly their (1) size and (2) origin.

1. To penetrate the cortex of the hair shaft effectively, protein hair conditioners must contain **substantive proteins.** Substantive proteins have been made or processed. They are **very small.** The size of the molecules that form the protein helps determine how well a conditioner will work on the hair; substantive proteins work best. Conditioning the hair can be compared to repairing a crack in the plaster wall of a building. Cement cannot be used to repair it because it has sand and stone particles that are much larger than those of plaster. Using a similar mixture of plaster, however, will fill the crack so that it will not be noticeable. In the same way, a hair conditioner **must** contain proteins **small** (substantive) enough to penetrate the hair's cuticle layer and to adhere (stick) to the damaged part of the hair.

Describe the use of proteins in conditioning hair.

Some people have used milk, egg whites, beer, and other foods containing proteins to condition the hair. In their **natural state,** these items are not very effective conditioners because the size of their protein molecules is **too large** to penetrate the hair. Using them to condition hair is somewhat like trying to force a bowling ball into a grape—impossible! However, these proteins can benefit the outside of the hair.

2. The **origin of the conditioner's protein** is also important. Most protein conditioners are made from **animal** or **vegetable** materials, although a few come from minerals.

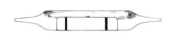

Some conditioners contain bovine serum, an **animal protein.** It contains refined and sterilized cattle tissues, such as blood and bone marrow. Bovine serum is diluted with buffering agents and water since pure animal protein can be used safely only in about 10 percent strength. The **placenta** (plah-SEN-tah) of female cattle and sheep is also refined and used in some hair conditioners. **Collagen** (KAHL-eh-jen) is another animal protein used to condition the hair.

Some conditioners contain vegetable proteins. **Vegetable proteins** are made from soybeans, balsam trees, tong beans, olives, wheat germ, and other high-protein plants. These ingredients are refined and formulated for conditioning the hair.

Both animal and vegetable protein conditioners are made in a very complicated way with many different combinations of chemicals. Only the **very basic** ingredients contained in these products have been mentioned.

A conditioner is often used **prior** to a strong chemical service to prevent hair damage; this application is called **preconditioning.** Conditioners **added** to products to improve or buffer their action on the hair **during** the service provide **in-process conditioning.** After a service, conditioners used on the hair are used to **recondition** the hair.

It **is possible to overcondition** the hair so that the conditioner stops the action of another chemical product applied to the hair. The hair can act like a saturated sponge if too many chemicals are applied. The hair can absorb just so many protein molecules; if its capacity is reached with the conditioner, there will be no room for cold-waving lotion (or other chemicals). Another example of overconditioning is the use of a very acid conditioner that closes the cuticle imbrications tightly against the cortex, preventing a tint from penetrating the cuticle to color the cortex. It is also possible to put so much oil on dry hair that it becomes greasy and unmanageable—even after rinsing!

Keep something in mind: conditioners are **not** magic! If the hair has been severely damaged or abused, a **series** of conditioning treatments may be necessary to return the hair to a normal state.

Cosmetologists are continually asked to buy this or that conditioner because the hair will be improved "miraculously" through some new scientific discovery. Although scientific product research continues to make valuable contributions, cosmetologists must judge products by studying the available facts and observing how well they actually work. You can use the following checklist in applying conditioners and assessing their effectiveness:

1. Did you carefully read and follow the label directions?
2. Did you consult your instructor or manager before you used the conditioner?
3. Was the condition (moisture, elasticity, porosity, texture, or appearance) of the hair improved?

If you chose the correct conditioner, used it according to the directions on the label, and followed the advice of your instructor, the hair's condition **should be improved.** If it is not, a series of conditioning treatments may be necessary, or a **different** conditioner may be needed.

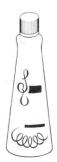

KNOWING SUBOBJECTIVE 3

There are so many hair conditioners available that you must know exactly what those used in your school or salon can and cannot do. There are five general types of hair conditioners.

Classify and describe the different types of conditioners.

1. **Instant conditioners** usually have a vegetable oil (for example, balsam) base, which benefits the hair by **restoring moisture** and **oils.** This type of conditioner often has an **acid** pH. The instant conditioner coats the hair and usually does **not** penetrate into the cortex to replace keratin in the hair shaft. This type may make fine hair too oily and limp and, thus, difficult to comb out.

Instant conditioners are applied to shampooed hair that has been towel-dried. When you use this kind of conditioner, let it stay on the hair for 1 or 2 minutes; then rinse the excess conditioner that has not been absorbed by the hair.

2. **Instant conditioning and setting aids** are mainly strong setting lotions that also have a little animal or vegetable protein. These conditioners are made to increase the diameter of the hair shaft. Parts of the setting aid have an **affinity** (attraction) for the cuticle of the hair shaft. Their pH can be

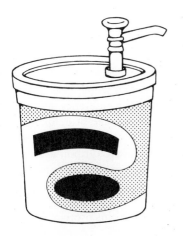
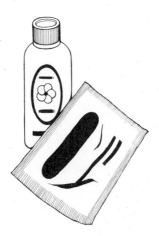

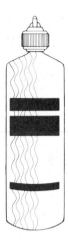

either acid or alkaline. This type of conditioner often is used between cold waves to make the hairstyle last longer. It has an **antihumectant,** which makes an antihumidity **barrier between the hair shaft** and the **moisture in the air** to help preserve the style of the hair. This type of conditioner is particularly good for fine hair. Most instant conditioning and setting aids are made in different **strengths** for fine, normal (not tinted or lightened), tinted, and bleached hair.

There are several important steps you should follow when applying an instant conditioning and setting aid. Apply it to the hair after you have shampooed and towel-dried it. **Always apply it immediately before setting the hair.** Do not rinse it away. After you have applied and combed it through the hair, spray water onto the hair and then comb it through. Water works as a carrying agent to assist the conditioner in penetrating the cuticle. If the hair dries out during the setting procedure, add **more water,** not setting lotion or conditioner. Some of these products make the hair feel "crisp" before combing.

3. **Protein conditioners** are those products that actually go through the cuticle of the hair shaft into the cortex to replace keratin that has been physically or chemically removed. This internal replacement results in **equal porosity** within the hair shaft, **greater elasticity,** and improved texture.

Because of the strength of substantive proteins, these kinds of conditioners are usually applied to hair that has been shampooed and then towel-dried. After a period of time and/or the application of heat, **protein conditioners are rinsed from the hair before setting!** This is the best way to use them. *You must carefully read and follow label directions and follow directions from your instructor or manager.*

4. **Normalizing conditioners** are made specifically to **neutralize** the **alkaline** effects of trace chemicals **after** such services as a tint, relaxer, cold wave, or lightener. Thus, the normalizing conditioner has an **acid pH.** If traces of alkali are not neutralized by these normalizing conditioners, the alkali may damage the hair or irritate the scalp. Two minutes after application they are rinsed.

5. **Nucleic** (NEW-klee-ik) **acid** is the newest, and scientifically, the best professional hair **reconstructor** (rebuilder) available. As you know, hair is made of hard protein, and this protein is made up of a combination of some of the twenty known **amino acids.** These amino acids each have a set of chemical "finger prints," which allows us to pick out one amino acid from the other—e.g., it gives each amino acid a name or identity. Scientists have given this chemical identification system a name, which is "RNA" (ribonucleic acid). The RNA system is so refined that the difference between amino acids that make-up hair protein and those that make heart muscle protein can be easily detected. The system for coding/copying (duplicating) the known amino acids is scientifically called DNA (deoxyribonucleic acid). It is this DNA duplicating system (called **protein synthesis**) that permits scientists to make the nucleic acid hair reconstructor, so that when it is applied to the hair, it replaces any amino acid(s) that the hair shaft should have, but does not. Animal and vegetable cells are used in this protein synthesis pro-

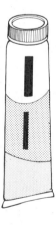

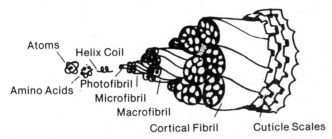

Breakdown of the hairshaft. Each hair shaft is composed of Atoms, Amino Acids, Helix Coils, and last but not least, Protein, which structure the hair in its orderly fibril make up

cess. **Micropolysaccharide** is the glue-like substance that cements the hair together. See pp. 48 and 49. This cement is like sap from a tree, only it is in your hair.

Therefore, nucleic acid conditioners rebuild damaged polypeptide (protein made of four or more amino acids) chains, hydrogen bonds, and sulphur bonds in the hair. These conditioners also protect hair from high alkaline services, such as, bleaching, tinting, and cold waving, etc.

The scientific facts are that nucleic acid is the best reconstructor for the hair because it: (1) restores moisture; (2) rebuilds the helix of the polypeptide chain; (3) penetrates the cuticle and cortex; (4) strengthens it without interfering (slowing down or diluting) with other chemical actions; (5) gives greater elasticity and shine; (6) adds body to hair for easier styling; and (7) remains in the hair longer. In short, nucleic acid does more for hair reconstruction than any other conditioner.

The exact way in which they work is not yet completely understood. Follow the advice of your instructor or manager so that you will be using this new product correctly.

DOING SUBOBJECTIVE 4

Supplies

- □ client release form
- □ shampoo supplies
- □ assortment of professional hair conditioners

Assess hair damage and select and apply the appropriate conditioner.

PROCEDURE

1. Drape the client and examine the scalp for scratches, abrasions, and general color.

2. If chemical services are not scheduled, brush the hair and then assess its condition.

RATIONALE

1. This is standard procedure.

2. Due to widespread physical and chemical abuse, almost 9 out of 10 clients in the salon have hair that requires some degree of conditioning.

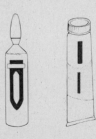

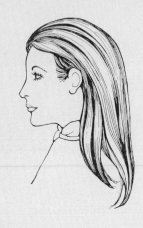

3. Note the luster or lack of luster in the hair as the light reflects from it.

4. Feel the hair to determine if it is smooth or rough to the touch.

5. Analyze the porosity and elasticity of the hair.

6. Shampoo and analyze the hair and explain the results of the analysis to your client.

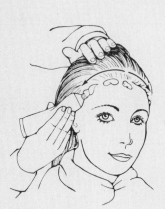

7. Recommend two different conditioners at two different prices to the client and explain how each will improve the condition of the hair. If a great deal of additional time will be needed to apply the conditioner, this should also be explained.

8. **An Example.** Ms. (Mrs., Mr.) Anderson, your hair needs conditioning. It seems to be dry. It lacks natural oils. This may be due to overexposure to the sun and wind, or it may have been caused by chemical abuse. I would recommend our Brand A or Brand C conditioner to restore oils to your hair so that it will have a beautiful shine. Brand A requires only three or four minutes and sells for $2. Brand C takes 10 to 12 minutes to apply and penetrates the cuticle of the hair shaft. It sells for $5.

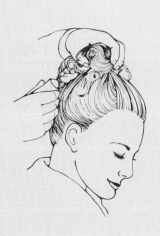

3. Luster indicates whether the sebaceous glands are functioning normally.

4. Dryness can be felt. To some extent, you also can feel the porosity of the hair if the cuticle imbrications stand away from the hair shaft.

5. This is standard procedure (explained in chapter 4).

6. It is good practice to analyze the hair twice, once when wet and once when dry. Always explain what the condition of the hair is.

7. Giving the client two choices of price and conditioner is good salesmanship. It puts the decision into an either/or instead of a yes/no category. The client has the right to know how the product will affect the hair and how long the application will take.

8. Clearly **identify the problem** for the client so that the condition of the hair is understood. Describe **what the hair lacks**. Explain **why the conditioner is needed**. Recommend **two** conditioners that will correct this hair damage so that client will have a **choice**. State the difference in the time required for each conditioner because the client may be operating on a tight schedule. The price difference also may be important to a client who has forgotten a checkbook and has only enough cash for the scheduled service. This should be standard procedure for recommending all salon services.

9. Apply the conditioner and work it through the hair. Then place protective plastic cap and then heating cap over the client's head.

9. The heat helps the conditioner penetrate the hair.

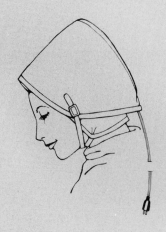

10. Ms. (Mrs., Mr.) Anderson, I have assessed the condition of your hair, and it is in very good shape. Although you have asked for a conditioner today, I honestly do not feel that your hair needs it now. If your hair needs conditioning in future visits to the salon, I will call it to your attention.

10. **Never attempt to sell a client an unneeded service.** The best way to win your client's confidence is to give honest, accurate, and professional advice. The reward for doing the right thing will be tenfold because it will enhance the client's trust in your technical competency.

GLOSSARY

Affinity   The attraction between chemicals or substances.

Animal proteins   One kind of protein in hair conditioners.

Antihumectant   A chemical that makes a barrier between the hair shaft and moisture in the air.

Appearance   Luster, sheen, or shininess of the hair.

Collagen (KAHL-eh-jen)   An animal protein used in some skin and hair cosmetics.

Elasticity   The degree to which a hair can be stretched without breaking.

In-process conditioning   Adding conditioners to products to improve or buffer their action during conditioning.

Instant conditioner   A conditioner with a vegetable oil base and often an acid pH that does not penetrate into the hair shaft.

Instant conditioning and setting aids   Strong setting lotions that also have a little animal or vegetable protein; can be either acid or alkaline.

Keratin (KER-eh-tin)   The basic protein that forms the structure of the hair shaft.

Manageability   The ease or difficulty with which a comb passes through the hair, whether wet or dry.

Micropolysaccharide (migh-kroh-pah-lee-SAK-e-righde)   A glue-like substance believed to cement the cortical fibers together.

Normalizing conditioners   Conditioners with an acid pH that neutralize the alkaline effects of trace chemicals after such services as a tint, relaxer, cold wave, or lightener.

Placenta (plah-SEN-tah)   The nutrient-providing organ in mammals—in this case, female cattle or sheep—that is refined and used in some protein hair conditioners.

Porosity   The amount of liquid the hair strand can absorb.

Preconditioning   Using a conditioner before a strong chemical service to prevent hair damage.

Protein conditioners   Products that penetrate the hair shaft to replace keratin that has been physically or chemically removed.

Reconditioning   Using a conditioner after the service.

Substantive proteins   Man-made or processed proteins.

Tensile strength   The amount of elasticity hair has.

Texture   The feel and diameter of the hair.

Vegetable proteins   One source of protein in hair conditioners. They come from high-protein plants, such as balsam trees.

QUESTIONS

1. Name the five characteristics that are used to describe the condition of the hair.
2. Using your own words, write the difference between instant conditioners and protein conditioners.
3. What is keratin?
4. Can you write a brief explanation for hair texture?
5. Do all clients need their hair conditioned?
6. When the hair is wet, what percentage of its length can it be stretched?
7. What is the term used to describe the ability of the hair to absorb moisture?

ANSWERS

1. Porosity, elasticity, texture, appearance, and manageability 2. Timing and effectiveness 3. The basic protein found in hair 4. The feel and diameter of hair 5. No 6. Almost 50 percent 7. Porosity

Giving Scalp Treatments 6

Scalp manipulations are a separate service offered in schools and salons. They can be given after a shampoo to help maintain a healthy scalp.

Purpose

Provided with information in this unit and practice under the supervision of your instructor, follow the proper steps to manipulate the scalp of a client after the shampooing service.

Major Objective

Use the proper steps for scalp manipulation in 30 to 40 minutes.

Level of Acceptability

1. Describe the benefits of scalp manipulations and explain when they can and cannot be given.

Knowing Subobjective

2. Give a scalp treatment.

Doing Subobjective

KNOWING SUBOBJECTIVE 1

Scalp manipulations are very beneficial. They stimulate the nerves, muscles, and glands in the scalp. They also increase the circulation of blood, which nourishes the scalp tissues.

Although there has never been scientific evidence to prove that scalp manipulations promote hair growth, you may observe that a client's scalp looks

Describe the benefits of scalp manipulations and explain when they can and cannot be given.

healthier after a scalp manipulation. It is true that a **healthy scalp** is more likely to have more healthy hair than an unhealthy one. Therefore anything, such as scalp manipulations, that contributes to a healthy scalp is an appropriate service. However, you **must not promise** hair growth to the client.

Safety Tip

Scalp manipulations are given immediately after the shampoo service. They should not be given, however, if the hair is to be cold waved, permanently colored, chemically straightened, or lightened during the appointment. (Don't give a scalp treatment before any chemical service.)

DOING SUBOBJECTIVE 2

Give a scalp treatment.

Supplies

☐ laundered towel
☐ scalp conditioner
☐ electric steamer or heating cap
☐ plastic under-cap

PROCEDURE

1. Ask the client what services are scheduled.

2. Determine the step-by-step procedures that you should follow; thoroughly wash your hands with soap and hot water.

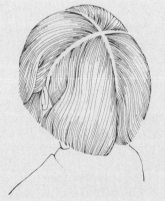

Divide the hair into four sections (quadrants)

3. Brush and shampoo the hair as described in chapter 4. Be sure to examine the scalp for any abnormal conditions. Then towel-dry the hair.
4. Consult your instructor or manager for assistance in selecting a scalp conditioner.
5. Part the hair into four equal sections.

RATIONALE

1. Shampooing, brushing, and scalp treatments vary according to services that follow.
2. Brush and shampoo the hair before scalp treatments unless chemical services (lightening, cold waving, permanent coloring, or chemical straightening) are to follow. You should not brush, and you should not give manipulations before these chemical services.
3. This is standard procedure.

4. Some conditioners are for oily scalps, while others are made for dry scalps.
5. This is standard procedure.

6. Squeeze a small amount of conditioner from the tube onto the back of your left hand near the thumb and index finger.

7. Apply the scalp conditioner in ½- to 1-inch horizontal subdivisions. Apply it from the crown to the nape and then into the sections on both sides of the head. Apply the conditioner with the middle finger of the right hand.

8. With the cushions of your fingertips, apply the conditioner to the scalp. Do not scratch the scalp with your fingernails.

9. Firmly apply the conditioner evenly in a circular movement across the scalp.

10. Check the evenness of application and add conditioner where needed.

11. Basic Movement 1-A. Stand behind the client. Place the middle and ring fingers of each hand on each side of the client's neck just above and in front of the trapezius (tra-PEE-zee-us) muscles. Press firmly for 4 seconds. Rotate your fingers counterclockwise (c.c.w.) 3 times. Move your middle and ring fingers upward 1 inch on each side of the neck. Press your fingers against the scalp; then rotate them c.c.w. 3 times. Continue the manipulating at 1-inch intervals toward the area just below the lobe of each ear.

6. This is the most convenient place to keep the conditioner while you apply it to the scalp.

7. These subdivisions of hair are the easiest to handle, and they insure even distribution of the conditioner.

8. This application procedure is safest for the client.

9. This is standard procedure.

10. This is standard procedure.

11. This movement increases circulation in the blood vessels leading to the scalp and stimulates the nerves in the path to the scalp.

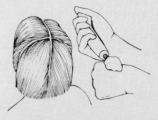

Apply scalp conditioner to back of hand

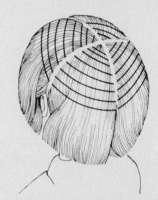

Part and apply conditioner along subsections

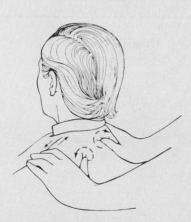

Rotate thumbs along trapezius muscle

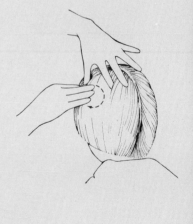

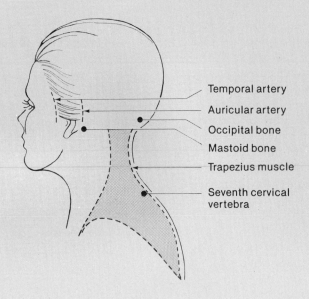

Temporal artery
Auricular artery
Occipital bone
Mastoid bone
Trapezius muscle
Seventh cervical vertebra

12. Basic Movement 1-B. Slide the same fingers from the sides of the client's head to the posterior auricular (pah-STIR-ee-ehr aw-RIK-yeh-lehr) arteries. Press firmly; then rotate clockwise (c.w.) 3 times.

12. This procedure continues to stimulate circulation at key points.

13. Basic Movement 1-C. Slide your fingers to the anterior auricular (an-TIR-ee-ehr aw-RIK-yeh-lehr) arteries. Press firmly; then rotate c.w. 3 times.

13. Same as step 12.

14. Basic Movement 1-D. Slide the same fingers to the temporal arteries on each side of the head. Press them against the scalp and rotate c.w. 3 times. Repeat **Basic Movement 1-A through 1-D** 3 times.

14. Same as step 12.

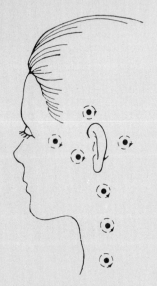

Pressure points

15. Basic Movement 2-A. Stand behind the client. Place your thumbs next to each other at the base of the occipital (ahk-SIP-eh-tahl) bone. Place the middle and ring fingers of each hand at the temporal arteries. Press with your thumbs and then with your fingertips. Rotate your thumbs c.w. 3 times. Now rotate the middle and ring fingers c.w. 3 times. Repeat these manipulations in an upward direction at 1-inch intervals, covering the center area from the occipital bone through the crown, both side sections, and the top of the head.

15. This movement continues to stimulate the blood supply and the important nerves, promoting a pliable, healthy scalp.

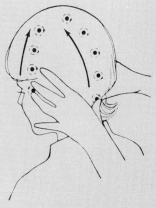

2-A. Press with thumbs, then rotate to next point

16. Basic Movement 2-B. Spread your thumbs in the crown area next to the path just completed. Slide the middle and ring fingers of each hand toward the center of the top of the head. Press and rotate your thumbs and then fingertips c.w. 3 times. Manipulate the scalp in a downward direction at 1-inch intervals toward the mastoid (MAS-toyd) bones. Repeat **Basic Movement 2-A and 2-B** 3 times.

16. Same as step 15.

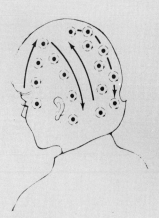

2-B. Press with fingertips, then rotate

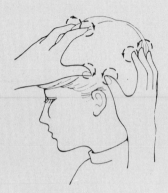

3-A. Use cushions of fingertips to massage across nape

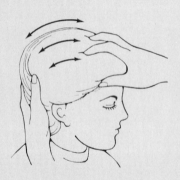

4-A. Support nape of clients head with one hand

17. Basic Movement 3-A. Stand at the client's left side. Spread the cushions of the fingertips of your left hand across the left front side of the client's scalp. Spread the cushions of the fingertips of your right hand across the left nape and lower crown areas. Rotate your left thumb and fingers c.w. while rotating your right thumb and fingers c.c.w. Repeat each position 3 times. Work your hands toward each other at 2-inch intervals until they meet. Reverse this procedure on the right side.

18. Basic Movement 3-B. Repeat **Basic Movement 3-A** 3 times.

19. Basic Movement 4-A. Stand by the client's right side. Provide support by placing your left hand across the back of the client's head in the nape area. Slide the fingertips of your right hand into the front hairline. Press moderately and slide fingertips in a straight line from the hairline through the crown and back again. Continue until the entire top section of the head has been manipulated. Repeat **Basic Movement 4-A** 3 times.

17. Same as step 15.

18. Repeating the movements provides a beneficial amount of stimulation.

19. This movement helps to loosen the scalp. In addition, it continues the stimulation of circulation and nerves.

20. Basic Movement 4-B.
Stand behind the client. Slide the fingertips of each hand through the hair in each side section at the front hairline. Manipulate the scalp firmly in straight lines. Work from the top to the bottom of the section and repeat manipulations, working from the hairline toward the crown section. Repeat **Basic Movement 4-B** 3 times.

21. Basic Movement 5.
Stand by the client's left side. Spread the thumb and index finger of your left hand across the client's forehead to support the head. Place your middle and ring fingers at the seventh cervical vertebra (SEHR-vi-kehl VUHR-teh-brah) (at center base of the shoulders). Press firmly; rotate c.c.w. 3 times. Repeat at 1-inch intervals, manipulating toward the occipital bone. Repeat **Basic Movement 5** 3 times.

22. Basic Movement 6-A.
Stand behind the client. Place palms of each hand on the left and right mastoid bones. Spread your fingertips toward the crown. Quickly draw your palms toward your spread fingertips. Repeat 3 times. This is a kneading action. Continue to knead at 2-inch intervals through the side and crown sections. Repeat each hand position 3 times.

20. Same as step 19.

21. This movement stimulates cervical (neck) nerves and blood supply, which leads to the scalp. It also provides stimulation of the occipital muscle.

22. Kneading provides a deeper stimulation of muscles, nerves, and circulation than do most other types of manipulations. Like other basic manipulations, it helps normalize the sebaceous glands.

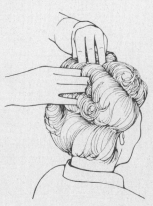

4-B. Massage from the top to bottom of section

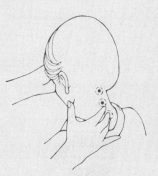

5. Support client's head by placing one hand across forehead

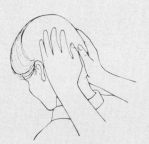

6-A. Use palms to massage scalp

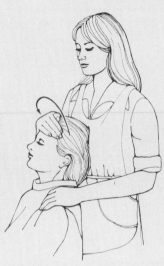

Firmly draw fingertips
across forehead

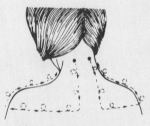

Movements along
trapezius muscle and
back

Safety
Tip

23. Basic Movement 6-B.
Stand at the client's left side.
Support the head by spreading
thumb and index finger across
forehead. Using your right
hand, knead through the center
of the nape, crown, and other
areas of the scalp. Repeat **Basic
Movement 6-A and 6-B** 3
times.

24. Basic Movement 7.
Stand behind the client. Place
the client's neck on the headrest
of the chair. Draw the fingertips
of your left hand from the right
side of the forehead to the left
side. Draw the fingertips of
your right hand from the left
side of the forehead to the right
side. Using your palms, press
and rotate temples c.w. with
your right hand and c.c.w. with
your left hand. Repeat **Basic
Movement 7** 3 times.

25. Basic Movement 8.
Stand behind the client. Place
one hand on the edge of each
shoulder. Rotate your right
thumb c.w. and your left thumb
c.c.w. along the trapezius
muscles of the shoulders toward
the neck. Repeat **Basic
Movement 8** 3 times.

26. Place a steamer or a plastic
cap over the hair and then
position the heating cap. **Do
not leave the client during
this procedure** (see page 97).

23. This movement provides
the deep stimulation of
kneading throughout the head.

24. This movement provides
beneficial stimulation of blood
supply and nerves in the
frontalis (forehead).

25. This movement stimulates
circulation of blood in the
shoulders and lower neck.

26. The application of heat
and/or steam is not only
beneficial to the scalp but also
relaxing to the client, **if heat is
not too high. Be careful not to
burn client's scalp!** Note:
either the heating cap is used or
an electric steamer, but not
both.

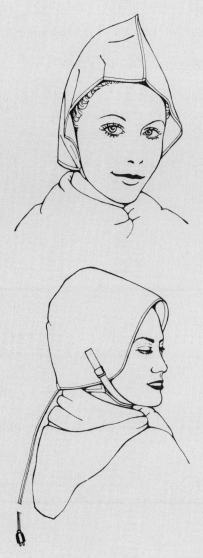

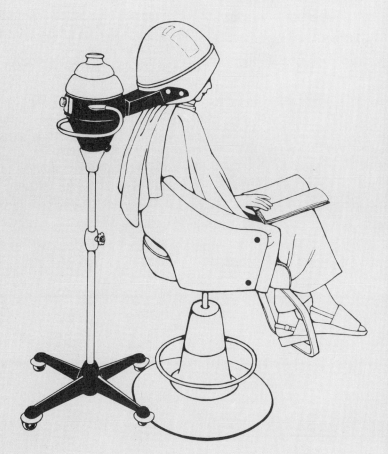

Steamer. Regulate temperature carefully

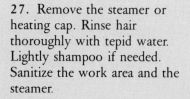

Heating cap

27. Remove the steamer or heating cap. Rinse hair thoroughly with tepid water. Lightly shampoo if needed. Sanitize the work area and the steamer.

27. Perspiration and sebum are brought to the scalp's surface during this steaming procedure. Rinsing and/or shampooing will remove them.

GLOSSARY

Anterior auricular (an-TIR-ee-ehr aw-RIK-yeh-lehr) arteries   Arteries located toward the front part of the ear.

Cervical vertebra (SEHR-vi-kehl VUHR-teh-brah)   The part of the backbone located at the center base of the shoulders.

Mastoid (MAS-toyd) bones   The bones behind the ears.

Occipital (ahk-SIP-eh-tehl) bone   The bone located at the back of the skull.

Posterior auricular (pah-STIR-ee-ahr aw-RIK-yeh-lehr) arteries   The arteries located near the rear part of the ear.

Temporal (TEM-peh-rehl) arteries   The arteries located at the temples.

Trapezius (tra-PEE-zee-uhs) muscle   The muscle that raises and rotates the shoulders and draws the head back and to the side.

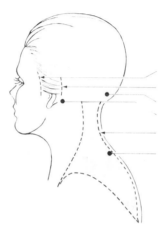

QUESTIONS

1. On the drawing, label the mastoid bone.
2. Indicate on the drawing where the seventh cervical vertebra would be located.
3. Identify the auricular artery.
4. Label the occipital bone.
5. Now label the approximate location of the temporal artery.
6. Should you give a scalp treatment before the application of a hair lightener?
7. How many sections should you divide the hair into for a scalp treatment?
8. Will a scalp treatment grow hair?
9. Write the benefits of a scalp treatment using your own words.
10. Where is the trapezius muscle located?

ANSWERS

1-5. Answers on page 92 6. No 7. Four 8. No 9. Increases the flow of blood 10. Neck and shoulders

Finger Waving the Hair 7

After you have shampooed the hair and, if necessary, conditioned it properly, you are ready to go on to the first stage of developing your hairstyling ability.

This first stage is **finger waving. Finger waving** is the art of combing the hair in alternating parallel arcs that have well-defined ridges. Cosmetologists call them **waves.**

Practicing finger waves before going on to a more complicated style has two advantages. First, it will give you experience working on the curved surfaces of the head to create designs and patterns in the hair.

Second, it will give you the opportunity to create a hairstyle that has become popular in recent years. This basic, fairly simple, tight, curly hairstyle will be a good way to get started on an important part of the cosmetologist's work. This style has a basic pattern that will help you direct your more imaginative and creative efforts.

By mastering effective finger-waving techniques, you will develop the dexterity, coordination, and strength that you will need to make hair shapings, sculpture curls, and roller placements used for more advanced hairstyles.

Major Objective

Comb, then brush, all of the client's hair in even, alternating rows of finger waves.

Level of Acceptability

Using a styling comb and the proper setting lotion, comb even and alternating waves that have well-defined ridges that are parallel to each other. Design all the hair (length permitting) in finger waves in 30 minutes. Score 75 percent or better on a multiple-choice exam on the information in this chapter.

Knowing Subobjective

1. Describe the parts of the finger wave and identify waves, shapings, sculpture curls, and base-directed hair.

Doing Subobjectives

2. Part off the 5 styling sections of the head.
3. Set and comb 3 alternating rows of horizontal finger waves in the crown section of the client's head.

KNOWING SUBOBJECTIVE 1

Describe the parts of the finger wave and identify waves, shapings, sculpture curls, and base-directed hair.

A finger wave is hair combed in alternating parallel semicircles. The hair between two parallel wave ridges is called the **wave trough**. A good finger wave must have the following characteristics:

1. A wave pattern, or "SS," must appear in the hair.
2. The hair in a given semicircle must be parallel to the hair on each side of it. If one pattern looks like this S the pattern before and after must be parallel to it: SSS.
3. The ridges must also be parallel to each other.
4. The wave troughs must have the same width.

Sculpture-wave patterns generally have wider or softer troughs between their ridges, and the ridges themselves are not as sharply defined as they are in the finger wave. Otherwise, sculpture-wave patterns are almost the same as finger-wave patterns. Before sculpture curling, comb some of the hairs into a parallel, semicircular (half-circle) design. These designs are called **hair**

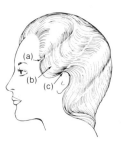

Parts of a wave (a) ridge, (b) trough, (c) ridge parallel to (a)

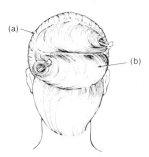

Wave shapes (a) counterclockwise, (b) clockwise

shapings. These shapings make waves that can be combed in either a clockwise (c.w.) or counterclockwise (c.c.w.) direction.

Hair direction usually describes how a strand or section of hair is combed as it applies to the overall hair strand or section from the scalp to the end of the hair shaft. (See p. 100.)

The **base direction** of a hair strand is the movement or direction of the hair as it grows from the scalp. Base direction refers to the first inch or two of a hair strand as it leaves the follicle in the scalp. The **first** half of a semicircular shaping is the base direction.

DOING SUBOBJECTIVE 2

Supplies

- □ two styling combs
- □ mannequin
- □ mannequin clamp

- □ two laundered towels
- □ water applicator bottle
- □ duck-bill clips

Part off the 5 styling sections of the head.

PROCEDURE

1. Fold a towel over the edge of the styling station and secure the clamp tightly. Place the mannequin on the clamp spindle.

2. Begin applying water in the nape section. Hold the applicator in your left hand and spray the section. Comb the water through the hair with your right hand. Apply water in this manner until all hair is wet and easy to comb.

3. Hold the bottom of one comb in a vertical position along right cheekbone and hold another comb horizontally, just behind the hairline.

RATIONALE

1. This protects the laminated surface of the styling station. The mannequin is now in place.

2. The hair must be wet for any styling procedure because the water breaks the hydrogen cross-bonds in the hair, causing it to stretch. These bonds will re-form naturally, with the new design in the hair, as the hair dries.

3. These combs will form a right angle. The vertically placed comb will be one side of the right angle and the horizontally held comb will be the other side of the right angle.

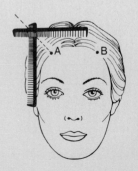

Finding points to divide the top from the side sections

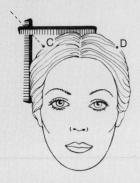

Finding points to divide the top from the crown section

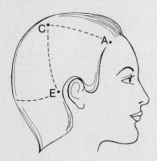

Lines AC, CE, and the hairline enclosing the side section

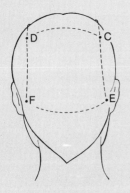

Crown section

4. Imagine a straight line that divides the right angle formed by the two combs into two equal parts. The point where this line meets the hairline is A. Use this procedure to find corresponding point B on left side.

5. Place a comb in a horizontal position along the side of the head and align the comb with point A. Hold another comb vertically at the back of the head. Divide the angle that the combs form as you did in step 4. The point where the line dividing the angle meets the surface of the head is C.

6. Repeat these steps on the left side of the client's head to find point D. Imagine a line connecting points A, C, D, and B.

7. Part the hair from point C to point E, which is 1 inch behind the right ear.

8. Part the hair on the left side in the same manner, working from point D to point F, which is 1 inch behind left ear.

9. Part the hair in a slight arc from F to E through occipital nerve point (at the top of the nape).

10. You can use this exercise to find the 5 styling areas on any head size.

4. The top profile of the head forms an arc. If you divide the right angle placed on the arc, you will get the approximate middle of that arc. This exercise is not absolutely accurate, but it will help you estimate the lines that divide the top from the two side sections.

5. Same as steps 3 and 4.

6. The area enclosed by the lines that connect these points is the top section.

7. This completes the division of the side section. The area enclosed by lines AC, CE, and hairline is the right side section.

8. This completes the division of the side section. The area enclosed by lines BD, DF, and the hairline is the left side section.

9. This establishes the crown and nape sections. Lines connecting C, E, F, and D enclose the crown section. Line FE and the bottom hairline enclose the nape section.

10. Considerable practice on a mannequin is helpful before working on a client.

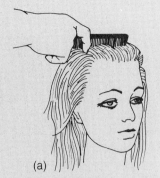

(a)

Comb hair away from
hairline

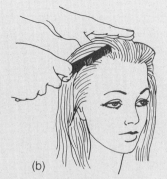

(b)

Push hair from crown—
forward

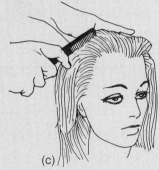

(c)

Watch for natural split
of hair

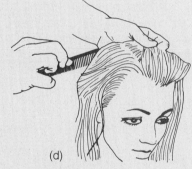

(d)

The natural part

DOING SUBOBJECTIVE 3

Supplies

- ☐ finger-waving lotion
- ☐ finger-waving comb
- ☐ laundered or paper towels

- ☐ duck-bill clips
- ☐ mannequin and clamp
- ☐ hair-setting tape

Set and comb 3
alternating rows of
horizontal finger
waves in the crown
section of a
mannequin or client.

PROCEDURE

1. Assemble all supplies and
implements in work area.

2. Beginning in the nape,
carefully brush or comb tangles
from the mannequin. Comb or
brush from the ends of hair and
work toward the scalp.

RATIONALE

1. This practice will help you
work more efficiently.

2. It is easier to remove
tangles by beginning in the
nape area. It is very difficult to
remove tangles from wet hair. If
you remove tangles and back-
combing before wetting the
hair, it will be much more
manageable when you apply
setting lotion.

3. Wet the hair on the mannequin or client. Ask your instructor about the wetting method and application of creme rinse.

3. The hair has to be wet for shaping. Water helps break hydrogen cross-bonds in the hair so that the strands will conform to setting pattern. Mannequins may require only brushing and spraying with water, followed by a creme rinse, which increases manageability. A client may have to be shampooed and given a creme* rinse or conditioner.

4. Towel-dry according to directions from your instructor or manager and the directions on the label of the creme rinse product you will be using.

4. This is standard procedure.

5. Part the top and side sections and secure them with duck-bill clips.

5. In all finger-waving exercises and services, sections not to be waved should be clipped out of the way. In this case, this includes all sections except the crown. Duck-bill clips are used to hold large sections of hair.

6. Obtain finger-waving lotion from your instructor.

6. A special semiliquid waving lotion is used for finger waving because its thick, or heavy, consistency (viscosity) makes it easier to form wave ridges.

7. Pour the lotion onto the crown hair with your right hand. Cup your left hand beneath the hair.

7. You must pour finger-waving lotion onto the hair because it cannot be sprayed on with a pump applicator. The cupped left hand catches dripping lotion, protecting client's clothing and the floor. Water on the hair acts as a wetting agent to distribute the lotion onto the hair shaft.

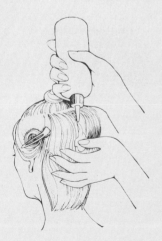

Apply finger waving lotion

*There is quite a variation in the use of the words "creme" and "cream" for products in the cosmetics industry. The spelling "creme," except in a few special cases, will be used in this text.

8. Comb the hair straight back and flat against the head after evenly distributing lotion. Deposit excess lotion on a laundered or paper towel.

9. Comb all crown hair downward and to right side of the head.

10. Hold the comb as shown at right.

11. Place the index finger of your left hand firmly across point A (see figure at right and on page 106). Hold your finger parallel to floor.

12. Place the fine teeth of the comb just below your index finger and perpendicular to the head. Insert the comb into hair at a 45-degree angle to your index finger.

13. To make the ridge, shift the comb along an imaginary line that is about 1 inch to the left of your index finger. Do not remove comb. Flip the comb downward, but do not remove it from shifted position.

8. You should comb the lotion evenly through the hair so it will dry uniformly. Combing it straight back and flat against the head also softens and stretches the hydrogen bonds in the hair. These bonds make the waving pattern firm and give it durability until the next shampoo. As the hair dries, it contracts, resulting in a bouncy setting pattern. The lotion gives body (surface substance) to the hair shaft.

9. These steps will give you the first half of the semicircular shaping that you will use to make a horizontal ridge pattern.

10. Holding the comb this way will make combing the ridges from the shaping easier.

11. Your index finger secures the base direction of the hair so that it will not move when you comb the first part of the ridge into the hair.

12. When the hair is shifted between the comb and index finger, the ridge begins to form. The fine teeth of the comb keep the strands closer together so that the hair will comb more smoothly.

13. If you remove the comb the ridge will relax and settle close to head. Placing comb flat gives you room to let your middle finger take position of your index finger, while you use your index finger to secure the hair immediately above the comb.

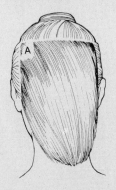

The hair combed down and to the right to begin semicircular shaping

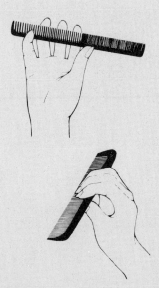

Correct way to hold comb for finger waving

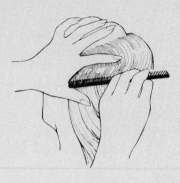

Move comb to left to make first ridge

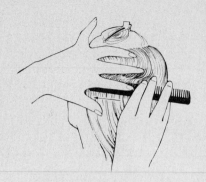

Shift finger position to secure ridge of wave

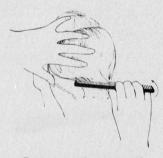

Rotate comb to smooth hair under index finger

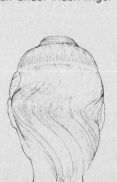

First wave shaping

14. Move the middle finger of your left hand to the position held by the index finger of your left hand.

15. Rotate the teeth of the comb to a flat position on the hair and place the index finger of your left hand across the lower half of the comb toward the head.

16. Push firmly against the head with your index and middle fingers; then shift the comb to the right. Rotate the comb away from the head and through the ends of the strand.

17. Repeat this procedure in 1-inch strands across the top crown of the head to form the first wave ridge.

18. Carefully comb through the hair as needed until the ridge is well defined.

19. Beginning on the right side of the head, repeat this procedure to form the second ridge across the middle crown.

14. This procedure secures the ridge before you reverse the direction of the comb.

15. Same as rationale 12. Placing the comb flat allows room for the index finger. Your middle finger takes the position that was occupied by your index finger to help hold the hair and form the ridge.

16. If you do not hold the hair firmly, the ridge will be disturbed and will flatten out.

17. A 1-inch strand seems to be the easiest size for adding to the ridge.

18. The shaping and ridge may have to be touched up a little to make all hairs in the shaping parallel to each other.

19. Be sure that the ridges are parallel and an equal distance from each other as you comb across from one side of the crown to the other.

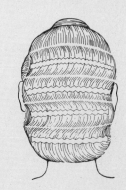

20. Start on the lower left side to comb the third ridge into the hair. Check the size of the wave troughs. Place hair-setting tape across the wave troughs and all loose hair. Ask your instructor for an evaluation.

21. Dry the hair thoroughly according to your instructor's directions. Remove and discard the tape. Comb or brush through the wave pattern. Repeat these procedures for all the hair.

20. Wave troughs should be about the same size from ridge to ridge. This first exercise must be correct if other waves are to be formed properly. The tape will not mark the hair (as clips will); but it is porous so that the hair will dry evenly. Also it helps define the ridges by bringing the wave troughs closer to the head.

21. If mannequins are used, your instructor may give you special instructions. To maintain sanitation, do not reuse tape. First, combing the hair will relax it. If the waves are too small, brush them to achieve more relaxation. The entire head must be finger waved.

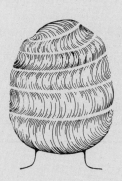

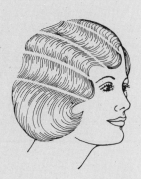

GLOSSARY

Base direction The movement or direction of the first inch or two of hair as it grows from the scalp.

Finger wave Hair combed in alternating parallel semicircles, or arcs, that have well-defined ridges.

Hair direction How a strand or section of hair is combed.

Hair shapings Combing some of the hairs into a parallel, semicircular design. These shaping designs make waves that can be combed in either a clockwise or counterclockwise direction.

Wave trough The hair between two parallel ridges.

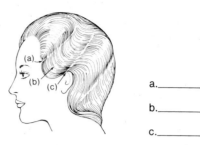

a._____

b._____

c._____

QUESTIONS

1. Label letter (a) on the drawing.
2. Label letter (b) on the drawing.
3. Label letter (c) on the drawing.
4. What kind of hair pattern results from combing the hair as shown in the drawing?
5. Write a definition for each part of the waves discussed in this chapter.
6. When hair is combed in alternating parallel arcs with a ridge in between, what is this formaiton called?
7. When hair is combed in a parallel pattern in a half-circle direction, what are these designs called?
8. What is the term used to describe where the hair is combed as it leaves the scalp?

ANSWERS

1. Ridge 2. Trough 3. Ridge parallel to (a) 4. Diagonal wave 5. Ridge, trough, alternating direction, "C" shaping, "S" shaping 6. A finger wave 7. Hair shapings 8. Base direction

Setting and Combing Sculpture Curls 8

Once you have mastered the basic techniques of finger waving, you can move on to master advanced hairstyling techniques.

Purpose

Your first two steps are basic, but very necessary, ones. First, you will need to know the basic hairstyling terms. Second, you will need to know and apply the basic principles used to create advanced hairstyles. There is a basic cause-and-effect relationship between the setting and combing patterns used for sculpture curls and the final style you wish to achieve. Thus, the results of a specific set of principles for setting and combing are quite predictable. If you want a particular pattern of curls, you simply need to use a certain principle of setting. Because this is true, you can apply basic hairstyling principles to unstyled hair and know that it will do what you want it to do.

In all cases, the key to good hairstyling is the mastery of these principles. High styling, or advanced styling, is simply a more advanced way of applying basic principles (with, of course, a little more imagination). When you master them, you will be able to create your own styles and give way to your imagination.

Using the proper implements, set all the client's or mannequin's hair in sculpture curls and comb it into place according to the proper styling principles.

Major Objective

Set the hair in 30 minutes, dry as necessary, and comb into place in 20 minutes. Score 75 percent or better on a multiple-choice exam on the information in this chapter.

Level of Acceptability

Knowing Subobjectives

1. List the setting and combing implements used to style the hair.
2. Identify hairstyling terms and define the 3 parts of a sculpture curl.
3. Describe the basic types of sculpture curls and their variations and give the 3 strengths of sculpture curls.

Doing Subobjective

4. Set and comb sculpture curls: (a) in horizontal wave patterns in the crown and nape sections of the head, (b) in one large semicircular formation in both side sections, (c) in alternating diagonal-wave formations in both side sections, and (d) in the top section to form an outside movement away from the head.

KNOWING SUBOBJECTIVE 1

List the setting and combing implements used to style the hair.

Like skilled workers in many fields, cosmetologists often are judged by the way they use and maintain their implements. Your skill as a cosmetologist is directly related to your implements. Always keep them sanitary and ready to use.

As a cosmetologist, you will use many different implements. You need to know which implement is needed to perform a particular task.

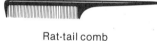

Rat-tail comb

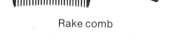

Rake comb

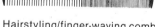

Hairstyling/finger-waving comb

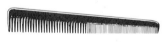

Barber comb

1. The rat-tail comb is often used for carving sculpture curls from their shapings or dividing the hair into sections for cold waving. It also can be used for applying chemical relaxers.
2. The rake comb can be used to apply chemical relaxers. It is also used to remove tangles by combing through the hair.
3. The styling comb is an all-purpose comb. It is used for all services except applying chemical relaxers.

The hair may be held in place by a variety of implements (see figure below).

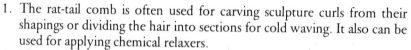

Hairpin   Bobbi pin   Single-prong clip

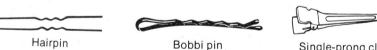

Double-prong clip   Duck-bill clip

KNOWING SUBOBJECTIVE 2

Setting and combing procedures for all hairstyles and designs are based on **geometric forms**. You will need a working knowledge of these geometric forms to work quickly and accurately.

The basic parts of a wave were given in chapter 7, so you are familiar with them. However, the parts of a sculpture curl have their own particular names. Every sculpture curl has three main parts, as shown at right: the base (A), the stem (B), and the circle end (C).

The **base** (or **base direction**) of a hair was defined in chapter 7. The base of the sculpture curl is the same thing. It is the direction the hair takes as it leaves the scalp to form a semicircle.

The term used in chapter 7 to describe the rest of the hair shaft was **hair direction**. For sculpture curls this is described in 2 parts: the stem and circle end.

Identify hairstyling terms and define the 3 parts of a sculpture curl.

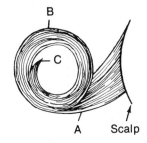

Base—scalp to A, stem—A to B; circle end—B to C

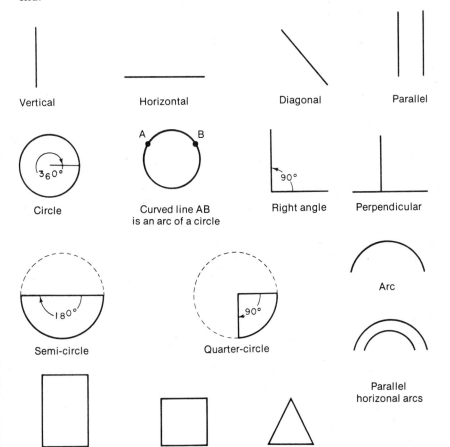

Vertical

Horizontal

Diagonal

Parallel

Circle 360°

Curved line AB is an arc of a circle

Right angle 90°

Perpendicular

Semi-circle 180°

Quarter-circle 90°

Arc

Parallel horizonal arcs

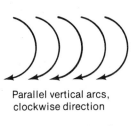

Parallel vertical arcs, clockwise direction

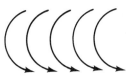

Parallel vertical arcs, counterclockwise direction

Vertical rectangle

Square

Triangle

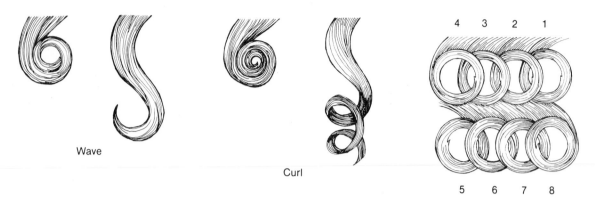

Wave

Curl

Alternating rows of curls to form wave

The **stem** (shown as arc AB) is that part of the curl that determines whether the **direction of the curl** will be **horizontal, vertical,** or **diagonal**.

The **circle end** is the round formation (part) of a sculpture curl. The **size of the circle end** (sometimes called the circle) and the number of turns in it regulate the size and strength of the wave. The **tightness** of a curl depends on how large or small the circle end is. Ordinarily, 1½ revolutions (turns) will result in a beautiful, uniform wave pattern.

If the ends are given more than 1½ turns, the wave pattern will be curly rather than wavy.

When making a sculpture curl, you should begin setting from the **open end** and let the circle end of the curl being made overlap the base of the **preceding** curl (the one before it). Note how the hair ends of curl 2 overlap the base of curl 1.

As is true for all sculpture curls, the kind of shaping designed into the hair and set in curls will decide what the finished hairstyle looks like. All the semicircular **base** shapings must remain parallel to each other; otherwise, the base direction of the shaping will be **disturbed**. The hair has to pivot (turn) from a point at the bottom of the shaping to retain the parallel shapings for the curls (see point A on figure on p. 111).

KNOWING SUBOBJECTIVE 3

Describe the basic kinds of sculpture curls and their variations and give the 3 strengths of sculpture curls.

Sculpture curls get their name from the way they are combed into the hair. A design is combed into the hair, and the curls then are secured close to the head. This is similar to the way a sculptor makes a statue. The sculptor works the general pattern (or blueprint) of his creation into the marble and then chisels in the specific details. The design combed into the hair for sculpture curls is called a **shaping**. (Sculpture curls are sometimes called **pin curls**, although the old-fashioned pin curl was not carved from a shaping.) Shapings should be combed in either a clockwise (c.w.) or counterclockwise (c.c.w.) direction. Once you comb the shapings into the hair, you can place single curls into it. However, you must not disturb the shaping after you have secured the curl with a clip.

The curl is carefully carved from the shaping in three different ways, which will determine how strong the curl will be when dried and combed into place. The **point** at which the curl is carved out of the shaping is called the **pickup line** or **pickup point**. The place in the shaping where the curl is picked up will determine the **kind** and **strength** of sculpture curl being set. The three types of sculpture curls are: no-stem, half-stem, and long-stem (see below).

The amount of **mobility** (movement) that a curl has depends on the type of stem that is used. The mobility indicates how tight, or firm, the curl will be. The **no-stem** curl produces the least mobility (tightest curl), and the **long-stem** curl produces the most mobility (loosest curl). The **half-stem** curl ranges between the other two.

A row of **secured** sculpture curls is correct only if:

1. The shaping was combed into the hair **before** the hair was set.
2. The parallel shapings next to the scalp are **not** disturbed or distorted.
3. The curls were set from the open end of the shaping and finished at the closed end.
4. The end of each curl has 1½ turns.
5. The end of each curl forms a perfect **circle**.
6. The extreme end of the hair used to make the curl is on the **inside** of the circle of hair.
7. The curl that has been secured is **overlapped** by the **following** curl.

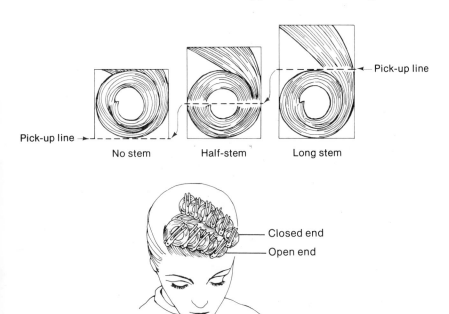

Pick-up line

Pick-up line

No stem   Half-stem   Long stem

Closed end
Open end

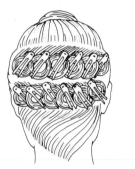
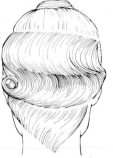
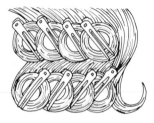

Alternating rows of scupture curls to produce wave

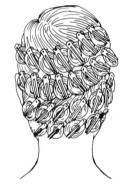

Soft wave setting pattern

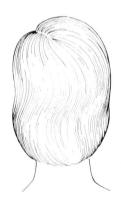

Soft wave comb-out

While all three stems offer some flexibility and a certain range of design possibilities, the half-stem curl offers the widest range of patterns and combinations because it is between the two extremes of the no-stem and long-stem.

The half-stem sculpture curl may be combed in either of **two** directions or in combinations of both. Depending on which combination you use, you will be able to get curls that are tight (a small amount of movement) or loose (larger movement).

You can make a **wave pattern** by using **alternating** rows of c.w. and c.c.w. sculpture curls (see above). These curls will have some movement, but it will be limited.

After you have secured a row of **c.w. sculpture curls**, it will be easy to figure out exactly where the **c.c.w. sculpture curls** should be placed. You can do this by carefully removing the clip from the last c.w. curl made and allowing it to unfold. The position of the hair **end** that forms the **last half** of that semicircle will determine exactly **where** the shaping should be made so that the c.w. curls will unfold into the c.c.w. curls.

Two rows of half-stem sculpture curls set in the **same** direction results in a **larger** movement (see figure at left).

Skip-waving patterns are made by using alternating **combinations** of unset hair shapings and sculpture curls.

Thus, make a row of sculpture curls, then a row of unset hair shapings, and so on. This pattern will produce a skip wave.

Stand-away (stand-up) curls usually are made when the style calls for the hair to move **away** from the head to achieve height or volume to silhouette or to frame the head in a particular way.

Several steps are needed to make these curls. First, comb the hair **away** from the head. Then comb the hair **into** the required design. Then **carve** the curl from the shaping and **secure** it in a **standing** position by using a **clip**. As with regular sculpture curls, you should pick the hair up from the **open end** of the shaping. The **base strand** for each of these curls may be **square, rectangular,** or **triangular**, depending on the desired results. You can avoid splits around the front hairline by using curls with triangular bases. Small puffs of cotton may be inserted in the standing circles so that they will not be disturbed under the dryer.

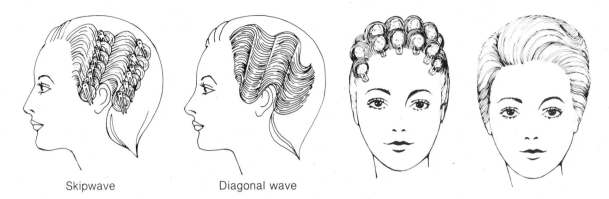

Skipwave   Diagonal wave

When larger strands are used to make stand-away curls, they sometimes are referred to as **barrel curls** and **cascade curls**.

When selecting the strength, or type (no-stem, half-stem, long-stem), of sculpture curl to be set, you should consider:

1. hair movement desired
2. location of the wave movement on the head
3. texture and length of the client's hair
4. setting lotion used to prepare the hair

1. Large, soft, flowing waves are made by a combination of half-stem and long-stem sculpture curls carved from perfectly designed hair shapings. Circle ends are wound about 1½ turns so that the hair will not become too curly.

2. Larger movements of hair are ordinarily desirable in the top, upper crown, and sides of the head, depending on prevailing hair fashions and the wishes of the client.

3. Hair texture and length are important considerations. Coarse or medium hair textures may also have a little natural curl, so **half-stem** and a **few long-stem** curls would be adequate for them. Fine hair may require the **exclusive use** of no-stem curls, and perhaps more of them, to preserve the hairstyle for even a short time. Long hair is usually set in rollers, which will be discussed in the next chapter.

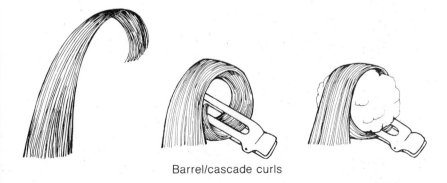

Barrel/cascade curls

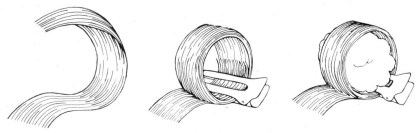

Stand-up curl

4. Some setting lotions make the hair crisp or stiff, usually producing a more durable hairstyle. Others make the hair soft and pliable, which may decrease the durability of the set, depending on the style. In using stiff setting lotions, more **half-** and **long-stem** curls and fewer **no-stem** curls are needed because these lotions do not allow the hair to relax as easily as the softer preparations do. Softer setting lotions generally require more no-stem and half-stem sculpture curls because the hair unfolds and relaxes more when combed.

DOING SUBOBJECTIVE 4

(a) Set and comb sculpture curls in the crown and nape sections of the head to form horizontal wave patterns.

Supplies

☐ combs (rat-tail and styling)
☐ brush
☐ setting lotion
☐ creme rinse
☐ water in spray bottle
☐ mannequin

☐ laundered towels
☐ cotton coil
☐ end wraps
☐ mannequin clamp
☐ duck-bill and double prong clips

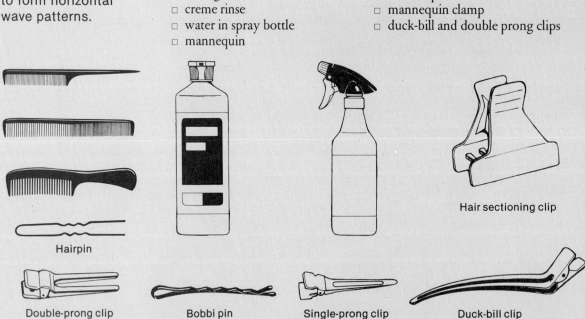

Hairpin

Hair sectioning clip

Double-prong clip

Bobbi pin

Single-prong clip

Duck-bill clip

PROCEDURE

1. Beginning in the **nape** section, carefully brush or comb tangles from mannequin. Comb or brush from the ends of the hair and work toward the scalp.

2. Wet the hair in the shampoo bowl. Shampoo the hair if necessary.

3. Towel-dry the hair and apply the creme rinse or conditioner that your instructor has recommended. Thoroughly rinse excess lotion from the hair according to the directions on the label.

4. Towel-dry the hair. Return to the styling area.

5. Comb all tangles from the hair. Begin in the nape area and comb toward the **front** of the head.

6. Part off both the **top** and **side** sections. Secure each section with a duck-bill clip.

7. Spray the crown and nape with **setting** lotion. Evenly distribute the lotion through hair. You can dilute the lotion by spraying **plain water** over the hair. Comb excess lotion and water onto a towel.

8. Determine whether a c.w. or c.c.w. horizontal shaping will be used in the crown. Consult your instructor for assistance.

RATIONALE

1. If you remove tangles or back-combing before you wet the hair, the hair will be much more manageable when you apply the setting lotion. It is very difficult to remove tangles from wet hair.

2. Shapings for sculpture curls cannot be designed (combed) into the hair unless it is wet.

3. The application of the rinse should remove any tangles that you might have missed when you brushed the hair. If you did not apply the creme rinse, the hair could be difficult to comb. This would cause loss of hair.

4. This will keep water from dripping on tiled or carpeted floor.

5. Tangles remove easily when hair is combed from the botton nape through the **top** and **side sections** of the hair.

6. The top and side sections will not be set, so you can clip them out of the way to make it easier to set the hair in the crown and nape.

7. Thorough saturation and combing are needed to stretch the hair. As the hair dries, it **contracts**. This gives a bouncy, durable setting pattern. The lotion adds body (surface substance) to the hair shaft.

8. This is standard procedure.

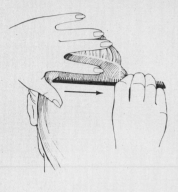

9. If you are going to shape the hair in a c.c.w. design, begin the **first half-base direction** of the semicircle by combing the hair to the left from the top parting (see figure at left). Hold the styling comb in your right hand.

10. Start forming the horizontal **stem** direction by firmly placing the index finger of your left hand in a horizontal position at the **open end** of the shaping, just above the point where you want the hair to change direction.

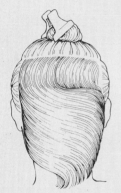

11. Place the comb **perpendicular** to the scalp and **slide** it along the index finger of your left hand. Shift the hair to complete semicircular shaping (see figure at left).

12. Move your index finger to the **left**, place the comb perpendicular to scalp, and continue to shift hair along index finger. Hold the comb in your **right** hand. Continue until shaping is complete.

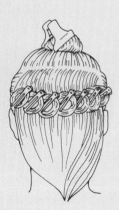

Row of c.c.w. sculpture curls. Note base direction of curls is undisturbed

13. Place the index finger of your **left hand parallel** to scalp at the **open end** and in **center** of the shaping; carve out a half-stem curl in the direction you want the design to go.

9. A horizontal wave pattern requires a series of **parallel**, vertical arcs. They should look like this (((. The first part of the arc moves to the left **before** you shift it to the right with the comb.

10. The index finger is firmly placed (nail up) on the hair to prevent the first part of the arc from being **disturbed**. Shapings have to begin at the **open end**.

11. By holding the comb perpendicular to the scalp and sliding it against your index finger, you can shift the hair easily and neatly to get the kind of wave pattern you want.

12. You should move your index finger to the left so that you can shift the next strand of hair out of the way. Each shift has to be made at the same distance from the top part, or the wave pattern will not be uniform. This has to be repeated until **all strands** are shaped into parallel arcs that are the same size.

13. Always carve the curl in the **same direction** that the curl will be set.

14. Being careful not to disturb shaping, lift the index finger and use the thumb, middle, and index fingers of both hands to manipulate the ends **inside** of the completed circle. Secure with a single- or double-prong clip from **right** side.

15. Put your index finger back on the shaping and carve the second curl. Lift your index finger (keep the circle end close to the head) and make the circle end **overlap** the first curl (from step 14). Secure this curl with single- or double-prong clip.
16. Fold an **end wrap** (paper) the long way into 3 equal panels. Carve out the curl as you have in the past; place the **circle end** in the center panel. Carefully fold the **right** and **left** panels **over the hair** and complete the circle as usual. Secure with a clip.

17. Carve out the next sculpture curl. Spread a ¾-inch piece of cotton coil the long way. Place the **circle end** in the **center** of the cotton across the **top** of the end, then fold the second edge of the cotton **over** the first and complete the sculpture curl. Secure the curl with a clip.

14. After you have carved the circle end of the curl from the shaping, you will need both hands to form the completed circle. Place the ends **inside** of the circle to maintain curl form and strength. Be sure to secure the curl on the **right side**. If you secure it on the left side, the clip will be in the way of the next curl.
15. If the fingers used to form circle end are not **close** to head, the shaping will be disturbed. If the curls do not overlap (the second curl over the first, the third over the second), the shapings will not be parallel to each other.
16. **Paper curls** are used on hair that is very short straight, coarse, or wiry. You can use them to help maintain circular forms in place and achieve stronger curls on hair that is otherwise very difficult to set. You must be careful not to disturb shapings or twist circle end when folding paper around curl.
17. A **powder-puff** curl basically achieves the same thing as a paper curl. Use a piece of cotton instead of an end wrap (paper) to make one. This works very well on bleached hair, which may be marked if it is held by a clip. Such a mark is sometimes called a **clip mark**. Consult your instructor for assistance.

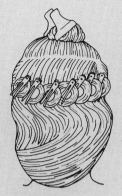

Row of c.c.w. sculpture curls. Note next section has been reshaped for carving

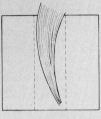

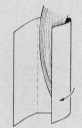

Paper curls

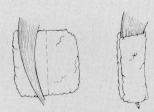

Powder puff curl

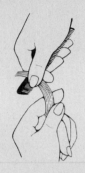

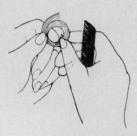

Ribboning the hair

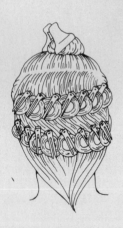

18. Carve out the next sculpture curl. Hold the beginning of the stem between the thumb and index fingers of your left hand. Insert the comb in the stem in front of fingers of your left hand. Rotate the comb ¼ of a turn and place the thumb of your **right** hand on the teeth of the comb. Slide the comb along the hair in a **circular** motion to a complete curl. Secure with clip.

19. Checklist: 1. Curls should follow a **perfectly parallel semicircular arc**. 2. Starting with the second curl, all circle ends should **overlap** the **base** of the **preceding curl**. 3. The circle ends should be perfectly **round, not oval**, and they **should not be disturbed** by clips.

20. Remove the last clip and carefully unfold the sculpture curl.

21. After you have decided where the c.w. shaping will be, put the curl back in place and hold it with a clip. Set all the hair in this shaping in sculpture curls.

22. Comb all unset hair from the scalp to the right side of the lower crown. Then, set all remaining hair in c.w. sculpture curls.

18. This procedure is called **ribboning** the hair. Its effect is similar to drawing the edge of a scissors against a piece of wrapping ribbon. This procedure causes the bonds in the hair to temporarily create a better circular form on the end of the curl. Ask your instructor for help.

19. The first row of horizontal c.c.w. sculpture curls should be checked.

20. This will help you see where the next shaping should be combed into the hair.

21. The curl has to be put back in place to complete the shaping.

22. The hair must be shaped again to set this row of sculpture curls.

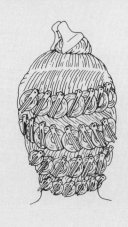

23. Set the rest of the nape hair in **no-stem** c.c.w. curls. Turn them 1½ times if the hair is long enough to do so. Use end wraps or cotton if necessary. If the hair dries out while you are setting it, **spray with water only**.

23. Since so little hair is left at this point, you should set it in the **same** direction as the shaping above it. There is not enough space to completely change the direction of hair. No-stem curls are used because the hair in the nape usually is subject to abuse from clothing collars and body heat. If the hair is quite short, cotton or end papers may be used. Water will reactivate the setting lotion that you already have applied. It is **not** necessary to apply more setting lotion. If you apply more lotion, **the hair may become sticky, stiff, or gummy**.

24. Check with your instructor to make sure you have set the hair correctly. If your instructor approves, then dry the set.

24. If the set is not correct, you should reset the areas that you did incorrectly. Because of the principles applied to a set, you should comb it out in a very predictable way.

25. Dry the set thoroughly by allowing the moisture to evaporate from the hair over-night or by using dryer on medium heat.

25. Mannequins are very expensive. They may be **damaged** if they are placed under dryer. Consult your instructor.

26. Remove all clips from the setting patterns and **make sure** that the hair is **dry**.

26. Any clips will interfere with brushing. If the hair is moist when you brush it, it will comb out straight rather than wavy.

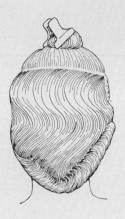

27. Comb through the curls with a clean, dry comb. This unfolds the setting pattern. Comb the hair in the same direction in which it was set.

27. Unfolding the hair with a comb causes the setting pattern to relax. If the set is too "tight," brushing may be needed to relax it.

28. You should not brush the hair straight down and flat against the head because it was not set that way. Brush it only in the direction in which it was set. Do not brush a long time because the hair may become too straight.

28. Brush the hair in the direction in which it was set, beginning at the open end of each wave and working toward the closed end.

29. Discuss the results of the combing with your instructor.

29. By checking with your instructor, you will be able to avoid repeating errors that you have made.

(b) Set and comb sculpture curls in both side sections to make one large semicircular formation.

(You will use the same principles for setting sculpture curls in the following subobjectives that you used in subobjective 4, except that the curls will be set in a different direction. If you feel confident that you have mastered the skills for setting sculpture curls, you may want to simply follow the illustrations. If you are not sure, ask your instructor for assistance.)

PROCEDURE

1. Prepare mannequin as described in previous exercise.

2. Part off and secure the top section, then proceed to set the side sections according to the pattern in the figures below.

RATIONALE

1. The mannequin's hair should be free of tangles and saturated with setting lotion and water.

2. Since only the sides will be set, other sections should be clipped out of the way.

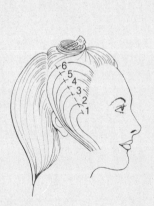
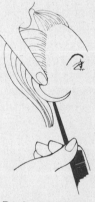
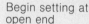

Begin setting at open end

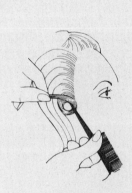

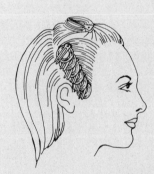

3. Follow the usual procedure to dry the hair.

4. After you have removed the clips, comb through both side sections of the hair, following the design of the shapings.

5. Compare your combed-out design to the one in the text.

3. This is standard procedure. If you feel that you need to refresh your memory, see subobjective 4 for the specific steps you should follow.

4. Always comb hair in the direction it was set. Combing the hair relaxes the setting pattern.

5. The illustrations shown should be similar to the setting and combing procedures you have just completed.

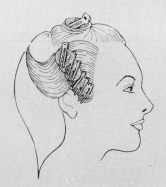

Diagonal column of c.c.w. curls

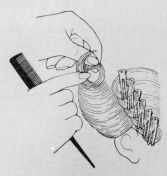

The end of each curl must be on the inside of each curl

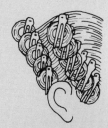

Completed rows of alternating c.c.w. and c.w. sculpture curls

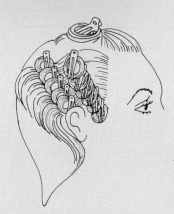

Always comb the shaping into the hair before setting the row of sculpture curls

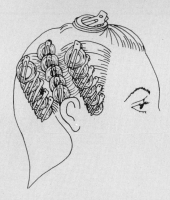

Completed pattern of diagonal sculpture curls

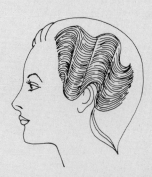

(c) Set and comb
sculpture curls in
alternating diagonal
wave formations in
both side sections.

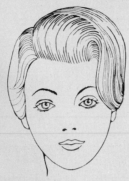

The shaping pattern is combed
into the top front section before
setting in sculpture curls

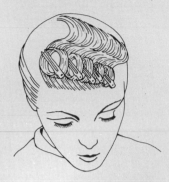

Setting pattern for first row of
c.w. sculpture curls. Begin
setting at point A

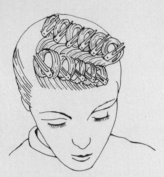

Alternating pattern of c.w. and
c.c.w. sculpture curls

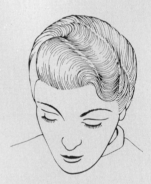

Finished wave pattern in top
front section

(d) Set and comb
sculpture curls in the
top section to form an
outside movement
away from the head.

(At this point you should have mastered the techniques necessary for setting
an entire head in sculpture curls. If you have any questions, look at the illustrations, review the previous subobjectives and ask your instructor for help.)

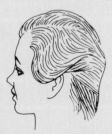

Comb in diagonal
wave shaping

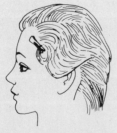

Begin at open end of
shaping; carve and
set sculpture curl

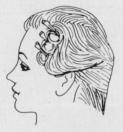

Continue setting curls in shaping

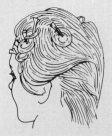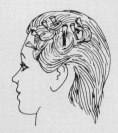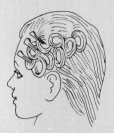

Begin at open end of c.c.w. shaping and proceed to set curls in shaping

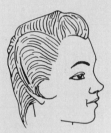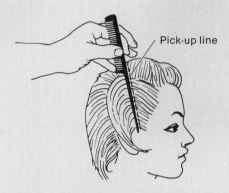

Pick-up line

Comb vertical shaping in side section in front of ear

Use end of tail comb to visualize pick-up line for making curls

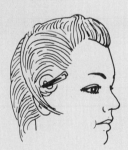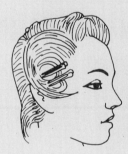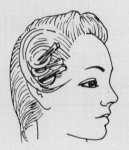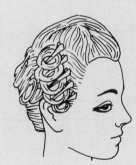

Begin by setting no-stem curl at open end of shaping. Complete setting curls in vertical shaping using c.c.w. half-stem and long-stem curls

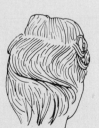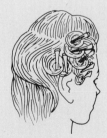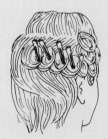

Comb horizontal shaping into crown section of hair. Set half-stem c.c.w. curls. Remember to start setting from the open end

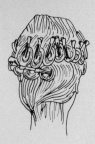 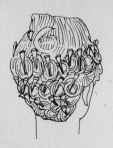 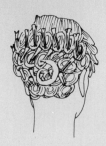

Comb c.w. shaping into hair, then begin setting from open end. Set c.w. curls to support the wave shaping. Dry the hair

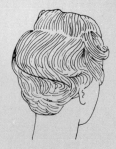 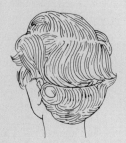 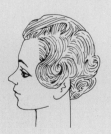 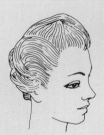

Remove clips and brush all the hair straight back and flat against the head. Brushing relaxes the degree of curl and blends the curls together. Use the brush to trace over the designs set into the hair

GLOSSARY

Barrel curls   Large stand-away curls. See also **Cascade curls**.

Base direction   The direction the hair takes when it leaves the scalp to form a semicircle.

Cascade curls   Large stand-away curls. See also **Barrel curls**.

Circle end   The round formation (part) of a sculpture circle that determines the curl's tightness; also called circle.

Half-stem curl   Halfway between a no-stem and a long-stem curl in mobility and tightness.

Long-stem curl (full-stem curl)   The loosest kind of curl. It has the greatest mobility.

Mobility   How tight or firm a curl will be.

No-stem curl   The tightest kind of curl. It has the least mobility.

Pickup line   Where the curl is carved out of the shaping.

Pickup point   See **Pickup line**.

Pin curl   See **shaping**.

Rake comb   A comb used to apply chemical relaxers and to remove tangles from the hair.

Rat-tail comb   A comb often used for carving sculpture curls, dividing hair into sections, and applying chemical relaxers.

Shaping   The design combed into the hair for sculpture curls or pin curls.

Skip-waving pattern   Alternating combinations of unset hair shapings and sculpture curls.

Stand-away curls   Sculpture curls that are clipped in a standing position to form a movement away from the head.

Stand-up curls   See **Stand-away curls**.

Stem   The part of the curl that determines whether the direction of the curl will be horizontal, vertical, or diagonal.

Styling comb   An all-purpose comb.

Wave pattern   Alternating rows of clockwise and counterclockwise sculpture curls.

QUESTIONS

1. Name the three basic types of sculpture curls.
2. In your own words, write a definition for the "open-end" of a shaping.
3. As in question No. 2, define "closed-end" of the shaping.
4. What is a "pick-up point"?
5. What type of curl bases should be used around the front hairline to avoid splits?
6. What is the strongest type of sculpture curl?
7. What type of sculpture curl has the least amount of strength?
8. If your sculpture curl set is too tight, how can you relax it?
9. If you try to brush the set and discover some wet sculpture curls, what will happen?
10. What will happen if too much setting lotion is used to set the hair?
11. During the setting process, where should the ends of each curl be set?

ANSWERS

1. No stem, half-stem, and long stem. 2. (Check text for accuracy) 3. (Check text for accuracy) 4. Where the curl is carved out of the shaping 5. Triangular-shaped curl bases 6. No-stem curl 7. Long-stem or full-stem curl 8. By brushing the hair 9. The wet hair will go straight 10. The hair will be stiff, sticky, or gummy 11. On the inside of the curl

Setting the Hair with Rollers 9

Do you have a hobby? Many people do. Many people like to work in their gardens. Some people seem to have "green thumbs." You may be one of these people. But could you run a 2,000-acre farm? Managing a farm—for a living—is a long way from raising some tomatoes and beans in your back yard.

The difference is simple. You are not a professional farmer or agriculturalist. A professional knows and uses all the "tricks of the trade" to perform quickly, efficiently, and productively.

The same thing is true for cosmetologists. Many people could set hair if they had to (not as many people think they could—in recent years cosmetologists have seen more and more cases of hair damage caused by the improper use of home-care products). But they would have to work very slowly, and they would not know what to expect.

As a professional you will learn to set hair efficiently (quickly but precisely), and you will be able to predict the outcome of your work.

One important skill in reaching that goal is the mastery of rollers. Rollers are basic implements that all cosmetologists use to design hairstyles.

Mastering the setting and combing principles involved in using rollers is useful for two reasons. You will be able to save time by using one roller instead of having to set several individual stand-away curls. You also will be able to set a wider (almost limitless) variety of designs and styles.

You will be tested on the material in this unit, but the real test will be when a client (maybe a potential "amateur") sees the results of your work and realizes, "You can only get professional results from a professional."

Use the proper roller-placement principles to set all the mannequin's or client's hair in rollers and comb the style into place.

Major Objective

Level of Acceptability

Set the hair in rollers in 15 to 25 minutes and (after it is dried) comb it into place in 20 to 30 minutes. Score 75 percent or better on a multiple-choice exam on the material in this unit.

Knowing Subobjectives

1. Explain the basic materials from which rollers are made and describe their shapes and sizes.
2. Describe the basic principles used to decide the correct roller diameter in relationship to the hair's length and define inside and outside movements of hair.
3. Explain the purpose of no-stem, half-stem, and long-stem roller placements.

Doing Subobjectives

4. Set and comb roller curls in 4 different patterns in the top section of the head.
5. Set and comb roller curls in 3 different patterns in the top, sides, crown, and nape sections of the head.

KNOWING SUBOBJECTIVE 1

Explain the basic materials from which rollers are made and describe their shapes and sizes.

Over the years many different kinds of rollers have been used in beauty schools and salons. Today, 2 basic kinds of rollers—**plastic** and **nylon**—are used most often by professionals. They are especially popular because they are **magnetic**. Wet hair will cling to them. Both have small ventilating holes on their surfaces that help dry the hair more quickly.

Although plastic and nylon rollers are similar in some ways, the differences between them are greater than you might think. **Plastic rollers** are heavier than nylon ones and have a tendency to warp with continued exposure to dryer heat. If they warp, you must throw them away. **Nylon rollers**, on the other hand, are much lighter than plastic rollers and cost about the same. They hold their shape much longer than plastic rollers, but they become stained by temporary and semipermanent rinses.

Plastic and nylon rollers come in two shapes: **cylindrical** and **conoid** (cone-shaped). Most plastic and nylon rollers are also made in various lengths and diameters. Short rollers are called **filler or directional rollers**.

The wire mesh/brush roller is basically a wire cylinder covered with mesh netting with a circular brush inserted into the hollow part of the roller's frame. For many years, nearly all cosmetologists used brush rollers. Finally it was realized that they quickly become unsanitary with salon use so that they needed to be sanitized every day. However, it is not practical to thoroughly sanitize them daily. There also was evidence that the tips of brush bristles can puncture and damage the hair as the hair strand dries (contracts).

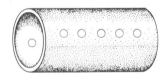

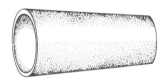

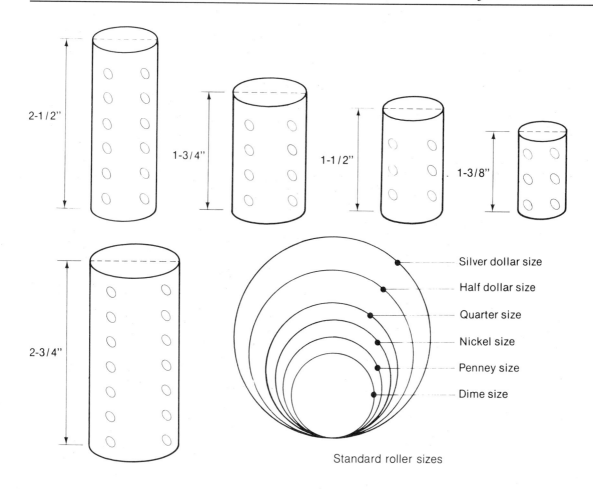

Standard roller sizes

KNOWING SUBOBJECTIVE 2

At this point you should have mastered the principles that apply to setting sculpture curls. If you have learned those principles, you are well on your way to mastering the principles used for setting with rollers.

1. The hair must be **shaped**.
2. The shapings must be **parallel to each other**, and the hair must be combed and wound smoothly on the roller.
3. Rollers are **set** into a shaping **from the open end** toward the closed end.
4. All the hair placed on a roller should form **all or part of a perfect circle**.
5. Rollers are set in **no-stem**, **half-stem**, and **long-stem** placements.
6. Probably the most important principle is that the hair should be wound 1½ to 2 turns around the roller (depending on the desired effect and hair texture).

Describe the basic principles used to decide the correct roller diameter in relationship to the hair's length and define inside and outside movements of hair.

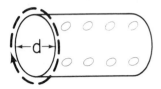

Roller circumference
(distance around the roller)
and diameter (d).

This last principle deserves more explanation. The number of turns needed will tell you what roller diameter to select. Roller diameters vary from about ½ to 1½ inches.

Here is a simple problem to work out. If the hair strand is 6 inches long, what roller diameter should you use?

You can use a combination of common sense and trial and error to arrive at the answer. You know that a large (1-to 1½-inch diameter) roller could **not** be used to set a strand of hair that is 1 inch long because the distance around that roller is 4½ inches. A simple rule of thumb to remember is that the **shorter** the hair is, the **smaller** the roller diameter must be for the ideal wrapping of 1½ turns.

All of this figuring and choosing among types and sizes of rollers has one basic purpose: to make a wave in the client's hair. There are 3 basic wave formations you will use rollers for.

Although there is an almost limitless number of styles and designs, all of them are made up to two basic kinds of roller movements. A pattern that gives height and volume, bringing hair away from the head, is called an **outside movement** of hair. A pattern that brings hair close to the head is called an **inside** or **indentation** movement (see figure below).

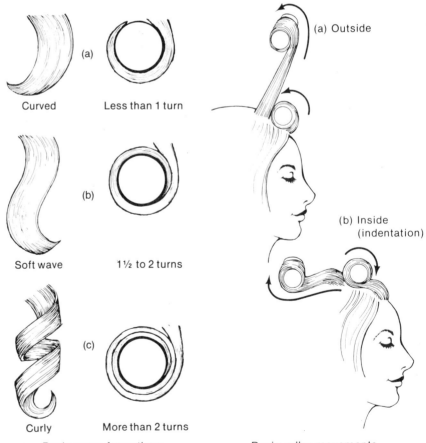

(a) Curved — Less than 1 turn

(b) Soft wave — 1½ to 2 turns

(c) Curly — More than 2 turns

Basic wave formations

(a) Outside

(b) Inside (indentation)

Basic roller movements

The **strength** of the curl produced by the roller depends on whether the roller is set in a **no-stem, half-stem,** or **long-stem** placement. You should remember these terms from chapter 8, which was about sculpture curls. The direction that the hair strand is combed and held before the roller is placed (see figure below) decides where the base for the roller will be.

The 3 types of roller placement are:

1. Directly on the base of the strand for a **no-stem** type.
2. Half on and half off the base of the strand for a **half-stem** type.
3. All the way off and usually below the base of the strand for a **long-stem** type.

The size of the section of hair to be wound around a roller also affects the strength of the curl. The section of hair to be wound should **not** be wider than the diameter of the roller. The hair should not cover more than **80 percent** of the **length** of the roller (see figures below).

When you want hair that is 6 inches or shorter to make an inside (indentation) movement, the width of the section should be larger than the diameter of the roller and the strand should be located entirely above the subsection (see figure bottom right). The width of the subsection should be **50 percent** larger than the **diameter** of the roller.

Explain the purpose of no-stem, half-stem, and long-stem roller placements.

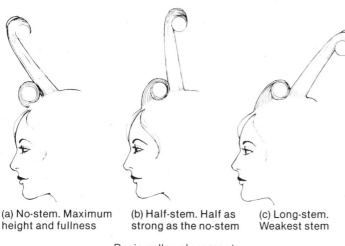

(a) No-stem. Maximum height and fullness

(b) Half-stem. Half as strong as the no-stem

(c) Long-stem. Weakest stem

Basic roller placements

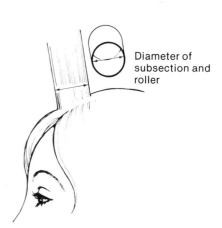

Diameter of subsection and roller

Width of roller section

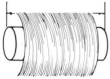

Correct length of roller section

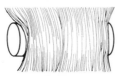

Incorrect

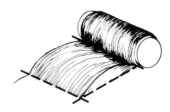

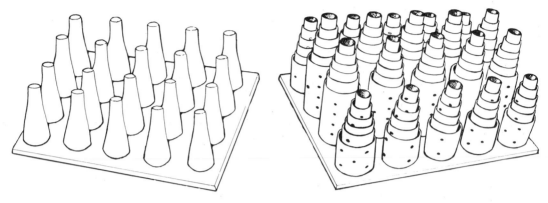

Roller rack

DOING SUBOBJECTIVE 4

Set and comb roller curls in 4 different patterns in the top section of the head.

Supplies

- □ shampoo supplies
- □ roller rack
- □ roller pins
- □ double-prong clips
- □ end wraps
- □ mannequin and clamp
- □ setting lotion
- □ spray applicator bottle for water

- □ rat-tail comb
- □ styling comb
- □ cushion brush
- □ neck strips
- □ protective comb-out cape
- □ hair spray

Top Setting Pattern 1-Half-Bang

PROCEDURE

1. Prepare mannequin for setting. Wet the hair. Apply setting lotion to hair with your left hand and comb it through the hair with your right hand.

2. Comb all hair straight back and flat against the head. Keep the hair wet at all times with water, not setting lotion.

3. Comb the hair at the hairline in the top according to the natural growth. Comb the hair in a half-bang design.

RATIONALE

1. Apply setting lotion to wet hair because the water helps to distribute it onto the cuticle of the hair. Always spray the lotion carefully.

2. This breaks the hydrogen cross-bonds in the hair. It also stretches the hair so that it will be easier to set on magnetic rollers and will dry to a longer-lasting hairstyle.

3. **Always** follow any **natural wave** or **cowlick** (hair standing upward, usually in a circular pattern) whenever possible. By doing so, the hairstyle will last much longer.

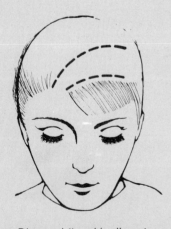

Diagonal "working" part

4. Part off the hair that will be set first.

5. Set the first strand of hair on a filler (short) roller to produce a no-stem curl.

6. Rollers 2, 3, and 4* should be set in triangular sections of hair on long cylinder rollers.

7. Standing behind the head, part across each strand. Catch the strand between the middle and index fingers of your left hand. Recomb the hairs of the strand next to the scalp and through the ends until the strand is smooth. Keep the strand tense by holding it tightly with your left hand. Lay the strand **evenly** across the roller and begin to turn the roller toward the head. Keep the strand tense until you have secured the hair. Place the clip where the roller meets the head.

4. This is the best way to begin setting rollers. Parting the hair makes the panel of hair easier to set.

5. Since other rollers will be set toward the crown and right side of head, a split in the style may occur if a long roller is placed right on the hairline. Most rollers (but not all, depending on the hairstyle) in the top section are set on their bases (no-stem) because this results in maximum height or volume (fullness) and durability when the hair is combed into place.

6. The panel of hair to be set is curved to conform to the contour of the head. To follow the curved part, you must use triangular sections of hair.

7. This is the easiest way to set the hair. You must comb the hair smooth to stretch the strand so that it easy to place on the roller. Clip the strand where the roller meets the head to maintain the tension you placed on it as you wound it. As the hair dries and contracts, the hydrogen cross-bonds re-form around the roller. The degree to which this takes place depends on the amount of tension you put on the strand of hair as you wind it around the roller toward the scalp. **The tension affects the degree of curliness.**

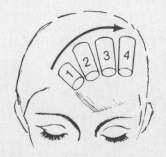

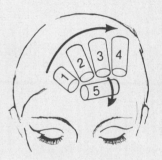

Half-bang set

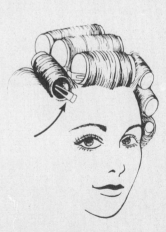

In any roller setting pattern, the clip is inserted where the roller touches the head. Generally only one end of the roller needs to be clipped

---

*Roller and curl will be used interchangeably in the context of **roller number** in the pattern.

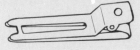

Roller clip

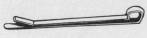

Roller pin

8. Place one double- or single-prong clip in the roller or use a roller pin or clip.

9. Pick up the roller with your right hand and place it beneath the middle finger of your left hand, which is holding the strand. Slide the strand between the middle and index fingers of your left hand while pushing the roller with your right hand. Spread the hair evenly across the roller. Hold the comb in the palm of your right hand **at all times**. Use a rolling action with your left hand to lay the hair across the roller. Using the thumb and fingertips of your left hand, place the strand neatly on the roller.

10. Set roller 5 half-stem or no-stem.

8. Rollers may be clipped into place with single- or double-prong clips or roller clips or pins. Roller clips or pins are usually more expensive than single- or double-prong clips, but using any of the items stated above is correct.

9. This motion makes the hair cling to the magnetic rollers. The strand is spread across the roller so that it will dry evenly in a circular form. If you place the comb on the styling station, you will waste a lot of time reaching back and forth as you set the rollers. With practice, it becomes easy to set the hair while holding the comb throughout the procedure.

10. Since this hair will be combed down onto the forehead, you might want to use a half-stem roller. Do not use a long-stem placement because it may cause a split between the panel of hair on rollers 1 through 4 and the hair on roller 5.

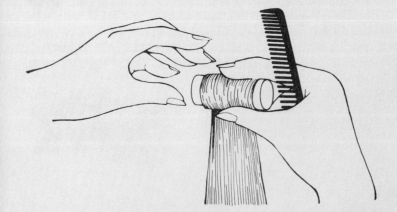

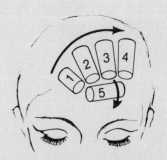

Half-bang set

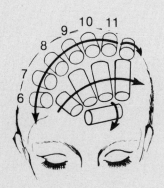

Half-bang set

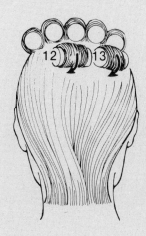

11. Shape the hair behind the first panel of hair from the left to the right (see above). Set rollers 6 through 11 in triangular-shaped strands of hair and on the **next-to-largest-size** rollers. Use a filler roller for curl 6.

11. Always comb the design into the hair before you set the rollers. This procedure will give a more defined, natural movement of hair. To give the hair dimension and form, the rollers in the top section that are **not** on the hairline are larger (by one size) than those used right on the hairline. This is done because the hair is longer toward the crown than around the hairline. You should seldom vary from this rule of thumb: as the hair becomes shorter, select the next smallest roller diameter. Do not vary the diameter of rollers 2 or 3 sizes from one section of the head to the next.

12. Set rollers 12 and 13. Ask your instructor for evaluation and drying instructions after you have set the rollers on the top of the head.

12. It is easier to see and correct setting errors **before** you have dried the hair. It is also easier to learn to relax, back-comb, back-brush (or tease), and control the style of the hair when only one section is used.

13. If you are working on a classmate or client, position the neck strip and shoulder cape.

13. Since the same shoulder cape may be used on everyone, a neck strip must be placed between the neck and the cape.

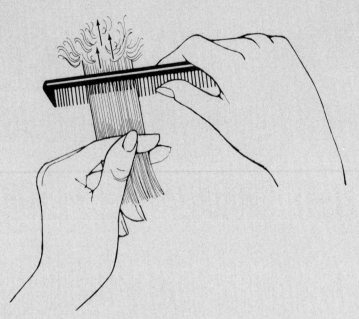

Back-combing the hair

14. Comb the hair through; then brush as needed to unfold and relax the setting pattern.

14. Combing and brushing relax and unfold the pattern. The more the hair is brushed, the more is relaxes.

15. Back-comb the hair by panels in the same order they were set.

15. This is the easiest place to begin. Back-combing supports the height of the style and also further relaxes the hair to blend roller sections.

16. Repeat the back-combing until all panels are lightly packed.

16. This supports the hairstyle.

17. Using your left hand, very carefully guide the hair into place. Hold the comb in your right hand. Clean up the back-combing with the wide teeth of the styling comb.

17. This procedure arranges the hair and removes visible back-combing from the surface of the hairstyle.

18. After your instructor has evaluated the comb-out of the top section, brush all back-combing from it.

18. It is important to spot-check so that you can catch any errors as soon as possible.

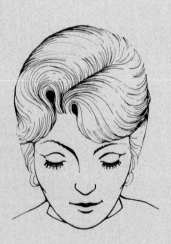

Half-bang comb out

Top-Setting Pattern 2

PROCEDURE

1. Comb a few curls onto the forehead from the hairline. Use long cylinder rollers in half-stem placements in the front top section along the hairline. Use hair-setting tape on bang hairs.

2. Set the entire head if the hair is long enough for this style. Use long cylinder rollers in half-stem placements for curls 5 and 6. Use a long cylinder roller in the no-stem position for curl 7.

3. Set rollers 8, 9, and 10 as in step 2.

4. Set curls 11 through 15 with long cylinder rollers in half-stem placements. Drape the center crown hair into filler rollers that are turned upward. Use rollers that have progressively smaller diameters as you move down toward the nape hairline.

5. Comb through or brush the hair if necessary. The hair should be back-brushed slightly. If you have difficulty, ask your instructor for help.

RATIONALE

1. Since very little back-combing will be needed because the hairstyle is not extremely bouffant (high) in the top section, long cylinder rollers set half-stem will produce the desired effect. Tape will keep bang hairs in place under the dryer.

2. Hair that is long enough for this set will be difficult to comb if only the top section is set. In this situation, it may be easier to set all the hair. Follow the directions of your instructor.

3. Same as step 2.

4. If the filler rollers are turned upward, the hair will flip upward. Draping the hair in the center crown brings the movement of the hair close to the head, which is the way you want the hair to move.

5. This unfolds and relaxes set into the hairstyle. Back-brushing will make the hair easier to control.

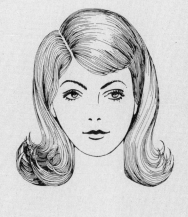

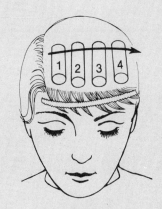

Full bang set

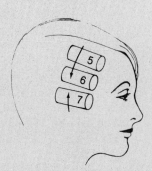

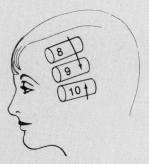

Set for flipping ends of hair

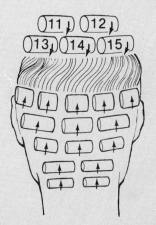

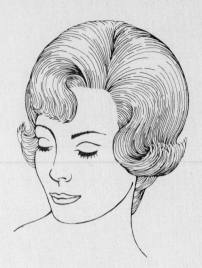

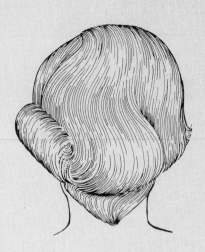

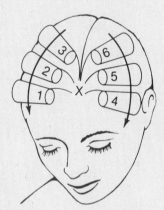

Pivotal half-bang set

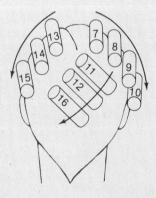

Top-Setting Pattern 3

PROCEDURE

1. Comb the design into the top section of the hair.

2. Note the pivot point marked "X" in figure at left. Set long cylinder rollers or filler rollers as indicated by the illustration. Use long-stem roller placement for rollers 1, 2, 3, 4, and 5. Set the rest of the top in half-stem roller placements.

3. Set the crown, side, and nape sections if your instructor tells you to.

4. Dry the hair after your instructor has evaluated the set.

5. Remove rollers and clips when the hair is thoroughly dry. Back-comb or back-brush as described in setting pattern.

RATIONALE

1. This is standard procedure.

2. The pivot point is a central point around which the hair movement flows. Long-stem roller placements are used because the hair will be combed close to, but **not** flat against, the head. Half-stem placements are used to complete set in the top section because only medium, rather than maximum, height is desired.

3. Your instructor may want you to set the entire head. If so, your instructor will give you additional directions.

4. It is easier to correct errors before the hair dries.

5. Back-combing and back-brushing techniques are the same, regardless of the top-setting pattern. The only thing that changes is the arrangement of the hair.

Top-Setting Pattern 4

PROCEDURE

1. Use rollers in no-stem placements for curls 1 through 6.

2. Use a filler roller in a no-stem placement for curl 7. Set long cylinder rollers no-stem for curls 8 through 11.

RATIONALE

1. Filler rollers in no-stem placements give maximum height and mobility to hair. It may be easier to comb the hair in different directions if you use filler (short) rollers rather than long rollers. In this set it is easier to comb hair around either side of forehead on hairline.

2. A filler-size no-stem is used for roller 7 so that there will not be a split in the hair between roller 1 and roller 7. Setting roller 7 (filler) at a slight angle will make combing the hair onto the forehead easier than using a long roller. Curls 8 through 11 are set no-stem with long cylinder rollers so that there will not be a split in the style. The direction of the style changes between the rollers set away from the hairline (1–6) and the rollers set downward (8–11). If you did not use long cylinder rollers in a no-stem placement, the style could split.

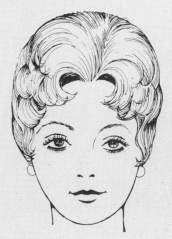

Classical Italian top comb out

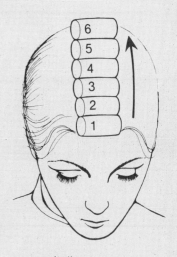

Italian top set

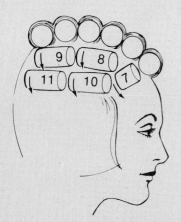

Italian top setting pattern

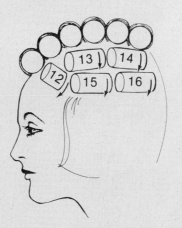

3. Use a filler-size roller to set roller 12 in a no-stem placement. Use long cylinder rollers to set curls 13 through 16 in no-stem placements. (Do not count rollers exactly.)

3. Same as step 2. Do not count rollers because the head size of the mannequin and the length of the hair may change the actual number of rollers used. Just use roller numbers as a **guide**. The direction the hair will be combed and the stem direction of the rollers are important things you should remember.

4. Unfold the setting pattern and comb or brush as necessary.

5. Arrange the hair in the top section according to the style shown at the beginning of this pattern.

4. This is standard procedure.

5. Unless the hair is extremely long or short, the top section should look like the illustration shown at the beginning of this setting pattern.

DOING SUBOBJECTIVE 5

Set and comb roller curls in 3 different patterns in the top, sides, crown and nape sections of the head.

Setting Pattern 1

PROCEDURE

1. Set rollers 1 through 12 according to the pattern described in subobjective 4.

RATIONALE

1. This is standard procedure (see figure at left)

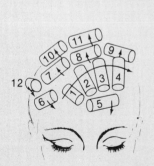

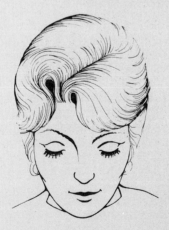

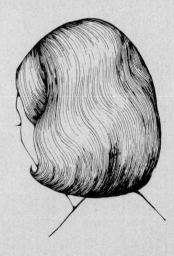

2. Clip hair strands for rollers 14, 15, and 16 out of the way. These will be set in no-stem filler rollers; set curl 13 on a long cylinder roller in a no-stem placement. Use filler rollers with **larger** diameters when you set curls 14, 15, and 16.

3. Repeat this procedure on the left side of the head.

4. Use long cylinder rollers at a slight angle in half-stem placements throughout the upper crown section.

5. Complete the set as shown in figure at bottom right. Dry your set, then comb out the hairstyle.

2. Roller 13 is set no-stem so that it will blend easily with the filler rollers above it. You should use rollers with larger diameters because hair lengths are longer toward the back of the head. Filler rollers are used for better hair control. The better the setting design is, the less back-combing or back-brushing will be needed.

3. By duplicating the set, the style will be **symmetrical** (the same on both sides).

4. Setting the hair this way creates the inside movement of the hair between rollers 10 and 11; the result will be a wave pattern. Hair from the top half of the roller will unfold in a c.w. direction, while hair from the lower half of the roller will unfold in a c.c.w. direction. Using half-stem placements and the slight angle makes the hair wave more easily.

5. This is standard procedure.

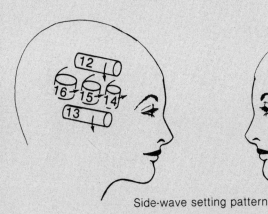

Side-wave setting pattern

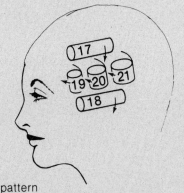

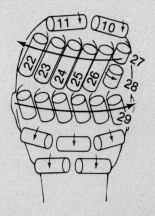

Setting Pattern 2

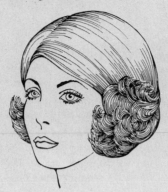

Finished hairstyle for setting pattern 2

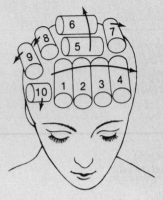

Set rollers in numerical order form 1 through 10

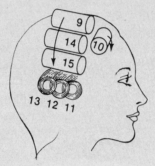

Clip hair to be set in rollers 14 and 15 to roller 9. Set c.c.w. sculpture curls 11 through 13. Place rollers 14 and 15

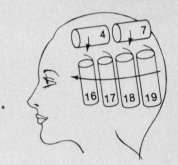

Complete setting pattern on the left side as shown

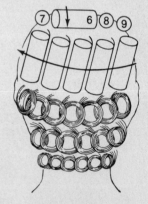

Beginning at the open end (tip of arrow) of the shaping set c.w. rollers in crown section.
Complete set with a row of c.c.w. sculpture curls, then finish nape section with 2 rows of c.w. curls

Setting Pattern 3

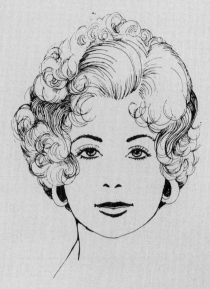

Finished hairstyle for setting pattern 3

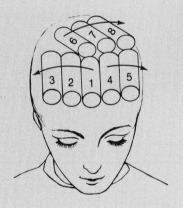

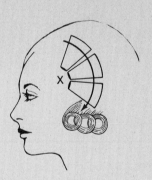

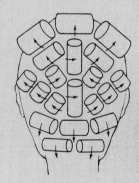

Half-stem roller placement   Placing rollers half on and half off the base of the strand.

Inside movement (indentation)   A hair pattern that brings hair close to the head.

Long-stem roller placement   Placing rollers all the way off and usually below the base of the hair strand.

Natural wave or cowlick   Hair standing upward, usually in a circular pattern.

No-stem roller placement   Placing the rollers directly on the base of the hair strand.

Outside movement   A hair pattern that gives height and volume, bringing hair away from the head.

GLOSSARY

QUESTIONS

1. What is the roller's circumference?
2. What is the roller's diameter?
3. How many turns to the head must the hair be rolled to get soft waves?
4. To achieve a curly look, how many turns must the hair be rolled?
5. What determines the strength of the curl produced by the roller?
6. When setting with rollers, what determines the curliness of the hair?
7. Normally, the diameter of the subsection used to set a roller should be what size?
8. Where should the clip be placed to secure the roller?
9. Is tension on the hair important when winding the roller to the head?
10. Does back-combing give height to the hairstyle, or bring the style close to the head?
11. Is an Italian-top setting pattern wound toward the face?

ANSWERS

1. Distance around the roller 2. Half of the roller's circle size (twice its radius) 3. 1½–2 turns 4. More than two turns 5. The stem placement 6. The number of times the hair is wound around the roller 7. The same diameter as roller 8. Where the roller touches the head 9. Yes 10. Gives height 11. No

Selecting Hairstyles 10

Purpose

Hairstyling involves arranging the hair to complement the features of a client's head, face, and body.

Have you ever bought something that you had to assemble yourself and, as you were almost finished putting it together, realized that a piece was missing? That missing piece was probably one little nut, or screw, or bolt–just one piece! But without that one piece, your bicycle was just a jumble of metal parts or your bookcase was little more than a pile of sticks. You had to have that piece.

Selecting a hairstyle is important in the same way. You might perform all of the necessary services perfectly. As you stand back to look at the finished product, you realize that something is wrong: the style doesn't suit the client. If you know what to look for when selecting a style, it shouldn't take much time. But it is very important because if your client does not like the hairstyle you choose, he or she probably will not be confident in your ability and will not ask for you to perform more expensive services.

In the past, cosmetologists did not learn these skills until they were on the job, after they were already working in salons. Learning from experience may be the best way to develop your ability to select the proper hairstyle, but you can learn much right now to develop these skills.

Major Objective

Correctly identify the facial shapes of six clients and recommend for each an appropriate hairstyle that demonstrates the principles stated in this unit.

Level of Acceptability

Given the information contained in this chapter, in addition to classroom instruction and practice, plan each hairstyle to create the illusion of an oval facial shape. Score 75 percent or better on a multiple-choice exam on the information in this chapter.

Knowing Subobjectives

1. Identify the ideal facial and head features.
2. Describe 6 facial shapes and ways to create the oval illusion for them.
3. Describe 3 common profiles.
4. Identify 6 other things to consider in hairstyling.

KNOWING SUBOBJECTIVE 1

Identify the ideal facial and head features.

It is easier to style the hair for a client who has an oval face. The oval type of face is considered the standard, and facial shapes that vary from the standard require more planning in the setting and combing stages.

First, a clear understanding of how to identify the standard oval is necessary. If you look at an oval face from the front, you should be able to see the 3 main and equal divisions of the face:

1. Chin to the bottom of the nose.
2. Bottom of the nose to the top of the eyebrows.
3. Top of the eyebrows to the forehead (hairline).

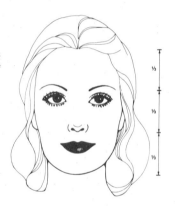

Proportions of the ideal facial type

The head that conforms to this description is easier to style because it does not have features that must be played down to improve the appearance of the client. A variety of hairstyles can be attractive on the client who has this kind of face.

In addition to facial shapes, you should be interested in the profile and silhouette of the hairstyle. The **profile** is the outline of the hair and head when viewed from the side. The **silhouette** (sil-eh-WET) is also an outline formed by the hair and head, but it may be viewed from any position, including the side.

In terms of overall appearance of the client, the hair is noticed first, then the eyes, and finally the clothes. The fashionable client will attempt to achieve a "total look":

1. Eyes are made up.
2. Hair is styled.
3. Clothes are coordinated.

Although the hairstyle is not everything, it is very important. The most attractive and expensive clothes will not complement the client unless the hair has been styled attractively. (Eye makeup will be discussed later in the text.)

Describe 6 facial shapes and ways to create the oval illusion for them.

There are six generally accepted facial shapes that differ from the ideal oval type. They are **diamond, heart, square, oblong, round,** and **pear.**

It is important to identify these problem facial shapes so that you will be able to create an optical illusion, making the face appear oval. This must be considered in planning, setting and arranging the final profile and silhouette.

Problem 1   **The diamond-shaped face** is characterized by a narrow chin and forehead and wide cheekbones.

Solution   To achieve an attractive oval look, fullness or width is needed in the forehead hairline and the lower cheekbone areas of the face. Fullness is not needed in the area of the upper cheekbones. The hair should be styled close to the head in that area. The hair should be styled with a fringe or bang to disguise the narrow forehead and with fullness around the jawbone on the face to complete the oval illusion.

Problem 2   **The heart-shaped face** is characterized by a large, wide forehead (often with a widow's peak), and a narrow chin.

Solution   To remedy the heart shape, some hair is brought onto the forehead to reduce the area across it. A pageboy-type style is good for the lower sides of the face because the hair is close to the head at the eyes, where narrowness is needed, but the hair is slightly full toward the face around the jaw and below and in front of the earlobes, where width is needed.

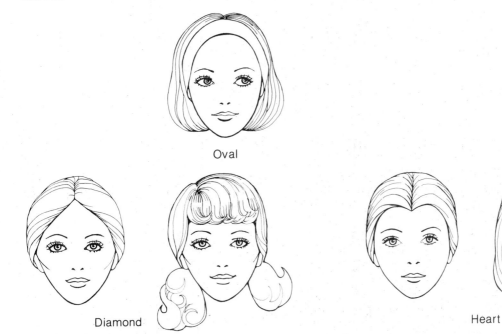

Oval

Diamond

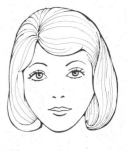

Heart

Problem 3   The square-shaped face is characterized by a wide hairline and jaw.

Solution   Bringing the hair forward and close to the face just below the cheekbones and setting and combing the hair off the forehead creates an oval illusion by adding the appearance of height to the face. Hair combed onto the sides of the face helps break the wide, straight lines common to the square face.

Problem 4   Oblong facial shapes are characterized by a very long and narrow bone structure. The client who has an oblong facial shape often also has a long, thin neck.

Solution   A fringe or half-bang across the forehead should be accompanied by soft waves or curls in the crown and nape areas. This flatters the face and neck by creating the oval illusion.

Problem 5   Round facial shapes are characterized by a wide hairline and fullness at and below the cheekbones. The contour moves from each cheekbone through the jawline and chin. The client may be overweight, and the neck may appear short.

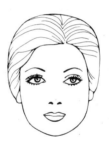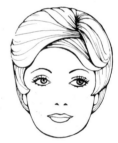

Square

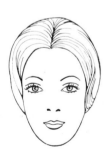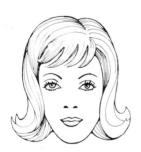

Oblong

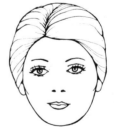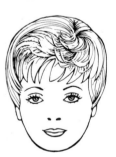

Round

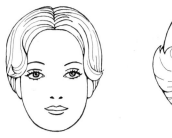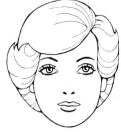

Pear

Solution   Setting and combing height in the top and crown sections of the style tends to diminish some of the roundness. Setting and combing the hair close to the head on the side and nape sections also helps.

Problem 6   **Pear facial shapes** are characterized by a small or narrow forehead and a rather large pouchy-appearing jawline.

Solution   Setting and combing the hair to add width from eye level through the crown of the head is helpful. Hair in the side and nape sections should be set and combed in a pattern close to the head.

KNOWING SUBOBJECTIVE 3

There are 3 common profiles: **straight**, **concave**, and **convex**.

The straight profile is characteristic of the ideal facial shape–the oval. The nose profile is in normal proportion to the forehead and the area below the lower lip.

The concave profile is characterized by the forehead and chin almost meeting a natural vertical line drawn perpendicular to the nose.

The convex profile is characterized by the nose, mouth, and chin protruding beyond the natural vertical line of the forehead.

Describe 3 common profiles.

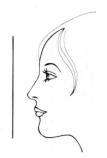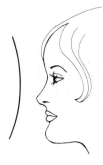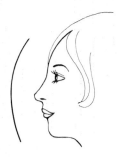

Straight   Concave   Convex

KNOWING SUBOBJECTIVE 4

Identify 6 other things to consider in hairstyling.

Facial shapes and profiles are the most basic considerations you will take into account when you style the client's hair, but they are not the only things that determine how the hair will be styled. Other factors are distinctive physical characteristics; personal choices; occupation; special occasions; personal habits; and hair color, texture, curliness, and shaping.

Physical imperfections, such as scars or large ears, may have to be camouflaged by arranging the hair in a certain way to cover them.

Personal choices, such as the client's desire to have a half-bang on the right side of the forehead rather than the left, or no bang at all, must be considered.

Occupation often dictates the style chosen. Statistics indicate that more than 50 percent of all married women work outside the home. For them, weekly visits to the beauty school or salon are usually considered a necessity rather than a luxury. The client's job also determines the type of hairstyle to some extent. Very long hair may create an unsanitary environment unacceptable in foodservice work. Hair, which is a collection point for germs, may fall into the food. Long hair also may create a hazard in a machine shop. The hair may get caught in a drill press and cause an injury.

Special occasions, such as weddings, anniversaries, graduations, birthdays, office parties, bowling banquets, and holidays, are also times when professional hairstyling services are requested. A casual or formal style should be chosen according to the occasion.

Personal eccentricities (distinctive behaviors or ideas) of clients sometimes affect hairstyling. Occasionally, a client will insist on a hairstyle that you know is unbecoming. For example, the client may insist on a fringe or half-bang on the right side of the forehead when the natural growth direction indicates the half-bang should be on the left side. In such a case, even if you have explained why the left side would be better, the bang should be set and combed on the right side! You should advise the client what is best, but give him or her what is requested.

Hair shaping, color, texture, and curliness also determine how the hair is styled. If the hair lengths are not correct for the style requested by the client, the hair should be shaped. If the hair is already too short, the client should be advised to allow it to grow to the correct length. The hair shaping must be correct for the desired hairstyle. If you are unsure of the relationship between the hairstyle and the hair shaping, ask your instructor for help.

Certain hairstyles also look better if they are done in certain colors–in some cases lighter, in other cases darker.

Some hairstyles can be achieved on fine hair that cannot be done on coarser hair textures, and vice versa.

The curliness or straightness of the hair can also be important factors in selecting a hairstyle. Straight hairstyles are difficult to form on very curly hair unless it has been chemically relaxed. On the other hand, curly hairstyles are difficult to form on hair that has not been cold waved (chemically waved) or does not have natural curl.

Profile   Outline of the head and hair as viewed from the side.

Silhouette (sil-eh-WET)   Outline formed by the hair and head as viewed from any angle.

QUESTIONS

1. On a separate sheet of paper, sketch and label six basic facial shapes. (Use a pencil.)
2. Write out the solution for a diamond-shaped face.
3. Write out the solution for a heart-shaped face.
4. Write out the solution for oblong facial shapes.
5. Is a heart-shaped face characterized by a large, wide forehead?
6. On the heart-shaped face, should hair be set and combed (styled) onto the forehead?
7. For a heart-shaped face, is it better to style some of the hair toward the face or away from the face?
8. For a square-shaped face, should the hair be styled away from the face?
9. Does a concave profile protrude outward?
10. Does a convex profile slope inward?
11. Would one characteristic of a pear-shaped face be a small, or narrow forehead?
12. Does a person's occupation have anything to do with a person's hairstyle? If yes, write an explanation in your own words.

ANSWERS

1. (Refer to text for comparison) 2. (Refer to text) 3. (Refer to text) 4. (Refer to text) 5. Yes 6. Yes 7. Toward the face 8. No, toward the face 9. No, inward 10. No, outward 11. Yes 12. Yes (with student's comments)

Shaping the Hair with Scissors, Razor, and Electric Clipper

11

Hair shaping (hair cutting) is one of the most important services performed in the salon because it affects so many other services. For example, if the hair isn't cut evenly from one subsection to the next, it will be very difficult to set on rollers. The same problem would occur in wrapping unevenly cut hair around permanent wave rods for chemical waving or curl reformation. Of course, you might have a real styling disaster if the hair hasn't been properly cut. In short, if the hair shaping is not done well—none of your other hairstyling services will be successful.

Like other tasks a cosmetologist must perform, hair shaping is a matter of doing many small tasks accurately, rather than doing a few large tasks well. You must be able to shape the hair correctly to do other tasks within the program.

Since the whole family—mom, dad, and the children—comes into the salon now, it is important that you learn how to shape hair for men as well as women. The texture, condition, color, degree of curliness or straightness, and growth pattern of the hair will determine the overall appearance of your hair shaping.

Since most of the cutting implements you will be using have extremely **sharp edges** and almost **needlelike points, be careful not to cut, snip, or pierce the client's eyes or skin around the ears, nose, or neck.** Public safety is an important part of your job. Be particularly cautious when giving a hairshaping to small children because they tend to move their heads without warning.

Major Objective	Using hair-shaping implements and supplies, cut the client's hair for the hairstyle requested.
Level of Acceptability	Use the proper hair-shaping techniques and safety precautions to cut the client's hair in 15-25 minutes with the razor, or 25-40 minutes with scissors. You will also be able to do some basic procedures with the electric clipper/trimmer/edger. Score 75 percent or better on a multiple-choice exam on the information in this chapter.

Knowing Subobjectives

1. Describe hair-shaping implements and basic cutting movements.
2. Explain the differences between razor shaping, scissor shaping, and electric clipper shaping.
3. Locate the basic parting sections of the head.
4. Define terms used in hair shaping and list safety precautions.

Doing Subobjectives

5. Give a basic scissor shaping on a female client.
6. Give a basic scissor shaping on a male client.
7. Give a basic clipper shaping on a female client.
8. Give a basic clipper shaping on a male client.
9. Give a basic razor shaping on a female client.
10. Trim a beard and a mustache.

KNOWING SUBOBJECTIVE 1

Describe hair-shaping implements and basic cutting movements.

You should be able to identify and describe hair-cutting implements and their individual parts in much the same way an artist can explain why a certain brush is used for a particular purpose.

1. **The double-edge scissors** is probably the most frequently used implement for shaping hair in the salon. Scissors are made in a variety of sizes ranging from about 4 to 8 inches from the **finger tang** (a little finger brace) to the tip of the cutting edge (point). They are also made without a finger tang; it depends on what hair-cutting technique the scissors will be used for.

The two most popular sizes of double-edge scissors are the 5½-inch and 7½-inch types. The 5½-inch type is ordinarily used to cut wet hair straight across (blunt or club cut), while the 7½-inch scissors are used to cut dry hair. The 7½-inch scissors are used generally in a sliding (slithering or effilating) movement to shorten and thin hair. Double-edge scissors may be purchased in both left-hand and right-hand models.

2. **Double-notch scissors** are used to thin the hair (remove bulk), but they are not used to remove length. They are also called **thinning scissors (shears)**.

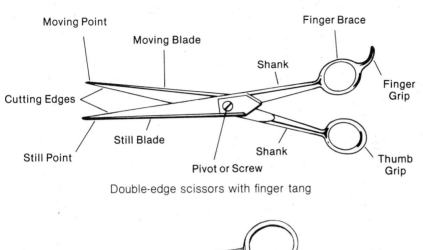

Double-edge scissors with finger tang

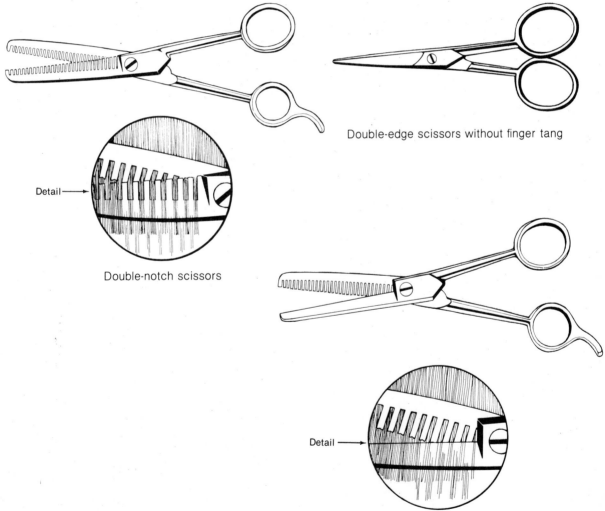

Double-edge scissors without finger tang

Double-notch scissors

Single-notch scissors with finger tang

3. **Single-notch scissors** are used to thin, or remove, bulk rather than length from the hair, but they remove or thin **more** hair than double-notch scissors do. Single notch scissors are also called **thinning** scissors.

4. The **single-edge** safety **razor** is also called a hair **shaper.** This implement is used to shorten and thin the hair. It is always used on **wet** hair.

5. The **styling comb,** which is 7 inches long, has both fine and coarse teeth. It is used to control the hair during the shaping service.

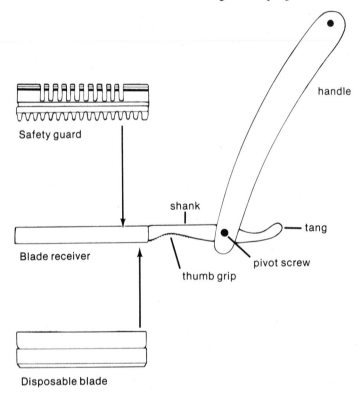

Safety guard

Blade receiver

shank

tang

pivot screw

thumb grip

handle

Disposable blade

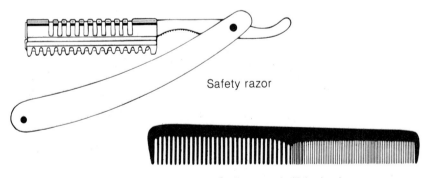

Safety razor

Styling comb (7 inches)

Top blade

Lower Blade

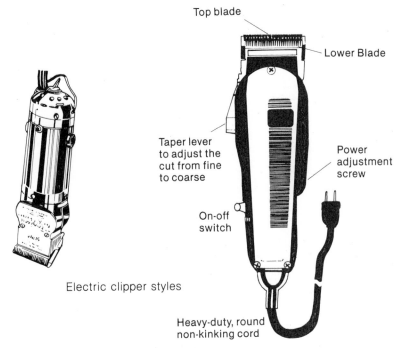

Taper lever
to adjust the
cut from fine
to coarse

Power
adjustment
screw

On-off
switch

Electric clipper styles

Heavy-duty, round
non-kinking cord

Size 0000
Close to shave,
hair length
1/250″

Size 000
Very close,
hair length
1/100″

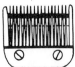

Size 0A
Close,
hair length
5/64″

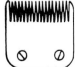

Size 1
Full tooth,
hair length
1/8″

Size 18
Skip tooth,
hair length
1/8″

Size 1A
Medium,
hair length
5/32″

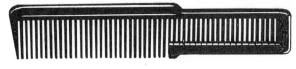

Clipper comb

Size 1-1/2
Medium full,
hair length
3/16″

Size 2
Full,
hair length
1/4″

Size 3-1/2
Fullest,
hair length
3/8″

Assortment of electric clipper blades

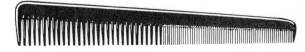

Barber comb

Cutting Movements

When you are shaping hair, either with a razor or scissors, you will need to make two basic kinds of motions with your cutting implement: **slither cutting (effilating)** and **blunt (club) cutting.**

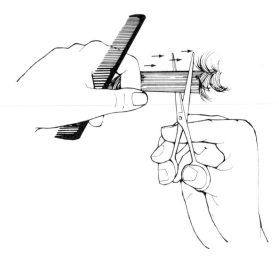

Slither cutting (effilating)

Slither cut the hair by sliding the cutting implement against the hair. If you are using scissors, close them **partially** as you slide them along the hair. This will give the hair a tapered, or "graduated," shape. **Do not** close the scissors completely. Slither cutting (effilating) is used to thin the hair, not to chop it off. If you close the scissors completely, you will cut the hair off completely. This will leave cutting **"marks" on the hair.**

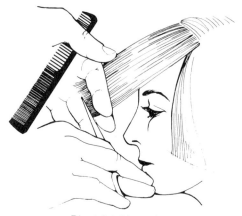

Blunt (club) cutting

Blunt, or club, cutting is cutting the hair straight off the strand without slithering or thinning it. This movement will give the hair an even, well-defined ("blunt") edge or line.

Hair shaping is a much better description of the hair-cutting task because the professional cosmetologist does much more than simply "cut" lengths of hair from the client's head. **Hair shaping takes into account the natural growth patterns, texture, condition, facial features, head structure,** and finished style of the hair. Although you may cut, and therefore shorten, hair in some areas of the head, you actually are shaping the hair to suit the hairdressing needs of a hair stylist client.

Although a skilled cosmetologist can use either implement for most hairstyles—individual practitioners often have strong preferences for one or the other—it is more practical to use one implement instead of the other for some styles. This is because certain hairstyles can be cut or combed into place faster if you use one implement rather than the other. For example, if the client desires a bouffant, teased (back-combed) hairstyle that is very high in the top and crown areas and requires rollers with a few sculptured curls, the razor is probably the better choice. For this style, the hair could be slither cut with scissors and thinned with single- or double-notch scissors, but it probably would be easier and faster to do it with a razor. On the other hand, blunt cutting is needed for some styles, and it is easier to do with scissors, even though a razor can produce similar results.

For some hairstyles, however, scissor cutting is a must. Hair to be air waved and/or curled with a curling iron to give fullness in the region of the eyes and a low top and crown should be shaped with scissors only. Therefore, your choice of a scissors or a razor is determined partly by what styling principles will be used after the hair shaping.

Explain the differences between razor shaping, scissor shaping, and electric clipper shaping.

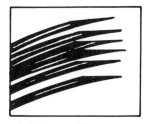

Hair cut with razor

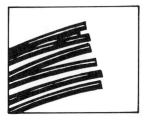

Hair cut with scissors

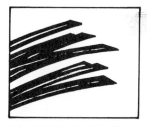

Hair cut with electric clipper

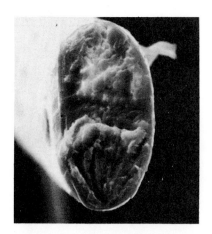

Scissor cut. Note how the action of the scissors squeezes the hair (Courtesy of 3M Company)

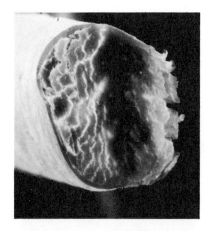

Razor cut. Note the edge of the outer cuticle (Courtesy of 3M Company)

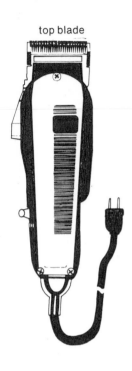

top blade

Some stylists do the entire haircut with the electric clipper because they feel it is faster. Your instructor will assist you in determining the best cutting implement for the clientele in your area.

Super-curly hair should be **cut dry.** Razor shaping is not recommended for this type of hair. It should be blunt cut or slither cut with scissors. Thinning shears are seldom, if ever, used on super-curly hair.

Precision or geometric haircuts are usually cut with a small scissors on wet hair. For example, a 5- or 5½-inch scissors without a finger tang can be used (it is difficult to turn the wrist to hold an implement at the correct cutting angles if it has a finger tang and longer blades). For this kind of style, the hair is always club or blunt cut, and the hair is not thinned very much, if at all.

The **electric hair clipper** is a cutting device made up of two closely-spaced serrated (like the teeth of thinning scissors) blades. The cutting blade (called the **top blade**) is driven by a small electric or magnetic motor to vibrate the blade back and forth against the still blade (**lower blade**). A portable, battery-operated clipper is also available. The hair caught in between the serrated blades is "sliced off" in much the same way as the hair is cut by the closing action of one scissors blade against the other.

Hair clippers come in different sizes. Some have an adjustable lever on the side that allows blunt cutting, much like scissors, or varying degrees of tapering, something like a razor. The **smaller clipper** model is sometimes called a **trimmer, outliner,** or **edger** because it is used mainly around the hairline to shorten the hair around the side burns, ears, or neck. The trimmer/outliner/edger is sometimes used to trim beards and mustaches. **Clipper shaping is generally done on dry hair to avoid the possibility of electric shock,** although a special model for cutting damp hair may be purchased from many different manufacturers. **Remember,** if wet hair

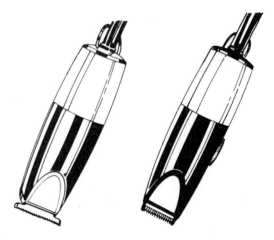

Examples of trimmers, outliners, or edgers used around hairline, and to outline beards, mustaches, etc.

hasn't been towel-dried, water may drip into the clipper causing the user or the client to get a hazardous **electrical shock!**

Since there are many good methods for parting and sectioning the hair for a hair shaping, consult your instructor about which method you should use.

Because each person's head is a different size and slightly different shape, it is important to have a clear picture in your mind (a mental image of design line) of how the head can be parted and sectioned. You probably have some idea already from the exercise in the Finger Waving chapter, doing subobjective 2.

So, the rectangle formed by points A, B, C, and D form the **top section.** The area on the head formed by points A, C, and G make up the **right side section.** Points B, D, and H make up the **left side section.** The rectangular area made up of points D, C, E, and F form the **crown section** of the head. The **crepe section** of the head is the area between the crown and the nape sections. It is made up of points F, E, G, and H on the drawing. The **nape section** is the area in the back of the head above the neck. It begins with the hairline, and goes up to the occipital bone. It extends across the lower-back of the head from ear-to-ear.

Sectioning of the hair is needed because the hair is easier to "handle" in small sections, particularly if the client has long and/or very dense hair. Generally, the accuracy of the hair shaping is better when a sectioning method is used.

Locate the basic parting sections of the head.

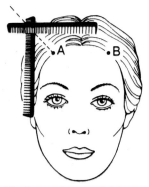

Finding points to divide the top from the side sections

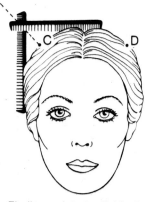

Finding points to divide the top from the crown section

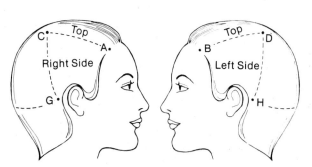

Lines AC, CG, and the hairline enclose the right side section. Lines BD, DH, and the hairline enclose the left side section

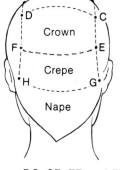

Lines DC, CE, EF, and FD enclose the crown section; lines FE, EG, GH, and HF enclose the crepe section, and the nape is below line GH from ear to ear

KNOWING SUBOBJECTIVE 4

Define terms used in hair shaping and list safety precautions.

There are quite a few words (terms) used in the hair-shaping service that are not normally used in everyday conversations. In order for you to communicate with your instructors and other professional stylists, it will be necessary for you to learn these new terms. A list of the basic terms follows: **guideline, hanging length, basic hairshaping, high elevation, low elevation, graduation, taper (layer), steps** or **marks, shingling, tailored neckline, feathering, angle, undercut, bi-level, finger-work, scissors-over comb, clipper-over comb.**

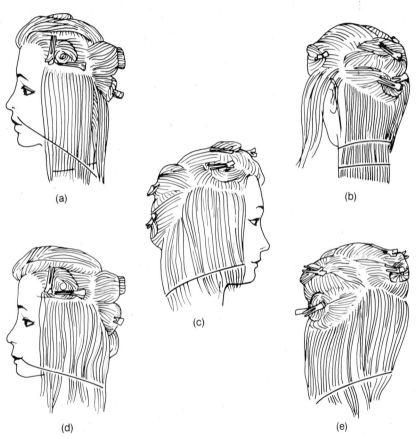

(a)

(b)

(c)

(d)

(e)

Black lines indicate possible shape for cutting the length of the **guideline**

Guideline   The guideline is one or more subsections (strands) of hair cut around the hairline or crown of the head. The purpose of the guideline is to give you **a measurement for cutting** the remaining hair. It is the yardstick by which you will cut the hair, a few strands at a time.

Hanging Length   The hanging length is the bottom length of the hair as it is combed downward. The hanging length is the longest hair around the bottom of the hairstyle.

Basic Hairshaping   A basic hair shaping is a general term used to describe a hair shaping that can be waved, blown, and styled in many different ways. Oftentimes, a basic hair shaping is a shorter hairstyle in the range of 3½ to 4½ inches in length (but may extend to as much as 6 inches in length). This type of cut can be easily wrapped on cold wave rods, set on rollers, set with an iron, blow combed, or set in sculpture curls. Particularly in a school setting, this is a good yet versatile hair shaping that will allow you to practice many of the different techniques already learned.

High Elevation   A high-elevation hair shaping is achieved by cutting subsections of hair held in an upward direction toward the crown or top of the head, rather than downward toward the nape of the head.

Low Elevation   A low-elevation hair shaping is achieved by cutting subsections of hair held in a downward direction toward the nape, rather than upward toward the crown or top of the head.

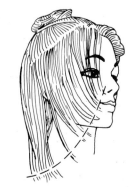

Dotted line shows length of hair after shaping—the **hanging length**

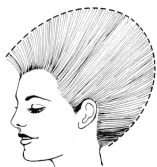

Proper distribution of hair lengths for a **basic haircut**

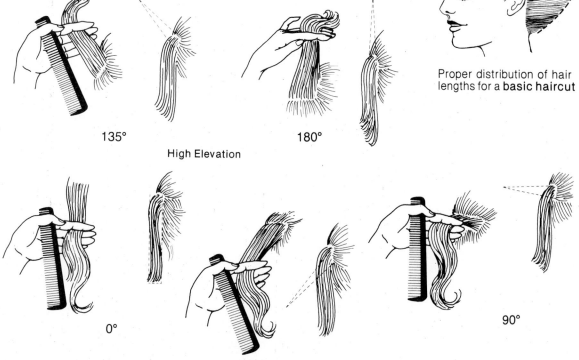

135°   180°

High Elevation

0°

Low Elevation   45°   90°

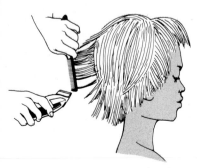

Graduating (layering) hair
lengths with electric
clipper

Graduation and Taper Graduation and taper mean about the same thing. Both terms refer to a shaping technique in which the hair is cut in layers. This is sometimes called layering, which is like the overlapping shingles on a roof, except closer together. For example, if the guideline on the bottom nape were cut in one length, the layer of hair above that is graduated, or cut **slightly** shorter. And the layer above that would be cut **slightly** shorter than the one below it.

Steps or Marks Steps or marks on the hair refer to a definite line(s) of demarcation from one layer of the hair to the layer below. This is the result of cutting the upper layer too short in relationship to the layer directly underneath it. When the guideline isn't followed, steps or marks can be easily seen, particularly on lighter hair colors, or hair that is naturally very straight or coarse.

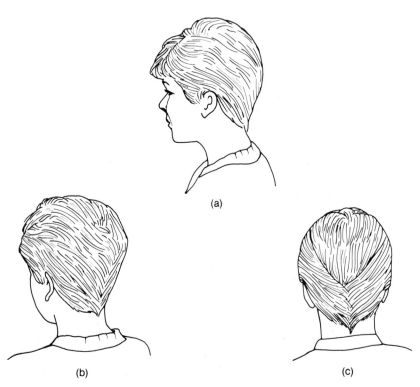

(a)

(b)   (c)

Shingling or tailored neck line shaping

Shingling and Tailored Neckline These terms are used interchangeably; they usually refer to a hair shaping that is very short in the nape of the neck. If the hairline in the nape grows toward the center of the nape, the hair is graduated into a "V" shape in the nape area for women. However, men tend to have their nape shaped into a more squared-off design.

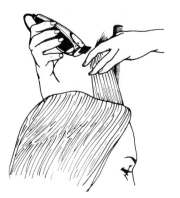

Feathering hair with electric clippers

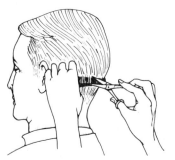

Example of cutting a "**feather edge**" for a male hair shaping. For safety, keep comb between client's head and scissors

Feathering   Feathering and the words "feather edge" are sometimes confused. Feathering is a term clients use to explain a shaping that is short and layered around the face (top, and both side sections). The length is about 3½ to 4½ inches, and it is styled away from the face, so that the ends of the hair can be seen. Feather edge, on the other hand, generally refers to the nape area of a man's hair shaping in which the hair is gradually layered down the neck until it seems to disappear into the skin.

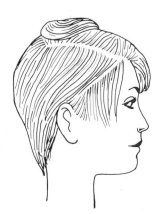

Hair is parted and cut parallel on a diagonal *angle*

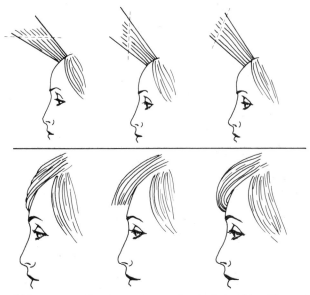

Different results shown for cutting hair held in different positions (angles)

Angle   An angle can refer to different hair-shaping situations. For example, to cut an angle in the front side section refers to parting the hair diagonally and parallel to the hairline to establish a cutting guideline. Angle may also refer to a design cut in the hanging length, or how the hair should be held when it is cut.

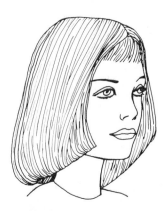

Note how hanging length of side sections are cut on an angle

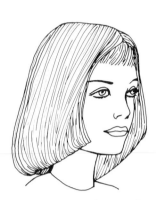

Hair gracefully flows under in nape and side sections because of **undercut** technique used for cutting hair

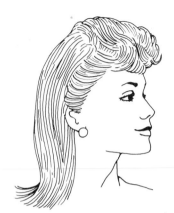

Bi-level. Hair is very short in front side sections, but hanging length is much longer

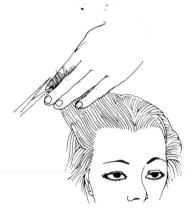

Finger-work (finishing) blends subsections together for a "finished look." (See end of first haircut procedure for illustration)

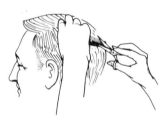

Scissors-over-comb technique often used after clipper for blending certain hair textures

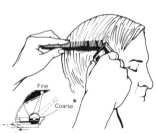

Using **clipper-over-comb** technique to blend top and side sections. Clipper adjustment lever should be in the lower position as shown by *

Undercut   Undercut is a term used to describe longer hair lengths that are all one length on the bottom of the hairstyle. In this hair shaping, the nape guideline is cut and then the client's head is tipped forward as far as is comfortably possible. The sections above the guideline are brought down one at a time and evenly cut on top of skin along the bottom of the hanging length. The same principle can be used for an undercut for shoulder-length hair.

Bi-level   A bi-level hair shaping is one in which the hair is cut in two different levels. It is quite short in the front hairline area and the front top section. The hanging length at the ear is usually short (about in the middle of the ear or less). The top-crown, crown, and back sections are left long (at about collar or shoulder length), and usually all one length like an undercut.

Finger-work   Finger-work is a barber/cosmetology technique of using the comb and scissors to blend sections of hair from one area of the head to another. It is used in very short hair shapings.

Scissors-over-comb and Clipper-over-comb   These terms are used to describe a barbering/cosmetology technique in which the hair is lifted away from the head with a comb and then cut with either the scissors or electric clipper.

You should know that as hair fashions change, different terms and techniques will be used. Various regions of the country or provinces may also have different terms that are used instead of the ones in this subobjective. Your instructor will teach you the hair-shaping terms that are used in your particular area.

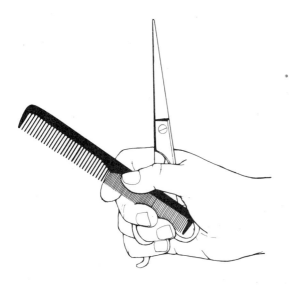

For safety, close scissors and rest them in palm when combing through the hair. Hold your scissors at all times during shaping

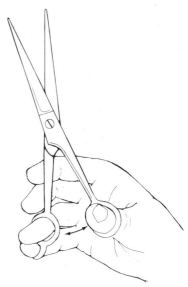

Correct way to hold scissors. Note position of thumb and ring finger

Be very careful not to cut yourself or your client during any hair-shaping procedure! The following is a checklist of things to remember in order to work safely!

SCISSORS SAFETY

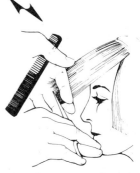

1. Always watch what you are doing. When not cutting, close scissors; palm them when combing through the hair.
2. Don't cut when you are talking to someone other than your client.
3. Never put scissors in uniform pocket, or you may severely cut yourself when reaching for them.
4. Keep your scissors sanitized when not in use.
5. If you have a small hand, it may be necessary to move along the strand by picking it up more than once.
6. **Use extra caution** when cutting hair in the area of the client's **eyes, ears, face, nose,** and **neck.**
7. **Be especially careful when shaping the hair of small children. A child may move his/her head quickly when you don't expect it. Try to anticipate a dangerous situation and avoid it.**
8. **Sanitize your scissors with alcohol after each hair-shaping service.**

Note fingers are placed between scissors and face to protect client's eyes and face

RAZOR SAFETY

1. **Don't attempt to change the blade of your shaper. Contact your instructor first for a demonstration.**
2. **Always use the guard on your razor.**
3. **Never put your razor in your uniform pocket. Reaching for a razor in your pocket could put you in the hospital with a serious injury!**

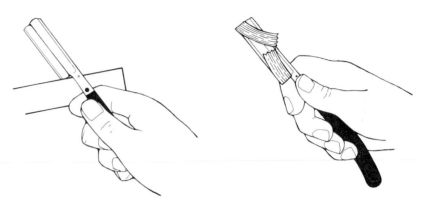

Removing an old razor blade

4. Don't use a shaper with a rusty blade because it could cause an infection if a cut occurred. Always use a sharp blade to avoid painful "pulling" of the hair.
5. Use a razor only on wet hair.
6. Be careful not to "nick" facial or neck moles, scars, or other skin lesions of the client!

CLIPPER SAFETY

1. Never use any electric (or battery-operated clipper) in the presence of water or other liquids. You or the client could get an electrical shock unless you have a special clipper with a waterproof case.
2. Use light clipper oil (one or two drops) daily to keep your blades working smoothly. Otherwise, the clipper may cause painful "pulling" of the hair.
3. Be careful not to "nick" facial or neck moles, scars, or other skin lesions of the client.
4. Adjust your clipper as often as needed.
5. Remove blades, if necessary, for cleaning.
6. Never use a clipper that has a broken tooth in either blade. Keep a spare replacement set of blades.
7. Align replacement blades correctly.
8. If you hear an irregular noise coming from your clipper, use a coin and turn the "power screw" counter-clockwise to "tune" the clipper for quieter operation. (Not all clippers have this feature.)
9. Never use a clipper which has rusty blades. Never submerge your clipper in water! If you do, you will cause an electrical shock!
10. Do not use a clipper if its case or power cord is cracked.
11. Never clean your clipper while the unit is turned on.

Always store all hair-shaping implements safely away from the reach of small children!

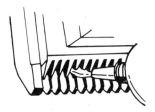

Oiling electric clipper blades

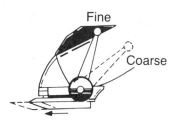

Taper adjustment lever

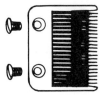

Removing blade for cleaning

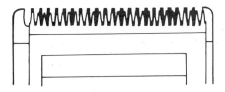

Correct alignment when changing electric clipper blades. Moving blade must *not* extend beyond still blade, or the client will be cut

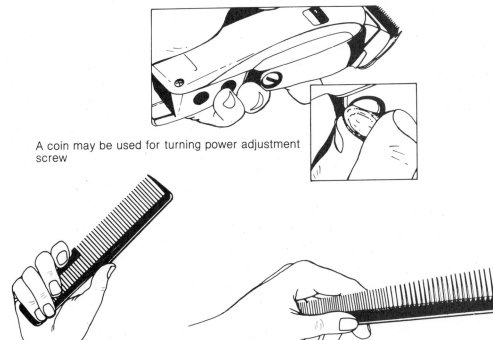

A coin may be used for turning power adjustment screw

Holding special barber comb

Holding comb for scissors-over comb or clipper-over comb cutting technique

DOING SUBOBJECTIVE 5

Give a basic scissor shaping on a female client.

Supplies

- ☐ talcum powder
- ☐ shampoo cape or chair cloth
- ☐ neck strips
- ☐ spray applicator bottle for water

- ☐ styling comb
- ☐ duck-bill clips
- ☐ double-edge scissors

Preparation

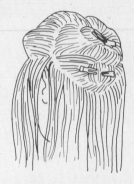

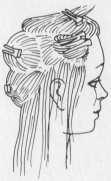

Part off sections of hair leaving guideline at bottom hairline

PROCEDURE

1. Drape the client with a shampoo cape and determine what services are to be performed.

2. Shampoo the hair and part off the top section and secure.

3. Part off each side section, but leave enough hair to establish a guideline on each side.

4. Part off the crown, crepe, and nape sections, but leave a strip of hair in the nape to establish a guideline.

RATIONALE

1. If the client will be having a certain chemical service, such as a tint or shampoo, a shampoo cape is necessary to protect their clothing from damage by possible contact with chemicals or water. Also, the hair would be tinted before either shampooing or shaping. For a hair shaping when no chemical services are given, including a shampoo, a chair cloth may be used for draping and will be more comfortable for the client as it is made of rayon or cotton or other woven fabric.

2. It is easier to begin in this section, and it is much better to work on clean hair. Shampooing removes hair oils, loose hair, spray, dust, etc.

3. The use of a guideline permits hair to be cut evenly from one subsection to the next.

4. It is more convenient to cut the hair in small sections, rather than trying to control all the hair at once.

5. **Ask many questions** of the client concerning the hairstyle desired. For example, how will the hair be styled–with a hot comb, hand dryer or rollers? Or will it be air-dried or finger waved?

6. Position your comb at different places around the hairline and try to imagine where you will be cutting the hair for various hair lengths.

5. You should develop a mental image of exactly what the client has in mind before cutting the hair.

6. Placement of the comb is helpful to you, and it allows the client to visualize how long or short the hair will be after the shaping.

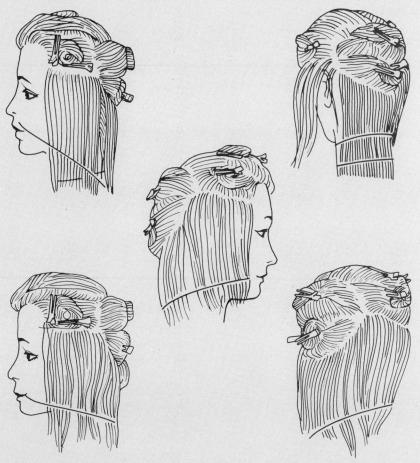

Possible imaginary guideline for cutting. Consult with client to determine desired length

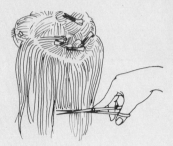

Begin cutting from center nape to next section

Shaping the Hair with Scissors

PROCEDURE

1. Begin cutting the hair in the left nape section.

2. Work forward from the nape to the front of the left side section.

3. Repeat steps 1 and 2 for cutting from the right nape section to the front of the right side section.

RATIONALE

1. This establishes a guideline in the nape section so that the subsections will be evenly cut from one section to the next.

2. Developing a system for working helps increase your accuracy and speed.

3. This is standard procedure.

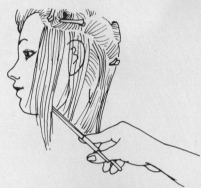

Continue cutting along imaginary guideline. Carefully cut hair on the skin. Holding hair to be cut in fingers causes it to become shorter

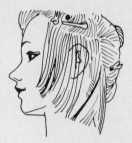

Hanging length of first guideline

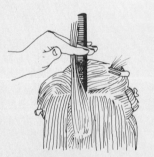

Hold strand and comb straight up from highest point on head. Half of the comb will leave 3½ inches of hair for guideline

4. Release the crown and crepe sections and comb them smoothly into the guideline. Hold your comb in a vertical position and comb a strand of hair alongside the comb. Measure the hair to "half the comb" (3½ inches +).

4. After establishing the "hanging length" in the nape and side sections, it is necessary to establish the longest length in the crown section. **If the hair is cut shorter than 3½ inches** (half the length of a styling comb), **you will have difficulty wrapping cold wave rods, setting,** and **iron curling the hair.**

5. Starting in the center back of the crown, pick up a thin vertical subsection. Comb the subsection into the guideline from step 4. Cut the hair that extends beyond the length of the guideline. Work from the center to the left ear until left crown has been cut. Repeat on right side of the center of the crown.

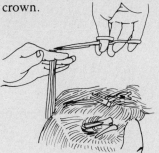

Cut guideline. Allow more length if client has a strong cowlick

6. Begin on the bottom of the crown section and part off a subsection of previously cut hair. Comb a thin, vertical subsection from the crepe section into your fingers. Cut the hair that extends beyond the crown guideline and the nape guideline. Work from center crepe to the left ear. Repeat by working from the center crepe to the right ear.

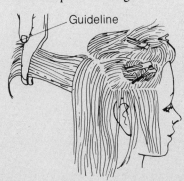

Note guideline at top of hair strand

5. Using these thin subsections and the guideline will give your hair shaping greater accuracy (evenness) throughout the hair.

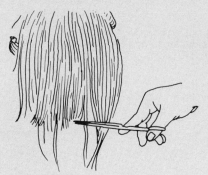

Cut crown/crepe sections even with hanging length

6. This will systematically allow you to complete cutting the entire crepe section.

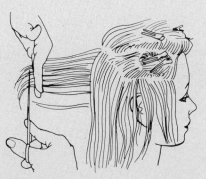

Use guidelines from top and lower nape to cut hair in between evenly

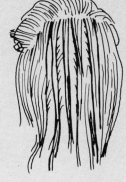

Use vertical partings to cut from guideline

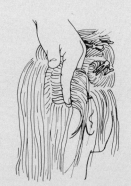

Cut from the center crown toward the right ear

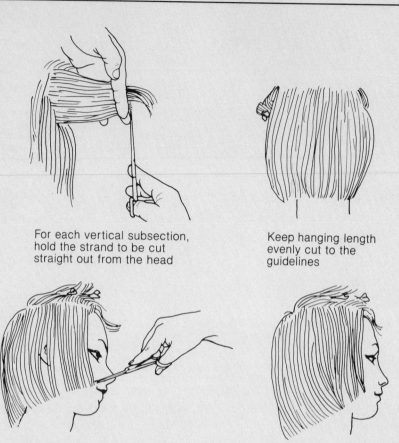

For each vertical subsection, hold the strand to be cut straight out from the head

Keep hanging length evenly cut to the guidelines

Carefully cut hair to guideline. Be careful of eyes and skin. Watch what you are doing

7. Go to the back of the right side section behind the ear. Part off a thin, vertical subsection from the sidesection. Comb it into the last subsection cut in step 6, then watch the hair as you gradually comb both subsections forward. Cut off the hair that extends beyond the guideline. Repeat until all subsections have been cut.

8. Repeat step 7 on the left side section. Begin behind the left ear.

7. This is standard procedure. Watching the hair closely as you comb it will allow you to see the difference between the guideline and the hair that needs to be cut.

8. This is standard procedure for cutting the left side section.

9. Release the top section. Part in the center and comb into each side section. Make a vertical parting from the center part to the hairline behind the ear. Starting at the bottom of the part, "walk" a subsection of hair to a horizontal position on top of the head.

10. The hair that extends beyond the guideline when the hair is held in a horizontal position should be cut. Repeat for each subsection. Comb each subsection into the one previously cut and then move your hand holding the hair forward before cutting.

9. This is standard procedure. You start combing behind the ear and combing the subsection to the top in order to "see" the guideline established in the hair that has already been cut.

10. It is important to use the guideline for measuring each subsection **before** it is cut. Moving the hair forward takes into account the natural curvature of the head as it gradually slopes forward.

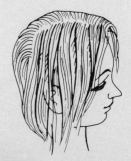

Release top section. Part hair in center

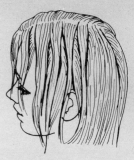

Use vertical partings to follow guideline toward front hairline

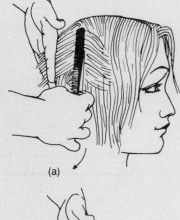

(a)

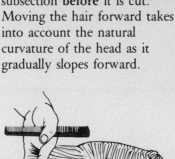

(b)

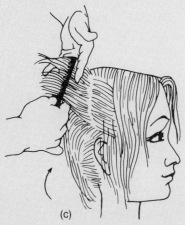

(c)

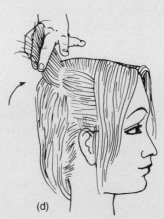

(d)

Keep raising your hand position to "walk" the strand to the top of the head

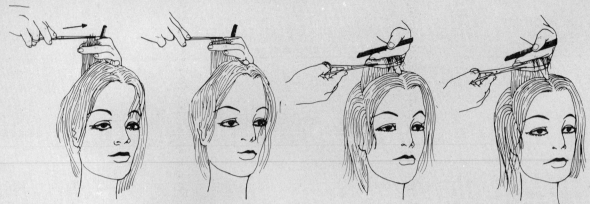

Cut hair that extends beyond guideline

Comb through again to make sure no hairs have fallen from strand you were cutting

As you work toward the front hairline, move your hand slightly forward to allow for the natural curvature of the head

Continue cutting toward the front hairline

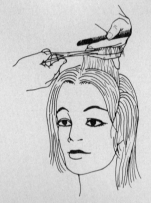

Cut left side to match right side. Use hair in right section as guideline

11. Repeat step 10 on the left side of the top section. Begin parting behind left ear and "walk" the subsection to the top of the head. Pick up a subsection of the hair cut on the right side of the top section and use it as a guideline to begin cutting the left side of the top section. Repeat until all subsections have been cut.

12. Check for hair that doesn't blend by systematically combing subsections between the top and side sections and trim as needed for evenness. Double-check hanging length for evenness and shape.

11. Since the right side of the top section is done, and you are reasonably sure it is correct, use a subsection from it as a guideline to cut the left side of the top section.

12. There will usually be a small "corner" of hair that doesn't fit into the haircut between the top and side sections. Neck hair tends to "creep" up a little, so careful combing is needed to make sure it is even and shaped correctly.

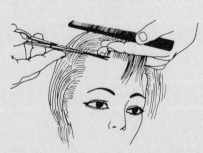

Remember to move your hand forward slightly to follow the shape of the client's head

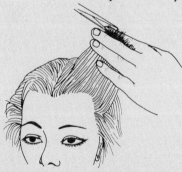

Checking hair lengths for "corners" between top and side sections

13. Using a small amount of talcum powder on a towel, thoroughly wipe hair clippings from client's face, neck, and clothing. Sweep, comb, or vacuum all hair from floor and work area. Dispose of hair clippings in closed container. Continue with next service. Sanitize and store cutting supplies and implements.

13. The powder allows the air to freely slide off the client onto the cape or the floor. Many states have laws requiring the removal of hair from the floor and work area immediately after the shaping. Cutting implements must be sanitized after **each** use.

DOING SUBOBJECTIVE 6

Give a basic scissor shaping on a male client.

Supplies

- □ talcum powder or hair vacuum
- □ shampoo cape or chair cloth
- □ neck strips
- □ spray applicator bottle for water
- □ styling comb
- □ duck-bill clips
- □ double-edge scissors
- □ barber comb
- □ electric clipper/outliner

NOTE: The basic difference between a shaping for a man and a woman is that the growth pattern is different around the hairline in front and the nape hairline at the back of the head. The shaping on the man will be somewhat more square around the sideburns and the nape of the neck. A shaping on a woman tends to be cut around the hairline with a more oval shape. The sideburns are angled more also, almost to a point for the female client. For the male client, the cutting procedure after the guideline has been established is nearly the same as specified in the previous subobjective. A man's hair shaping, however, is often cut much shorter. If a permanent wave or curl reformation is not scheduled, the guideline for the male client is usually 2 to 3 inches. Length of the guideline will also be determined by the texture and density of the hair, along with the wishes of the client.

Rationales for the steps of this subobjective have been omitted because they are essentially the same as those for subobjective 5.

Preparation

Repeat steps 1 through 6 of the Subobjective 5.

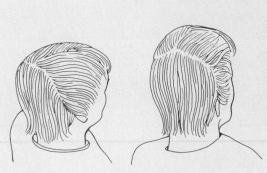

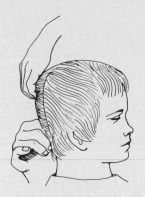

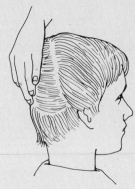

Section hair from top of crown section to behind each ear

If hair isn't too short, clip crown and crepe sections out of the way. Leave a strip of hair at the bottom of nape for cutting guideline

Side sections may be combed out of the way, or secured with a clippie or duck bill clip

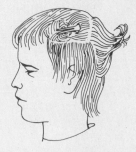

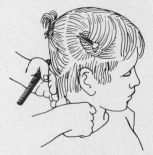

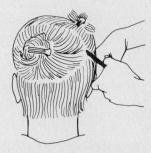

Secure side sections if hair is not too short. Leave guideline strip of hair over ears

Cut guideline in nape section

Continue to cut guideline from ear to nape along hairline

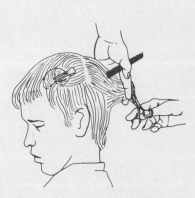

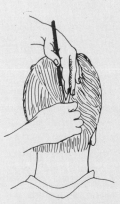

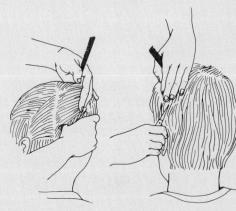

Use vertical sections to work nape guideline into crepe section of head

Continue to work into upper crown section of head

Cut the hair using vertical sections. Work from the center of the head to left and right ears

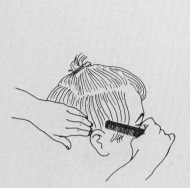

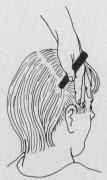

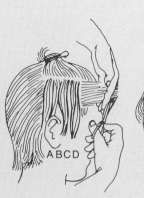

Part off hair at top of ear. Cut guideline on either side of ear

Consult client to determine desired length of hair over ears. Repeat on left side section

Use bottom guideline to cut hair in right side section and left side section. Hold hair straight out from head for cutting

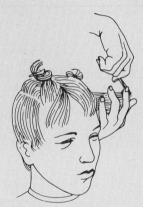

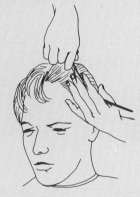

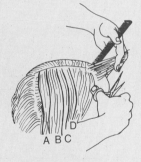

Move your hand slightly forward as you cut the hair to follow the curvature of the head

Begin at section "A," and "walk" the hair to the top of the head. Use guide from side section for cutting top section

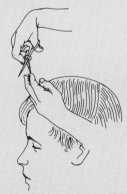

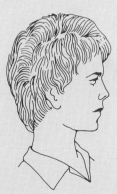

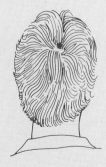

Repeat steps to cut left top section to match

DOING SUBOBJECTIVE 7

Give a basic clipper shaping on a female client.

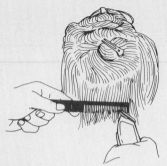

Section hair and cut guideline in nape section

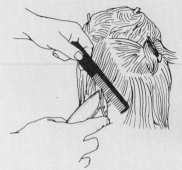

Work from center of nape toward left ear

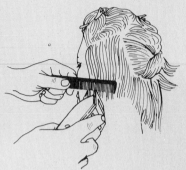

Cut side section guideline

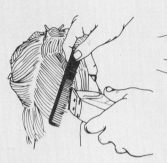

Work from center nape to right side section

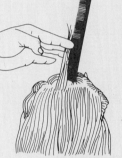

Establish crown guideline and cut

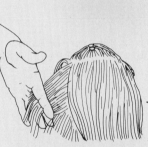

Use clipper to blend hair between top and bottom guidelines

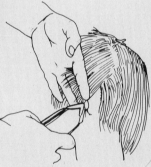

Cut between top and bottom guides using vertical partings

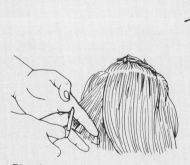

Blend top and bottom sections

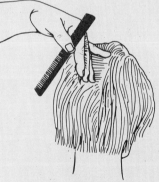

Work from center of crown toward right side using vertical subsections

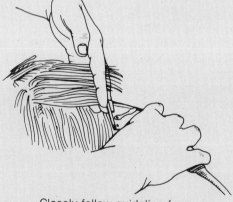

Closely follow guideline from previously cut section

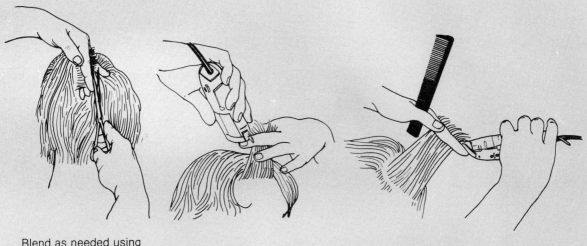

Blend as needed using
scissors

DOING SUBOBJECTIVE 8

**Give a basic clipper
shaping on a male
client.**

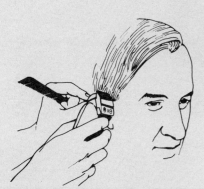

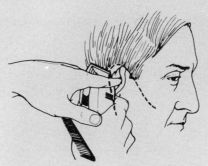

Give basic haircut with implement
of your choice. Then establish
guideline at side hairline

Fold ear out of work area to establish
shape of hairline. Do *not* cut into
natural hairline. Dotted line indicates
shape of short haircut for male
clients

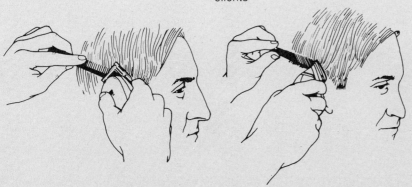

Use clipper-over comb technique to blend sides with hair above

DOING SUBOBJECTIVE 9

Give a basic razor shaping on a female client.

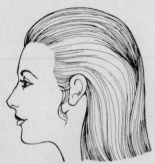

Bulky, untapered hair

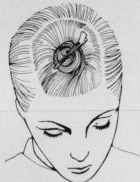

Part off the top section

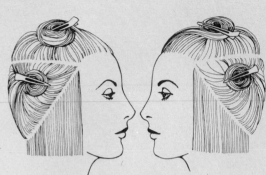

Part off the side sections

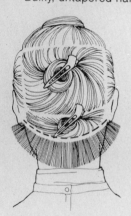

Part off the crown and crepe sections, but leave a strip of hair to cut the guideline at the bottom

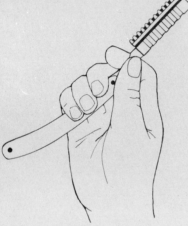

Manner in which the razor should be held

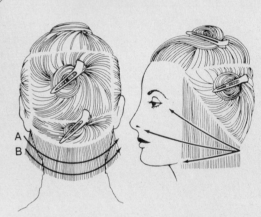

Decide guideline for hanging length A or B. Decide hanging length for both side sections

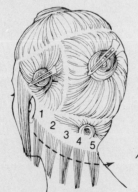

Begin cutting behind left ear to make guideline

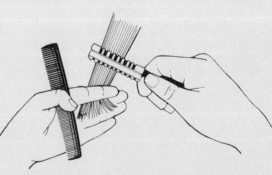

Hold razor almost flat against hair strand. Pressure of razor against hair will determine how much hair is removed

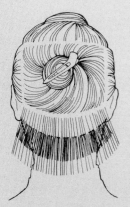

Bring down crepe section. Dark area shows guideline

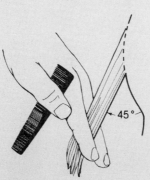

Hold hair at 45° angle. Slide fingers down strand until guideline begins to fall. Then begin cutting

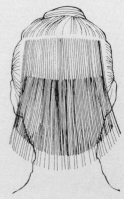

Divide crown section in half and bring down. Slide fingers down verticle strands until crepe guideline falls. Then begin to cut

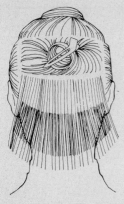

Bring down other half of crown and blend with lower half. Comb down both side sections and repeat procedure using bottom guideline

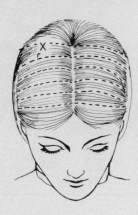

Make a center part. Begin at point "X" and use verticle parts to "walk" the hair to the top of the head and cut using your guide. Continue until all subsections are cut. Repeat procedure for other top section

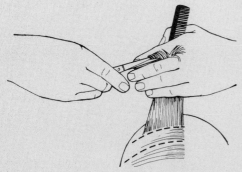

Check hair lengths from one section to the next

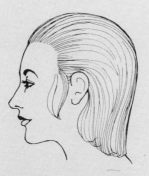

Properly tapered hair

DOING SUBOBJECTIVE 10

Trim a beard and a
mustache.

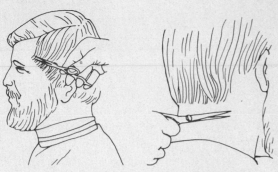

To begin, cut front and nape hanging length
guidelines

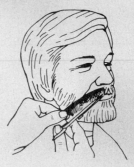

Use small, mustache
comb for trimming
mustache

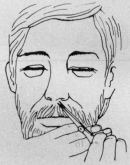

Use one hand to guide
scissors. Be careful *not*
to cut skin

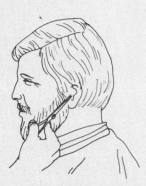

Trim outline of beard.
Be careful of ear

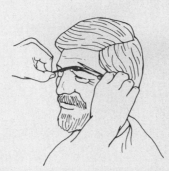

Use mustache comb to trim
eyebrows

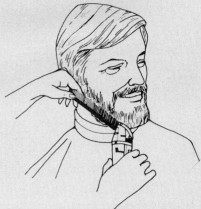

Use clipper-over-comb technique to
remove fullness from beard

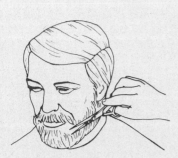

Overly-curly hairs can be trimmed
in shape using scissors

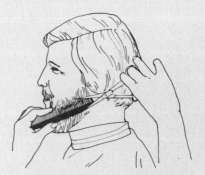

Use finger-work to remove
additional fullness from
beard

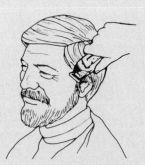

Use edger (trimmer) to
define border of beard

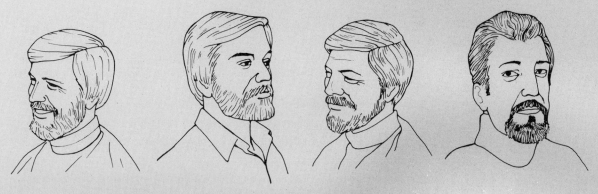

Finished beard shapings

Angle   A term which can be applied to different hairshaping situations in which the hair is cut on the bias.

Basic hair shaping   A hair shaping that can be waved, blown, and styled in many different ways.

Bi-level shaping   A hair shaping in which the hair is cut in two different levels.

Blunt cutting   Cutting straight across the hair.

Clipper-over-comb   The technique of lifting the hair away from the head with a comb and then cutting it with a clipper.

Club cutting   See **Blunt cutting.**

Crepe section   The area of the head between the crown and nape sections.

Double-edge scissors   A frequently used implement for hair shaping.

Double-notch scissors   Used to thin the hair (remove bulk rather than length).

Edger   See **Trimmer.**

Effilating   Slither cutting.

Electric hair clipper   A cutting device made up of two closely-spaced serrated blades.

Feather edge   The nape area of a man's hair shaping, in which the hair is gradually layered down the neck.

Feathering   A shaping that is short and layered around the face.

Finger-work   The technique of using the comb and scissors to blend sections of hair from one area of the head to another.

Graduation   A shaping technique in which the hair is cut in layers.

Guideline   One or more strands of hair cut around the hairline or crown to provide a measurement for cutting the rest of the hair. Also, a narrow strip of hair used on both sides of the head and nape to establish the hanging length of a hairstyle.

Hair shaping   Cutting the hair with scissors, razor, or electric clipper taking natural growth patterns, facial features, finished style, and other factors into account.

Hanging length   The longest hair around the bottom of the hairstyle.

High-elevation shaping A hair shaping achieved by cutting subsections of hair held in an upward direction toward the crown or top of the head, rather than downward toward the nape.

Low-elevation shaping A hair shaping achieved by cutting subsections of hair held in a downward direciton toward the nape, rather than upward toward the crown of top of head.

Lower blade The blade of an electric clipper, which does not move.

Marks The line of demarcation from one layer to the one below.

Nape section The area in the back of the head above the neck.

Outliner See **Trimmer.**

Scissors-over-comb The technique of lifting the hair away from the head with a comb and then cutting it with scissors.

Shaper Used to shorten and thin wet hair; **single-edge razor.**

Shingling A hair shaping that is very short in the nape.

Singel-edge razor Used to shorten and thin wet hair.

Single-notch scissors Used to thin the hair (remove bulk rather than length).

Slither cutting Cutting the hair by sliding the blade along the hair to give it a tapered shape; **effilating.**

Steps The line of demarcation from one layer to the one below.

Styling comb Used to control hair during shaping.

Tailored neckline A hair shaping that is very short in the nape.

Taper A shaping technique in which the hair is cut in layers.

Thinning Removing bulk during a haircut.

Thinning scissors See **Single-notch** and **Double-notch scissors.**

Top blade The blade of an electric clipper, which moves back and forth against the still blade.

Trimmer A small hair clipper, which is mainly used around the hairline.

Undercut Hair subsections from the crepe and crown sections are cut so they are longer than the nape guideline.

QUESTIONS

1. Write a short paragraph explaining the importance of hair shaping.
2. What is effilating?
3. Super-curly hair is generally cut with what implement?
4. On a separate sheet of paper, sketch the basic haircut taught in your school.
5. Write an explanation comparing a low-elevation hair shaping and a high-elevation hair shaping.
6. Which hair shaping implement is used to blunt cut and shape the hair around the sideburns of a male client?
7. Which cutting implement should only be used on hair that is wet?

8. On the electric clipper, which is the adjustable blade, the top or the bottom blade?
9. What is the name for the comb which is very tapered at one end that is used to cut short hair?
10. Which type of hair should not be cut with a razor?
11. Make a drawing, showing the sectioning divisions of the head.
12. Is the strand held upward for a high-elevation shaping?
13. What is the name for a shaping that is very short in the nape of the neck and cut in a "V" shape?
14. When not in use, should you store your scissors or razor in your pocket?
15. Is it cooler for the client to be draped for a hair shaping with a shampoo cape or cloth cape?
16. Should you shape the hair the way you think it should be cut or consult the client?
17. True or false. If the hair is cut at 2½ inches, it can be easily wrapped on permanent wave rods.
18. If the hair is very thick, what size subsections should you use?
19. Is a guideline really necessary in order to give an even hair shaping?
20. If you don't have a blower or vacuum, what is the easiest way to remove hair from the client's skin after a hair shaping?

ANSWERS

1. (Students' comments.) 2. Sliding the scissors along the hair strand to thin it 3. Scissors 4. (Students' sketches) 5. Text 6. Electric clipper 7. Razor (shaper) 8. The bottom blade 9. Barber comb 10. Super-curly hair 11. (Students' sketch) 12. Yes 13. Shingle or tailored neckline 14. No 15. Cloth cape (chair cloth) 16. Consult the client 17. False 18. Thin subsections 19. Yes 20. Apply a small amount of talcum powder to the corner of a towel and dust the neck

Air Waving and Blow Waving the Hair 12

Fashions, like the weather, are sure to change. Sometimes they seem to change almost as quickly as the weather does; other times they change more slowly.

Hairstyles are an important part of fashion, and like fashion, they change as "looks" change. Air waving and blow waving are two examples of new styling techniques that have become quite popular. The use of a hand dryer to produce special effects is not completely new, but the techniques and designs of hand dryers used for air waving and blow waving are new.

Special styles often require some kind of special treatment or special care. This is true for air waving and blow waving. If you use these techniques, you must be sure to give the hair a very good scissor shaping. With practice you will be able to master these skills.

Purpose

Using a professional air waver or blow waver, dry the client's hair in a current hairstyle.

Major Objective

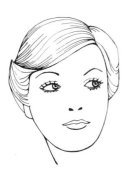 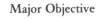 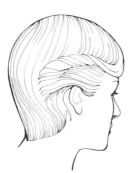

Level of Acceptability

The client's hair should be air waved (with air waver or blow waver) in 30 to 40 minutes. It should be thoroughly dried and arranged in a current hairstyle. Score 75 percent or better on a multiple-choice exam on the information in this chapter.

Knowing Subobjective

1. Explain "quick-service" hairstyling and describe the implements used.

Doing Subobjectives

2. Air wave the hair.
3. Blow wave the hair.

KNOWING SUBOBJECTIVE 1

Explain "quick-service" hairstyling and describe the implements used.

Air waving and blow waving are "quick-service" types of hairstyling. "Quick-service" hairstyling **saves time for the client.** After the hair is shampooed, it can be styled into place with an air waver or blow waver. Setting, drying, and combing the hair, which take quite a bit of time, are not needed.

Air waving uses electrically heated air from an **air waver (blow comb)** and combing techniques to dry the hair into **wave patterns.**

Blow waving is similar to air waving; it uses electrically heated air from a **blow waver (hand dryer)** and combing and brushing techniques to dry the hair. But there is one important difference: blow-waving the hair results in **larger wave patterns.** they can give the hair more volume (height) than air waving. Blow waving produces a more casual hairstyle than air waving. Appliances used for air waving and blow waving differ in several ways.

1. Law requires that the **electrical power** for both air wavers and blow wavers must be stamped somewhere on them. This power is stated in **watts.** The amount of power needed to run these appliances and the degree to which they heat the air vary. Their power ratings can vary from about **250 to 1350 watts.** The higher the rating, the **hotter** the appliance will heat the hair.

2. High-powered air wavers and blowers have from two to five heat settings (from hot to cold) that work best for particular hair types. Hotter settings are for normal and coarse hair that has **not been chemically treated.** As you flip the switches lower, you will get cooler temperatures for tinted, fine, and bleached hair.

3. In addition to the amount of heat, you also should be intersted in the speed (force) of the air coming from the air waver or blow waver. The **speed** of the heated air leaving the appliance determines how fast the hair can be arranged and dried into a hairstyle. Most professional air wavers have more than one air speed setting.

4. Air wavers and blow wavers can be bought with a variety of attachments, but the most useful ones are the **fine-tooth** metal comb for the air

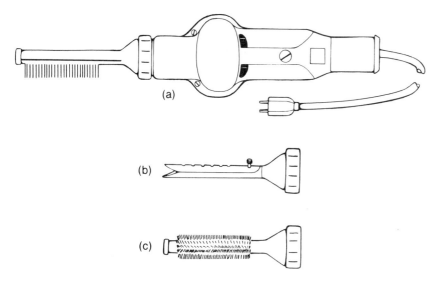

Air waving attachments (a) comb, (b) curler, (c) brush

waver (blow comb) and the **standard** nozzle (plastic or metal) for the blow waver.

To insure safety for yourself and your client, all air wavers and blow wavers used in the beauty school or salon must be **"U.L." (Underwriters Laboratories)** approved.

The **"U.L." seal means** that the waver has been tested and **judged safe.** It should not overheat or cause accidental electric shocks.

Supplies

Air wave the hair.

☐ Shampoo supplies
☐ electric air waver
☐ 28-tooth comb attachment
   for air waver
☐ hard rubber air-waving (styling) comb
☐ air-waving lotion

PROCEDURE

1. Shampoo and towel-dry the hair. Analyze and condition the hair, if necessary. Apply and comb air-waving lotion evenly through the hair.

RATIONALE

1. Special air-waving lotions are best for the hair and air-waving implements because regular styling lotions may stick to the air comb and styling comb.

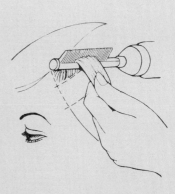

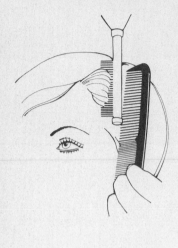

2. Turn on the air waver to low temperature and fast air speed. Subdivide the hair into strands about the same size as those used for a roller setting.

3. Hold the end of the strand with your left hand and place the metal air comb close to, **but not on,** the scalp. Moving your right wrist in a circular pattern, turn the comb attachment against the hair. Fasten dried hair with a clip until it has cooled.

4. Use a regular styling comb (hard rubber) on very short strands.

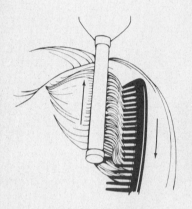

5. Slide the air comb close to the scalp toward the face at an angle that matches the desired wave pattern.

6. Insert the air comb into the hairline, shaping toward the crown. Insert the styling comb behind the air comb and the first ridge of the wave pattern. Slide the air comb upward toward the right while shifting the styling comb to the left.

7. Use your left hand to support the hair in the side section while flipping the ends there. Continue to dry the hair until a diagonal wave is formed in this section.

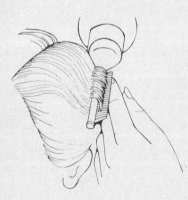

Direct flow of air away from scalp

2. Starting at a lower temperature helps prevent accidentally burning the client's scalp or face. Smaller strands are easier to control and dry quickly. Roller-size sections afford the most durable hairstyle.

3. Rotating the air comb gives height and strength to the base of each hair strand. The hair will relax into a straighter position if it is not clipped into place and allowed to cool at room temperature.

4. Hard rubber combs stand up to heat better than plastic combs. The large hard rubber air-waving comb is easier to use, except on very short hair.

5. This technique shapes the hair into the desired formation.

6. Gentle but correct use of the comb against the attachment gives the base and ridge of the wave their form. Be sure that the air does not blow on the client's face or scalp.

7. Using the fingers of either hand to assist the air-waving comb is often easier than using a styling comb (depending on the length of the hair).

8. Check that the wave has depth and is easy to see. Begin drying the hair in the top section. Direct the teeth of the air comb toward the part.

9. Holding the air-waving comb in your right hand, make a semicircular motion to support the shape of the pattern.

10. Repeat this procedure to form an "S" pattern in the hair.

11. Repeat steps 7 and 8.

12. Continue waving and drying until the style is finished.

8. The base direction should be partly circular, and ridges should be parallel to each other. Directing the teeth of the air comb toward the part helps to form desired wave patterns and their ridges.

9. The semicircular wrist motion gives the wave pattern its depth and helps the hair dry evenly so that the patterns curve and are parallel to each other.

10. This is standard procedure to form a wave pattern in the top section.

11. This is standard procedure to form a diagonal wave pattern in the side.

12. Be sure that the hair is **completely** dry.

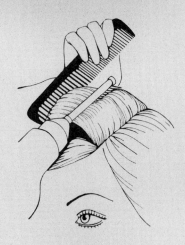

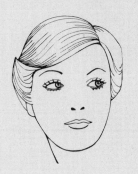

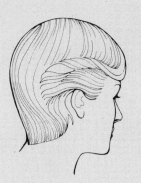

DOING SUBOBJECTIVE 3

Supplies

- ☐ shampoo supplies
- ☐ electric blow waver (hand dryer) with nozzle attachments
- ☐ boar bristle round brush
- ☐ styling comb
- ☐ hair spray
- ☐ blow-waving lotion

Blow wave the hair.

CAUTION: long hair may be drawn into the air intake of the dryer.

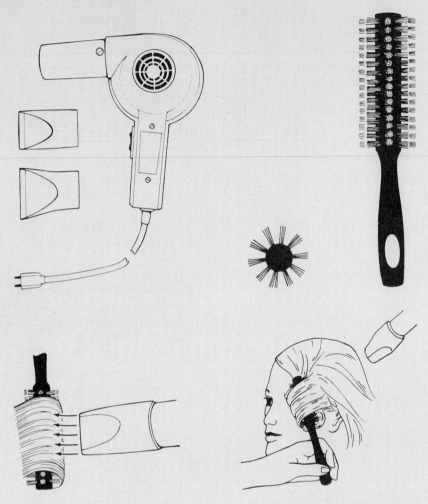

Curling the hair forward

PROCEDURE

1. Shampoo and condition the hair if necessary. Apply blow-waving lotion and comb it evenly through the hair.

2. Start the blow waver at a cool-to-warm temperature and direct the air at the left front side section. Direct the flow of heated air toward the base of the hair strand and styling bursh, **not** at the skin.

RATIONALE

1. This is standard procedure.

2. You must point the flow of warm or hot air at the base of the hair strand so it will dry at the desired height and volume. Always point the nozzle of the blow waver toward the brush to prevent the heated air from burning the skin.

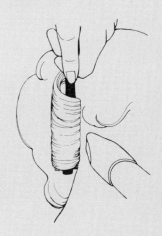

3. Turn the brush into the strand next to the scalp. As the hair dries, slide the strand through the brush.

4. Thoroughly dry and shape the hair from the front hairline to the center of the ear on both side sections.

5. As the hair dries, rotate the brush to help shape all hair next to the scalp.

6. Rotate the brush in a vertical horizontal, or diagonal position.

7. Dry and shape the hair ends in the nape, top, and crown sections into place. Dry and place all the hair.

8. Arrange stray ends with the styling comb as needed to complete the coiffure. Spray hair lightly.

3. This gives the hair an outside movement away from the scalp.

4. You must dry the hair thoroughly as it is styled to get a long-lasting style.

5. This procedure gives the hair curl as well as height and volume.

6. The way you hold the brush will depend on the section of the head you are styling and the style you are trying to create.

7. This is standard procedure for finishing the hairstyle.

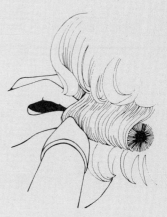

8. The ends may need arranging. The hair becomes too sticky if too much spray is put on it.

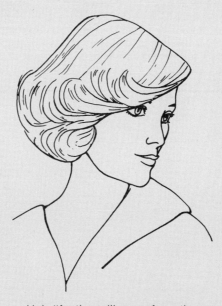

Hair styled forward, toward the face

Hair "feathered" away from the face

GLOSSARY

Air waver (blow comb)   An electrical appliance that blows heated air used in air waving the hair.

Air waving   Using electrically heated air and combing techniques to dry shampooed hair into small wave patterns.

Blow comb   See **Air waver.**

Blow waver (hand dryer)   An electrical appliance that blows heated air used in blow waving the hair.

Blow waving   Using electrically heated air and combing techniques to dry shampooed hair into large wave patterns.

Hand dryer   See **Blow waver.**

Watt   A measure of the amount of power needed to run hair-drying appliances.

QUESTIONS

1. Write a brief paragraph explaining the difference between air waving and blow waving.
2. What do the initials "U.L." stand for?
3. Why is it important to direct the flow of air in the same direction as the cuticle of the hair shaft?
4. In your own words, write at least two sentences explaining how a client could be injured with an air waver or blow comb.

ANSWERS

1. (Students' statement compared to text ref. p. 192) 2. Underwriters Laboratories 3. To prevent damage to hair 4. Flow of hot air directly on scalp; a burn from allowing hair to be sucked into air inlet vent of hand dryer

Applying Temporary Hair Colors 13

Purpose

Dyes, bleaches, frosts, tints, streaks, tips—you may have heard of some of these terms and you may know a little about some of them. Or you may not know a thing about any of them. All of these and many more have been used to make the color of the hair somehow different and better, and you will learn about them in the following chapters. Whether they were used to change the hair color or to highlight the natural color, men and women have tried to find new and different ways to give their hair more "exciting" or more "natural" looking color.

Giving temporary hair-coloring services is one of the five most profitable services salons offer. By mastering the skills shown in this chapter you will be able to improve your client's appearance and earn quite a bit of money.

Salons offer many different kinds of hair-color treatments. **This chapter shows** the techniques used for applying **temporary colors**. The chapters that follow will deal with other color treatments.

Major Objective

Use the proper steps to apply temporary hair color(s) to the client's hair.

Level of Acceptability

Using the proper safety precautions and following label directions, apply a temporary color to the client's hair in 3 to 5 minutes. Score 75 percent or better on a multiple-choice exam on the information in this chapter.

Knowing Subobjectives

1. Define temporary hair coloring and describe the early use and development of hair-coloring products.

2. Describe the advantages and disadvantages of different types of temporary hair colors.
3. Discriminate between primary, secondary, and tertiary colors.

Doing Subobjective

4. Select and apply temporary rinses.

KNOWING SUBOBJECTIVE 1

Define temporary hair coloring and describe the early use and development of hair-coloring products.

Any preparation that deposits color on or into the hair is called a **hair dye**. The dyes that color the hair from shampoo-to-shampoo are called **temporary rinses**. All hair colors should be applied immediately before the hair is styled. Temporary hair coloring is the process of changing the hair color by coating the clear cuticle of the hair with color pigment. Pigment is a substance that makes a color look the way it does. The number and color of particles of **melanin** (MEL-eh-nehn), a kind of pigment, in the hair determine what color the hair will be.

For thousands of years, people have changed their hair color. Hair-coloring products have been made from a variety of substances.

Vegetable dyes were among the earliest kinds of hair colors used. Temporary colors were made from certain vegetables and herbs. About four thousand years ago Egyptians used vegetable dyes called **henna*** and **camomile**

*As it is now made, henna is a semipermanent hair color. Semipermanent colors will be covered in the next chapter.

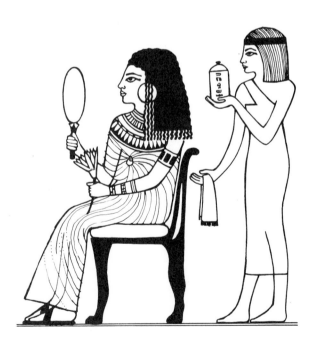

ARE YOU COLOR BLIND?

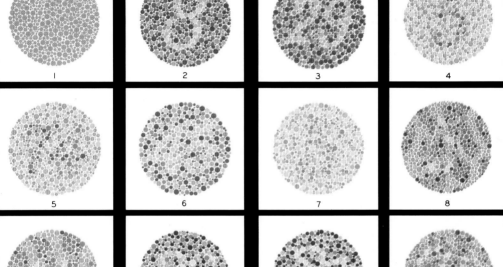

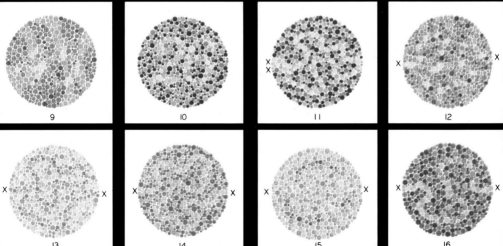

NO.	NORMAL EYE	COLOR BLIND EYE
1	12	12
2	8	3
3	29	70
4	5	2
5	74	21
6	45	NOTHING
7	5	NOTHING
8	NOTHING	5

NO.	NORMAL EYE	COLOR BLIND EYE
9	NOTHING	45
10	26	2 OR 6
11	2 LINES X TO X	LINE X TO X
12	NOTHING	LINE X TO X
13	LINE X TO X	NOTHING
14	LINE X TO X	NOTHING
15	LINE X TO X	NOTHING
16	LINE X TO X	LINE X TO X

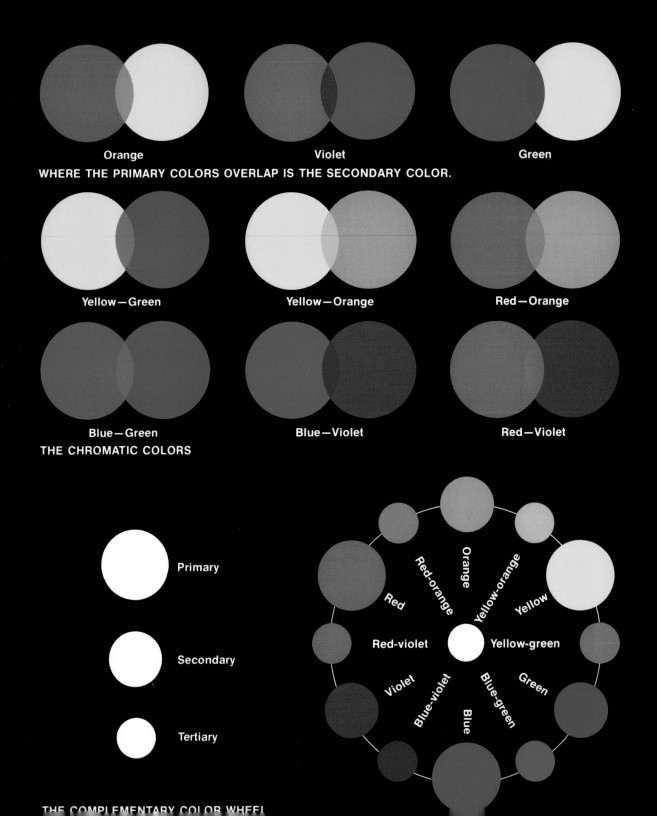

Orange

Violet

Green

WHERE THE PRIMARY COLORS OVERLAP IS THE SECONDARY COLOR.

Yellow—Green

Yellow—Orange

Red—Orange

Blue—Green

Blue—Violet

Red—Violet

THE CHROMATIC COLORS

Primary

Secondary

Tertiary

Red-orange

Orange

Yellow-orange

Red

Yellow

Red-violet

Yellow-green

Violet

Green

Blue-violet

Blue-green

Blue

THE COMPLEMENTARY COLOR WHEEL

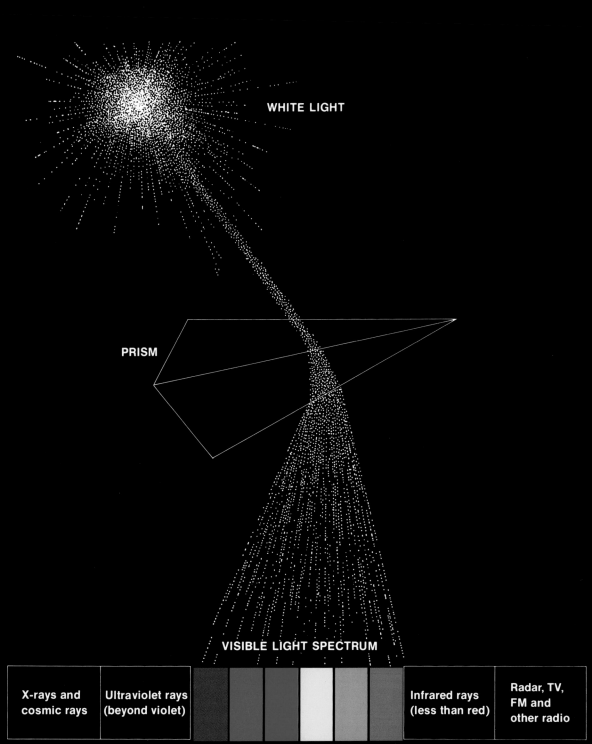

WHITE LIGHT

PRISM

VISIBLE LIGHT SPECTRUM

| X-rays and cosmic rays | Ultraviolet rays (beyond violet) | | | | | | Infrared rays (less than red) | Radar, TV, FM and other radio |

INVISIBLE SHORT WAVES

INVISIBLE LONG WAVES

pH CHART

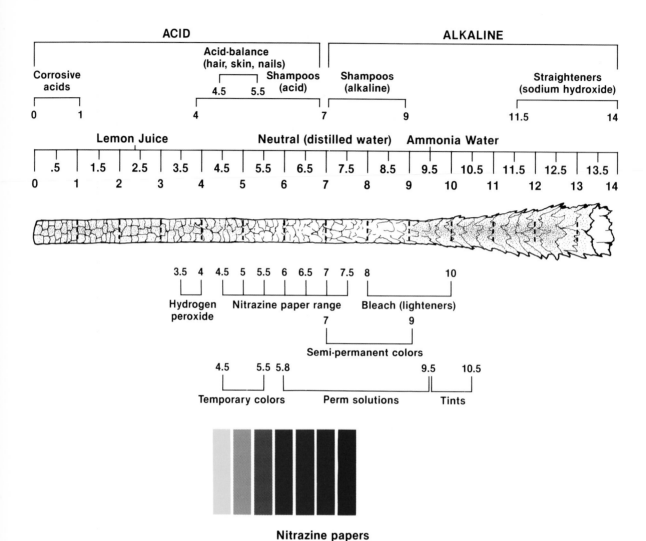

Nitrazine papers

pH RATINGS		
Substances or Products	pH	Acid/Alkaline
Lemon Juice	2.3	Acid
Hydrogen Peroxide	3.5–4.0	Acid
Shampoos (acid)	4.0–7.0	Acid-Neutral
Hair, Skin, and Nails	4.5–5.5	Acid-balanced
Temporary Colors	4.5–5.5	Acid
Neutral Wave Solutions	4.5–5.7	Acid
Acid Wave Solutions	5.8–6.8	Acid
Distilled Water	7.0	Neutral
Shampoos (alkaline)	7.0–9.0	Neutral-Alkaline
Semi-permanent Colors	7.0–9.0	Neutral-Alkaline
Bleach (lighteners)	8.0–10.0	Alkaline
Permanent (cold) Wave Solutions	8.5–9.5	Alkaline
Ammonia Water	9.5	Alkaline
Tints	9.5–10.5	Alkaline
Chemical relaxers	11.5–14.0	Alkaline

Plate 4

(KAM-ah-mighl). **Henna** (HEN-ah) colors the hair red, and **camomile** colors the hair blonde. Both of them **coat** (cover) the **cuticle** (outside) of the hair shaft. They are called **progressive dyes**, because with each application, they build up on the hair and make the color darker and darker. This build-up is called a **color buildup**.

Metallic salt dyes came into use later. They are combinations of copper, lead, silver, and other metals as well as **pyrogallol** (pye-roh-GAL-ol), a weak acid.

Over the years, **compound dyes** were developed. They are combinations of **vegetable** dyes and **metallic** salt dyes.

These dyes have serious disadvantages. Vegetable and herbal dyes coat the hair too much. The color tends to look unnatural, and it is difficult to remove. Metallic salt preparations can cause discoloration of the hair, and compound dyes cause a combination of these problems. The hair may feel brittle, and have a dull appearance.

Although some hair-coloring products for home use contain metallic salts and compound dyes, the salon products that you will use do not contain these substances.

Have you ever seen someone who had orange, green, or purple hair? He or she certainly wasn't born with it! This person probably used a home-care product that did not react properly with the one that was already on the hair.

The same thing is true for professional products. **Never cold wave, bleach,** or **permanently color** hair that already has a metallic salt product on it. Salon products do **not** combine well with metallic salts. They will cause unnatural hair colors.

Three types of hair-coloring products are used in the salon today: temporary, semipermanent, and permanent. Temporary coloring products only

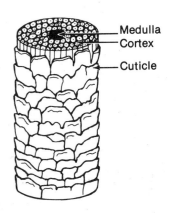

Imbricated cuticle layer of hair shaft

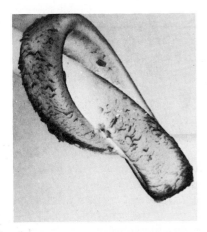

A knotted piece of hair. Note that as the hair is twisted the cuticle layers stand away from the shaft (Courtesy of 3M Company)

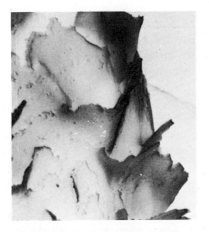

Cuticle layers of a hair as seen by a scanning electron microscope (Courtesy of 3M Company)

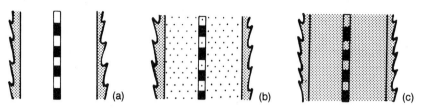

Action of hair-coloring products (a) temporary color coats cuticle; (b) semipermanent color partially penetrates cortex; (c) permanent color completely penetrates hair shaft

remain in the hair from **one shampoo to the next. Semipermanent** colors last from 4 to 6 weeks. Permanent hair-coloring preparations remain in the hair until the dyed hair grows out and is cut off.

These types have different chemical makeups, different effects, and different uses. This chapter will focus on temporary coloring and a few principles common to all three types. Semipermanent and permanent coloring follow in the next two chapters.

KNOWING SUBOBJECTIVE 2

Describe the advantages and disadvantages of different styles of temporary hair colors.

Temporary colors remain on the hair for a short time—only until the next shampoo. They thinly **coat** the hair cuticle but do not penetrate into the cortex because the molecules are too large. They are available as rinses, sprays, creams, powders, crayons, and shampoos. All, except powders, are in ready-to-use form.

The most commonly used forms of temporary colors are called **color rinses.** This is why temporary colors are often called **temporary rinses.** These rinses generally come in plastic applicator bottles. There are many kinds of rinses on the market. They can have different combinations of chemicals and colors, but they usually have water, **azo** dyes (a group of synthetic dyes), and colors made from vegetables and herbs. These products often are acid-balanced. The cuticle layer of the hair shaft (the one that protects the cortex) attracts rinses. The color settles into the scaly crevices of the cuticle and lightly coats it.

Spray colors come in aerosol cans. These aerosols contain water, color pigments, and a gas propellant called freon, which shoots the pigment from the can. They can be sprayed onto the hair after a shampoo or comb-out, depending on the kind used. They are used mainly to create unusual effects.

Creme colors come in small jars or tubes. They are used mostly by persons performing on stage, because they can be removed easily.

Powder colors need to be mixed with water before they are brushed through the hair. They are not ordinarily used in the salon.

Crayon hair colors, which look very much like tubes of lipstick, contain color pigments combined with a synthetic wax base. Crayons color the hair as they are rubbed against it. They are used to cover gray or blend in a new growth in permanently colored hair.

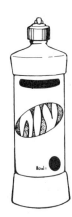
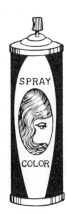

You probably have seen advertisements for "miracle" coloring products. You should keep one thing in mind: there are no "miracles" associated with any product. There are only advantages and disadvantages. Be cautious and be skeptical. By doing so, you will be doing yourself and your client a big favor.

Some of the **advantages** of temporary color rinses are:

1. The natural pH of the hair is not changed to any great extent, so that the condition of the hair remains the same.
2. Clients can highlight or darken natural color, cover gray, and improve off-shades, all with the convenience of quick removal by shampoo.
3. Unless specified by the manufacturer, a predisposition (allergy) test is not required.
4. Since temporary colors usually do not require time to develop, they are quick and convenient to apply.
5. Many ready-to-use colors are available.
6. Temporary colors may be mixed to achieve different colors: however, only products manufactured by the same company may be mixed. The color of Brand X may be mixed with another color of Brand X, but not with Brand Y.

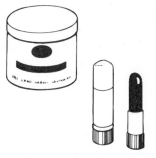

Temporary color rinses also have several **disadvantages**:

1. Some temporary rinses rub off on clothing and pillowcases.
2. Excessive perspiration from the scalp may carry color from hair onto clothing.
3. Temporary rinses **cannot lighten** natural hair color.
4. Temporary rinses may not evenly color the hair.
5. The color has to be applied after every shampoo.
6. Since it is a coating process, the color might not have the natural luster that semipermanent and permanent colors give the hair. For example, resistant hair may not accept very much color at all, and porous hair may accept too much color.

When deciding on a product, the first question you must answer is: What is the client's purpose or need? For example, a client who is cautiously experimenting with hair coloring may see quick removal as an advantage. On the other hand, a client who is already comfortable with coloring may see quick removal as a disadvantage.

KNOWING SUBOBJECTIVE 3

Discriminate between primary, secondary, and tertiary colors.

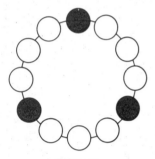

Primary

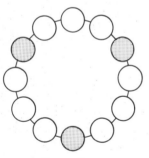

Secondary

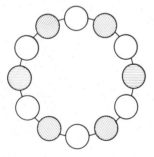

Tertiary

You need a basic knowledge of color and color mixing to master hair-coloring techniques.

Colors are divided into two types-chromatic and achromatic. Black, white, and gray are **achromatic** (ak-rah-MAT-ik) **colors**. All other colors are **chromatic** (kroh-MAT-ik). In addition to studying the mixing of chromatic colors, you must learn how to apply specific coloring principles to select or correct a client's hair color. Color plate 2 shows the principles of color mixing for selecting appropriate colors and correcting color problems.

Chromatic colors are divided into primary, secondary, and tertiary groups.

Primary (PRIGH-mehr-ee) **colors** are red, yellow, and blue. All hair colors can be mixed from these three.

Secondary colors (orange, violet, and green) are achieved by mixing equal amounts of 2 of the primary colors. Yellow and red mixed in equal parts make orange; red and blue make violet; blue and yellow make green.

A **tertiary** (TER-shee-ehr-ee) (or intermediate) **color** is made by mixing a primary and a secondary color. The 6 tertiary colors are made by the following combinations:

yellow and orange = yellow-orange
yellow and green = yellow-green
red and orange = red-orange
red and violet = red-violet
blue and violet = blue-violet
blue and green = blue-green

Complementary (kom-pleh-MEN-tah-ree) **colors** are directly opposite each other on the chart. These opposites (for example, yellow and violet) have a tendency to neutralize each other. Cosmetologists use these opposites to correct hair-coloring problems. For example, if a client has gray hair with unwanted yellow streaks, the cosmetologist would apply a violet-base color called a **bluing rinse. The violet neutralizes the yellow streaks**, and the client's hair appears consistently gray. Similarly, if hair has a green cast, a red-base color would be used to neutralize the green.

These 12 pure colors form the basis for hair-coloring products used in the salon. If they were used as pure colors, they would be unattractive, so manufacturers darken and lighten them. Pure colors are **darkened** by the addition of black, resulting in a certain **shade of a color**. For example, if blue is darkened by black, the result is navy blue. White added to a pure color produces a **tint of the color**. For instance pink is a tint of red. When a combination of black and white (in other words, gray) is mixed with a pure color, the result is a **tone color**. Rust is a tone of orange.

The federal **Food and Drug Administration** (FDA) labels as **certified** the pure colors used in professional temporary rinses. This means that the colors are safe for application on the scalp and do not require a predisposition (allergy) test.

Because color varies with its application on each client, **it is wise to make a strand test before applying any hair coloring to the entire head**. This testing of the color in a small area is especially important for semipermanent and permanent coloring. It is also advisable for temporary rinses.

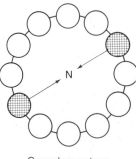

Complementary

DOING SUBOBJECTIVE 4

Select and apply temporary rinses.

Supplies

- ☐ shampooing supplies
- ☐ temporary-color chart
- ☐ temporary color rinse

PROCEDURE

1. Shampoo the hair twice and towel-dry.

2. Ask the client what services are desired. Use the color chart to help the client choose a color.

RATIONALE

1. This removes sebum, soil, sprays, and other residues. Water molecules adhere to cuticle layers, so you must be sure that the hair is fairly dry. Too much water will interfere with the color put on the cuticle. Do not use an acid rinse before applying temporary color because it will close the cuticle imbrications so much that color will not stick to the cuticle.

2. If the hair is to be shaped, it should be done before coloring. The client usually has a certain color effect in mind, but it is your responsibility to discuss color selection with client.

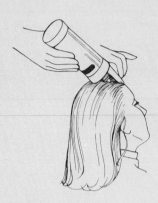

Apply rinse in chair, or at shampoo bowl

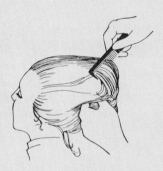

Evenly distribute rinse through hair

3. Ask the client to show you the choice on the color chart. If you feel another selection would be better, explain it to the client.

4. Select a color and read label directions.

5. Apply the selected rinse (according to directions) around the entire front hairline and **comb it through the hair toward the back of the head**. Towel-blot dripping color from crown area of head.

6. Apply a small amount of color across the nape area and comb it toward the bottom hairline.

7. Towel-blot dripping color and begin styling the hair.

3. You must know exactly which color effect the client has in mind. Not all clients know what a temporary color does to hair, so you may have to explain what the rinse can or cannot do.

4. Many temporary coloring products are available; they are applied differently, so you must read the label directions carefully. The label will indicate whether a predisposition test is required.

5. This evenly distributes color through hair and prevents color from dripping into client's eyes.

6. Applying small amounts makes it easier to evenly distribute color throughout hair.

7. Not all temporary colors are set in the hair. **Some must be rinsed** before the hair is styled. Follow the directions on the label.

GLOSSARY

Achromatic (ak-rah-MAT-ik) colors   Black, white, and gray.

Azo dyes   Synthetic dyes used in hair coloring products.

Bluing rinse   A violet-based temporary color used to neutralize yellow streaks in gray hair.

Camomile (KAM-ah-mighl)   A vegetable dye that colors the hair blonde.

Chromatic (kroh-MAT-ik) colors   All colors that are not black, white, or gray.

Color buildup   A darkening of the hair resulting from the use of progressive dyes which coat and recoat the hair with repeated applications.

Color rinses   The most commonly used forms of temporary hair colors, applied with an applicator bottle.

Complementary (kom-pleh-MEN-tah-ree) colors   Colors directly opposite each other on a color chart.

Crayon hair colors   Temporary hair colors that contain color pigments combined with a synthetic wax base and come in a tube. They are applied by rubbing againt the hair.

Creme colors   Temporary hair colors that come in small jars or tubes and are most often used by persons performing on stage because they can be removed easily.

Hair dye   Any preparation that deposits color on or into the hair.

Henna (HEN-ah)   A temporary vegetable hair dye that colors the hair red.

Melanin (MEL-eh-nehn)   A kind of pigment in the hair that gives it color.

Metallic salt dyes   Hair dyes made from combinations of copper, lead, silver, and other metals as well as pyrogallol.

Pigment (PIG-mehnt)   A substance that gives color to something, such as hair, skin, or paint.

Powder colors   Temporary hair colors that are mixed with water and brushed through the hair; not ordinarily used in the salon.

Primary (PRY-mehr-ee) colors   Red, yellow, and blue.

Progressive dyes   Hair dyes that coat the cuticle of the hair and build up with repeated applications, making the hair darker each time.

Pyrogallol (pigh-roh-GAL-ol)   A substance with weak acid properties found in metallic hair dyes.

Secondary colors   Orange, violet, and green, obtained by mixing equal amounts of 2 primary colors.

Shade of a color   The color obtained when a pure color is darkened by adding black.

Spray hair colors   Temporary hair dyes that come in aerosol cans and are sprayed onto the hair after a shampoo or comb-out.

Temporary rinses   Temporary hair colors applied with an applicator bottle. They coat only the cuticle of the hair.

Tertiary (TER-shee-ehr-ee) colors   Colors obtained by mixing a primary with a secondary color.

Tint of a color   The color obtained when white is added to a pure color.

Tone of a color   The color obtained when gray is added to a pure color.

QUESTIONS

1. What are the three layers of the hair?
2. How long do temporary rinses stay in the hair?
3. Do temporary rinses completely cover gray hair?
4. What are progressive dyes?
5. Is the cuticle layer on the outer or inner part of the hair shaft?
6. What are chromatic colors?
7. What are complementary colors?
8. What name is given to a hair color that lasts only from one shampoo to the next?

9. What is the name given to a product or substance that gives color to something else?
10. What layer of the hair does a temporary color cling to?
11. Can a temporary rinse lighten natural hair color?
12. What name is given to the color used in a temporary rinse?
13. Does a temporary rinse change the nautral pH of the hair?
14. Will a temporary rinse completely cover hair that is 70% gray?

ANSWERS

1. Cuticle, cortex, and medulla 2. Shampoo to shampoo 3. No 4. Those that build up on the hair and make it darker 5. Outer 6. All colors except black, white, and gray 7. Those opposite each other on the color chart; those opposite colors that tend to neutralize each other 8. Temporary color 9. A dye 10. The cuticle 11. No 12. Certified color (FDA approved) 13. No 14. No

Applying Semipermanent Hair Colors 14

Many of your clients who have had their hair colored many times in the past will have a fairly good idea of what they want. While they may still ask you for your advice, they probably will be much more comfortable with the whole idea of hair coloring. They will want a semipermanent hair color because it will last through up to 6 shampoos.

If you master the principles involved in applying semipermanent hair colors, you will be able to provide a service that is both fun and profitable.

Provided with an assortment of semipermanent hair colors and a hair-coloring chart, change the client's hair color by following the proper steps.

Using the proper safety precautions, evenly apply a semipermanent color to the client's hair in 5 to 10 minutes. Score 75 percent or better on a multiple-choice exam on the information in this chapter.

1. Define semipermanent hair color, compare it with temporary color, and list its advantages and disadvantages.
2. Identify the client's hair color.

3. Select and apply semipermanent hair colors.

KNOWING SUBOBJECTIVE 1

Define semipermanent hair color, compare it with temporary color, and list its advantages and disadvantages.

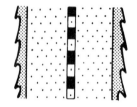

Cross-section of the hair showing cortex, cuticle, and medulla

Do you know what the prefix semi- means? It means half, or mid-way. Semipermanent hair-color rinses are about halfway between temporary and permanent hair colors. They partially penetrate the cortex and put some color inside the hair. But they do not completely penetrate the cortex, and they do not remain in the hair until the hair grows out. They usually last through 4 to 6 shampoos. These semipermanent colors are called 6-week rinses.

Semipermanent coloring products are longer lasting than temporary ones because of what they contain. Like temporary coloring products, semipermanent coloring products contain water, certified vegetable dyes, and azo dye. But they also contain various combinations of **sulfur** and **ammonium thioglycolate** (ah-MOHN-ee-uhm thigh-oh-GLIGH-kah-layt) **(thio)**, which enable the color to partially penetrate the cortex. Both raise the pH level to an alkaline range of 7 to 9. This alkalinity causes the cuticle to swell so that some of the color pigment can enter the cortex. The sulfur molecules contain the color pigment. These molecules attach themselves to the keratin (hard protein fiber) of the cuticle, and to some of the salt bonds in the cortex. The cuticle is **stained** and the cortex is also **partially** colored.

The physical and chemical actions of every shampoo cause semipermanent color to **fade**. Since the semipermanent color gives only partial penetration of the cortex of the hair, the color tends gradually to slip out of the cortex. Most of the color has faded between the fourth and sixth shampoos.

The U.S. Food, Drug, and Cosmetic Act requires a patch test before each application of all permanent colors and some semipermanent colors. This **patch test (predisposition test)** shows if the client is allergic to any ingredient in the product. This test is very easy to give. Apply a small amount of the chosen color to the client's skin at least 24 hours before the coloring appointment. If the client does not have an allergic reaction, such as skin irritation, nausea, or vomiting, during this period, you may use the product.

When a client does have an allergic reaction from the patch test (or later from the actual application of a coloring or cold-waving product), tell him or her to take the product box to a physician. The doctor can contact the local branch of the **Poison Control Center** for further information about the product. Most cosmetic firms furnish such information to these centers.

Because allergy may develop even after a product has been used with no reaction, **the test must be given before every** application of any product requiring it.

Semipermanent hair-coloring products have several **advantages**: (1) the color lasts longer than one shampoo; (2) many ready-to-use products are available; (3) the color will not easily rub off on the client's clothing; (4) retouching is not necessary; (5) it covers gray hair better than temporary color does; (6) colors may be used on decolorized (bleached or lightened) hair when frosting, streaking, or tipping; and (7) semipermanent colors manufactured by the same company may be mixed to achieve primary, secondary, or tertiary colors (in other words, Brand X with Brand X, not Brand X with Brand Y).

Semipermanent colors also have several **disadvantages:** (1) the Food and Drug Administration requires a predisposition test (patch test) for most semipermanent colors 24 hours before color application; (2) colors need time to develop—perhaps 10 to 15 minutes (or more); (3) semipermanent coloring is more expensive per application than temporary coloring; and (4) after 4 to 6 weeks, the color has usually faded so much that it must be applied again.

KNOWING SUBOBJECTIVE 2

Because semipermanent color partially penetrates the hair, it is important for you to have a better understanding of how to identify different hair colors. It is also important to learn new words to assist you in labeling different colors by their correct names, so it will be easier for you to communicate with other professional cosmetologists.

Identify the client's hair color.

Figuring out the client's hair color is a simple matter if you approach the problem with a system. If you think about it, there are only three hair colors possible: **Blonde, Brown,** and **Black.** Gray or white hair (canities) is not a color. Red hair is actually a color of brown. Differences within a certain color are called **levels.** In this system, numbers are given to the colors to indicate how much light each color reflects to the eye. Colors with small numbers are dark because they reflect only a small amount of light. Colors that have been given a larger number are lighter colors because they reflect more light.

For example, if you look around your classroom, you will soon discover that some classmates have dark brown hair, some medium brown hair, and yet others have light brown hair. These variations of brown are called **Levels of Color.** The chart will help you identify other color levels:

BLACK COLORS
1 dark black
2 medium black
3 light black

BROWN COLORS
4 dark brown
5 medium brown
6 light brown

BLONDE COLORS
7 dark blonde
8 medium blonde
9 light blonde

All hair colors should fall into one of these three categories.

In addition to color levels, hair color also has a "tone" level. The tone level shows differences from one tone to the next. The tone of the hair color is usually described as being a "warm tone," or a "cool or drab tone." **Warm tones** would include red, orange, or gold tones. Warm tones reflect light and tend to highlight the hair. **Cool or drab tones** would include **ash** or gray tones and have a blue or violet base. Cool, or drab, tones have no red or gold highlights. The following chart gives each tone a number:

COOL TONE LEVELS
1 ash
2 mauve (purple)

WARM TONE LEVELS
3 gold/yellow
4 copper (orange/red)
5 tobacco (red/gold)
6 auburn (red-red/brown)

Therefore, if your classmate has medium brown hair with a gold tone to it, you would describe the hair color as "medium golden brown." (Refer to color plate 5.) Another way to express this is with two numbers from the color level/tone level chart, or 5/3. The number 5 should tell you the color is medium brown, and the number 3 should tell you the tone is gold.

In addition to helping you identify natural hair colors, this system should aid you in comparing one hair color manufacturer's colors to that of another manufacturer. This would be true because you are learning the hair color names often used by many of the makers of hair colors. For example, if you are using a semipermanent color in a medium ash blonde made by **Professional Company** X, and run out of stock in that color, you could come up with a comparable color with **Professional Company** Y by using the color tone/level theory. And this theory would be the same whether you are using semipermanent hair colors or permanent hair colors.

DOING SUBOBJECTIVE 3

Select and apply semipermanent hair colors.

Supplies

☐ shampooing supplies
☐ gloves
☐ talcum powder
☐ timer
☐ color product
☐ color chart

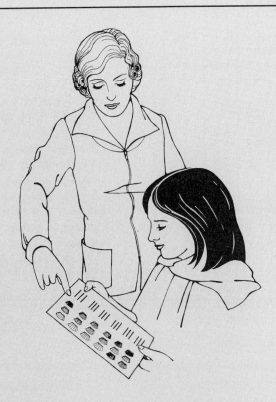

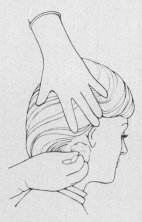

Cleanse test area

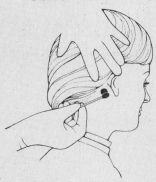

Steps for Selecting Color and Giving a Patch Test

PROCEDURE	RATIONALE
1. Show the client the color chart and tell him or her if a predisposition test is required.	1. Read label directions. **Most, but not all, semipermanent colors require a skin test.**
2. If the test is needed, pour ¼ ounce of the color into a small container and get a small, clean cotton swab from the dispensary. Explain the test to the client: the product to be used must be applied to the bend of one elbow or immediately behind the ear.	2. This is standard procedure. Note: **A positive patch test that inflames the skin is called dermatitis venenata** (VEN-en-ah-TAH).
3. Explain that the color must remain on the skin for 24 hours. Using a swab, apply a small amount of color to the bend of the elbow or behind the ear. Dispose of leftover supplies in a closed receptacle.	3. This is standard procedure.

Apply product to be used

Safety Tip

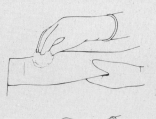

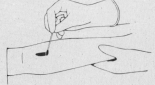

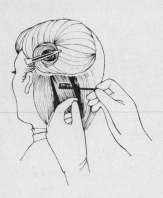

Strand test

4. Proceed to style the hair while explaining that the test site must be examined the next day. Inform the client what type of allergic reactions might occur.

5. **Advise the client to call the school or salon immediately if any discomfort occurs in the test area.**

6. Record the location of the patch test, the product used, and the date on the client's service form.
7. Perform and complete scheduled services.
8. Record the information for the client's appointment.

4. Possible reactions to any chemical service performed in the school or salon might include redness and swelling of skin, headache, nausea, and vomiting. Although some reaction can occur before 24 hours have passed, **the full time should be allowed for added protection**.
5. Depending on the reactions the client describes, the **school instructor or salon manager may ask the client to have the test site inspected by a doctor**.
6. Keeping accurate records is necessary to protect yourself against any possible legal action.
7. This is standard procedure.

8. This helps you to follow up the results of the patch test. Even a client who regularly uses the same color every time must be tested before each application of it.

Steps for Applying Semipermanent Coloring

1. Remove the client's service form from the file and inspect the patch test. Ask the client if there were any reactions.
2. Record the client's response on the service form.

1. Checking the form will help you remember the client and the product to be used.

2. Cosmetologists perform so many services for different clients that it is almost impossible to remember all the important facts about them. You must use the same product that was used for the patch test.

3. After examining the scalp, carefully **read label directions**.

4. Put gloves on both hands.

5. "Strand test" the color on 1 square inch of hair in the lower crown. Apply color from the scalp all the way through the ends of the strand. Allow material to remain on the test strand for approximately a third of the time specified for developing the whole head of hair. Blot with a clean, dry towel.

6. Apply color according to directions on the label.

7. Set the timer for half the time the directions say should be allowed for developing.

8. Test one or more strands when the timer rings. If the color is not ready, set the timer for the rest of the developing time stated on the label and apply color to hair that was used for initial strand testing.

3. Do not proceed if cuts, abrasions, or contagious diseases are present. Application procedures vary from one brand to another. **Some require shampooing** prior to color application, while **others do not**.

4. This will protect your hands and nails from direct contact. If a client can develop an allergy to the color, the cosmetologist can, too. The gloves also protect your fingernails from staining.

5. Always "strand test." This professional technique will help you see how a specific color will appear on a particular client's hair. If the strand test produces an unsatisfactory color, you will know that there may be a problem before you color the entire head. If necessary, a different color may be scheduled when the strand test indicates a problem.

6. Some colors are applied to shampooed hair that has been towel-dried. Other products combining hair color and shampoo are applied to dry hair.

7. Porosity of hair varies from person to person, so the developing time will not be the same for all clients.

8. This is standard procedure.

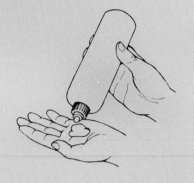
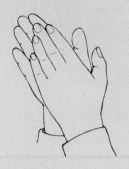
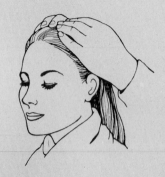

Application of normalizing rinse

9. When the timer rings at the end of the full developing time, remove the plastic cap (if the label said that one should be used) and strand test the color.

10. Thoroughly water rinse the hair until the water runs clear and the scalp is free of color.

11. Apply an acid or normalizing rinse.

12. Style the hair. Note color results on the client's service form and file it.

9. If the color is not dark (or light) enough, you may want to rinse the color off and dry the hair. Then, reapply the color.

10. No semipermanent hair colors will "set" into hair without being rinsed first. The client's scalp around the hairline should be completely free of color stains.

11. This restores the natural pH of the hair by neutralizing the alkali of the coloring product.

12. The form will provide information for future decisions on coloring.

GLOSSARY

Ammonium thioglycolate (ah-MOHN-ee-uhm thigh-oh-GLIGH-kah-layt) A chemical sometimes contained in semipermanent hair coloring that enables the dye to partially penetrate the cortex of the hair.

Cool (drab) hair colors Hair-color products that correspond to the cool secondary colors on the color chart. There are ash, silver, platinum, smoke, and steel gray.

Dermatitis Venenata A positive patch test that inflames the skin.

Drab tones See Cool tones.

Levels of color Variation within the three hair colors of blonde, brown, and black.

Patch test Predisposition test.

Poison Control Center   An agency that provides information about poisonous and potentially hazardous or allergy-producing products.

Predisposition test   A test for allergy to hair coloring given by applying a small amount of color to the client's skin at least 24 hours before the product is used on the scalp.

Semipermanent hair coloring   A hair dye that partially penetrates the cortex of the hair and lasts 4 to 6 weeks.

Sulfur   An element contained in semipermanent hair coloring that enables the coloring pigment to partially penetrate the cortex of the hair.

Tone level   The variation from one tone to the next, such as drab tones, warm tones, etc.

Warm tones   Color variations including red, orange, and gold.

QUESTIONS

1. What Federal Act requires a patch test for certain hair color products?
2. Using a dictionary, write a definition for the word "allergy."
3. Before applying a semipermanent color, what are you looking for when you examine the scalp?
4. Where are the two points on the body where patch tests are given?
5. Does the application of a semipermanent hair color require a predisposition test?
6. What two chemicals would be found in a semipermanent hair color?
7. Can you partially penetrate the hair shaft with a semipermanent color?
8. Is it necessary to give an allergy test before each application of a semipermanent color?
9. What are the three basic natural hair colors?
10. Is gray hair a hair color?
11. Is the color green a warm tone or a drab tone?
12. What tone is orange? Is it a warm or a drab tone?
13. Write a definition of dermatitis venenata.
14. Is it really necessary to keep a record on the color used, or can you simply remember the client's formula?
15. Do you need to wear protective gloves when applying a semipermanent color?

ANSWERS

1. The U.S. Food, Drug, and Cosmetic Act 2. (Students' answer) 3. Cuts, abrasion, or disease 4. Behind the ear and bend of the elbow 5. Yes 6. Sulfur and ammonium thioglycolate 7. Yes 8. Yes 9. Blonde, brown, and black 10. No 11. Drab tone 12. Warm tone 13. (Students' comments) 14. Keep a record 15. Yes

Permanently Coloring the Hair 15

The demand for permanent hair coloring has increased dramatically in recent years, and this demand will probably continue. As requests for this service have increased, so has the number of professional permanent hair-coloring products. New procedures to achieve unusually beautiful hair-coloring effects have emerged and so, of course, have problems. This means that mastering permanent hair-coloring techniques will be a continuing challenge and source of satisfaction for you.

Since permanent hair coloring is probably the second or third most profitable service in schools and salons, mastering basic scientific coloring principles and procedures will also be important to your financial success.

Purpose

Provided with permanent hair-coloring products and supplies, permanently change the client's hair color.

Major Objective

Using the proper safety precautions and following label directions, apply a permanent hair color to the client's hair in 15 to 20 minutes. Score 75 percent or better on a multiple-choice exam on the information in this chapter.

Level of Acceptability

1. Define permanent hair-coloring services, terms, and chemicals.
2. Describe the advantages and disadvantages and the safety measures needed when using permanent hair-coloring products.

Knowing Subobjectives

Doing Subobjectives

Use the proper steps and safety precautions to:

3. Test the hair for metallic salts.
4. Apply a virgin tint to lighten or darken hair.
5. Apply a tint retouch.

KNOWING SUBOBJECTIVE 1

Define permanent hair-coloring services, terms, and chemicals.

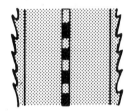

Cross-section of the hair showing cortex, cuticle, and medulla

Hair colors that permanently **penetrate** the cuticle of the hair and deposit color in the cortex of the shaft are called **penetrating tints**. Because of their chemical action within the hair shaft, they are also called **oxidizing permanent hair colors** or **oxidation tints**. When these products are given in one application, the process is called a **single-application** coloring service.

Another method of permanently coloring the hair is **double-application** hair coloring. **Bleaching and toning** are double-application methods of coloring because two different products are applied separately to the hair. First, the hair is bleached (decolorized), and then a toner is applied to achieve the desired color. Bleaching and toning will be discussed in chapter 16.

Hair that has not been overexposed to the sun or treated by tints, chemical straighteners, cold-waving solutions, or other chemical services is called **virgin hair**. The process used to color virgin hair is called a **virgin tint**.

As the tinted hair grows, the new growth of hair has to be colored. This is called a **retouch tint**, or a **tint retouch**. The purpose of a retouch is to touch up with color that hair that has grown from the scalp so that it matches the permanent color previously applied to the rest of the hair. This is normally done every 3 to 5 weeks, depending on how fast the hair grows.

Occasionally, a client will request that the hair's natural color be permanently highlighted, rather than drastically changed. This service, called a **soap cap**, combines permanent hair color with shampoo and hydrogen peroxide to **slightly change**, or **highlight**, the natural color. The soap cap is applied like a shampoo to dry hair. It is left in for 10 to 15 minutes (or as directed) before the hair is rinsed thoroughly.

The main chemical compound in the bases of most permanent colors is **para-phenylene-diamine** (PA-rah-FEN-l-een-DIGH-eh-meen), a synthetic (artificial) organic dye compound that scientists developed around 1900. It is an **aniline** (AN-ehl-ehn) **derivative** that comes from **coal tar**. Products containing this compound are called **tints**.

Tinting products work by the process of **oxidation**. It is the process of combining oxygen and a substance. The substance that supplied (or gave up) the oxygen is called the **oxidizer** (oxidizing agent). The substance that received oxygen is said to have been oxidized.

In most modern tinting products, the oxidizer is **20-volume* hydrogen peroxide**, commonly called peroxide or developer. The chemical symbol of

---

*Volume strength shows the amount of oxygen gas released from a certain amount of hydrogen peroxide; 20-volume peroxide is equal to a 6-percent solution of peroxide in water.

HAIR-COLORING TERMS

Accelerator.
Peroxide in powder form added to peroxide bleach mixtures to increase bleaching effect. Also called "activator" or "booster."

Bleaching.
Removal of some or all of the hair color, whether natural or previously applied. Also called "lifting" or "lightening."

Bleach Lotion or Oil.
See Lightener Lotion.

Conditioners.
Ingredients in color lotions, or applied independently to the hair, to improve its sheen, softness, and manageability.

Creme Colors.
An oxidation hair dye product that forms a thick creamy lotion when mixed with developer. It is applied to new growth by "parting and sectioning" and is then combed through the hair tips.*

Creme Rinses.
A rinse applied after coloring and shampooing to restore the initial condition of the hair, i.e., its normal acidity, softness, manageability.

Developer.
Hydrogen peroxide (usually 20 volume which equals 6 percent strength) supplied either as a clear liquid or cream lotion and used either to bleach hair or to develop the color of an oxidation dye.

Double Process.
Two-step process by which the hair is first bleached, usually drastically, and then re-dyed with a toner.

Frosting.
Bleaching and toning the entire length of random strands of hair over the entire head.

Gentle Lightener.
Mild peroxide formula which provides only a light bleaching effect.

Lightener Lotion.
The vehicle to which developer (peroxide) and accelerator are added to produce an effective bleach mixture. It is usually an ammoniacal soap solution and is often called "oil bleach."

Metallic Dye.
A hair dye product which contains metallic salts, usually lead acetate, as the active ingredient.

Oxidation Hair Dye.
A dye containing paraphenylenediamine and other hair dye intermediates that must be mixed with a peroxide developer just prior to application to the hair in order to develop the color.

Para Dye.
A hair dye product containing paraphenylenediamine as the primary hair dye intermediate. See Oxidation Dye.

Patch Test.
A test on the forearm, bend of the elbow, or behind ear to detect allergic sensitivity; by law it is required that a warning to perform such a test before each application of a hair color (unless the product contains only color approved by FDA for cosmetic use) appear on the product labeling.

Permanent Color.
See Oxidation Dye.

Prebleach.
Bleaching the hair before application of a hair color or toner.

Progressive Dye.
A dye that colors the hair gradually during repeated application, a metallic dye.

Restorer (Hair Color Restorer).
Euphemism for a metallic dye.

Retouching.
The process of bleaching or dyeing the new growth (roots) with a permanent dye; it requires parting and sectioning of the hair; subsequently the applied bleach or dye is combed through the entire hair.

Rinse (Color Rinse).
A temporary hair color of low strength which is in the form of a rinse. It is removable by one shampooing.

Semipermanent Color.
Color that lasts through several shampoos. Usually a nonoxidation type hair dye product.

Shampoo-in Hair Color.
Permanent dyes of the oxidation type that are applied like a shampoo. Also called color shampoo.

Single Process.
Bleaching and re-dyeing the hair in one step, as in the oxidation hair dyeing process.

Streaking.
The application of hair bleach to predetermined or random sections of hair.

Stripping.
Total removal of all natural and artificial color from hair with a soapy peroxide solution.

Temporary Color.
Color that is removed by the first shampoo.

Tipping.
Bleaching of predetermined or random tip ends of the hair.

Toner.
A light hair color applied to prebleached hair, usually an oxidation dye.

Vegetable Dye.
A color formed by applying only natural plant products, usually from the henna plant.

*This refers to products normally purchased for home use.

From *FDA Consumer*, November 1974 (reprinted), (Washington, D.C.: U.S. Department of Health, Education and Welfare).

hydrogen peroxide is H_2O_2. Peroxide is also called the developer. The tinting process produces color within the cortex of the hair. The para-phenylene-diamine dye bases (para dyes) have small molecules that easily pass through the imbrications of the cuticle **into the cortex**. After they have entered the cortex, the colored molecules of the dye base combine with oxygen from the hydrogen peroxide to make large molecules of dye. These newly formed molecules of dye are too large to pass back through the imbrications, so they are permanently held within the cortex. The cross-bonds that develop between the color molecules and keratin also hold the color in place. Hydrogen peroxide and the base (dye) must be kept in separate containers. The reaction (oxidation between the dye and hydrogen peroxide) takes 20 to 45 minutes. It begins when they are mixed, so you must keep them separated until you are ready to use them.

Hydrogen peroxide is an **acid**. It has a **pH of between 3.5 and 4**.

In most tinting products, ammonia is part of the dye base. This ammonia compound (an alkali) is the activator. That is, it helps start the tinting process in the following ways:

1. As an alkali, it makes the cuticle swell so that the molecules of tint base can easily pass into the cortex.
2. It creates the alkaline conditions needed to develop the color.
3. It causes the hydrogen peroxide (H_2O_2) to give up oxygen for oxidation of the para dyes.

The addition of the ammonia makes the ready-to-use coloring product alkaline. Most products have a pH of about 9.5 to 10.5.

Manufacturers have made great improvements in professional tints. Tints can **lighten** or **darken** the hair. Hair can be lightened by softening the cuticle. The coloring can be done in a single application of tint. Different products have different strengths, so the amount of lightening will vary with the product you use. Natural hair color also is an important factor. For instance, light brown hair can be lightened much more easily than dark brown or black hair.

KNOWING SUBOBJECTIVE 2

Describe the advantages and disadvantages and the safety measures needed when using permanent hair-coloring products.

As you know, you must protect your client and yourself when you are using products that might be harmful. Tints containing paraphenylene-diamine may be harmful to the client, so you must give the client a **predisposition** (pree-dis-peh-ZISH-ehn) **(patch) test**. This test should show if the client is **hypersensitive** (high-per-SEN-seh-tiv) (allergic) to the product to be used. Details on the patch test can be reviewed in chapter 14. The best way to protect yourself from allergies is to wear an apron and protective gloves whenever you mix or apply permanent hair colors.

All professional products used in the school or salon are required by the Food, Drug, and Cosmetic Act to have directions on the label or inside of the package. Professional hair tints are made to color **only hair on the head**. To use a tint in any other way may be very dangerous (for example, using a tint to color eyebrows or eyelashes **may cause blindness**). Never tint eyebrows or eyelashes with any product unless the label directions state that the product was made for that purpose!

Tints usually are packaged in amber-colored bottles, small boxes, or tubes because light alters their chemical makeup. If they are exposed to light, heat, or air, they may become ineffective—they should not be used. Always mix permanent hair coloring in a plastic or glass container. Do not use a metal mixing container for any oxidizing-type service. Peroxide reacts adversely with metal.

Permanent hair coloring has several advantages for the client.

1. Since it is difficult to cover resistant gray hair with temporary or semi-permanent colors, you soon realize that permanent color products (tints) are the most effective. Usually, tints completely **cover gray** hair.

2. Many persons experiment at home with cold-waving and coloring products, which frequently discolor the hair. As a result, many of them seek professional services to **restore their natural hair color**.

3. Cosmetologists are becoming extremely creative in employing new methods of producing **decorative** and **accenting** effects. These new coloring effects (and methods) are so much in demand that many salons are starting to specialize in them. These services include: framing, painting, frosting, streaking, and tipping. They will be discussed in chapter 17.

4. In America's youth-conscious society, many persons want to avoid gray hair—a sign of aging. Although cosmetology offers services to enhance the natural beauty of gray hair, many persons choose to cover it. For those who want to appear younger, permanent hair coloring is a valuable service.

5. Clients have discovered that if their natural hair color does not flatter their eye color or skin tones, they can use penetrating tints to do what nature did not. Generally, clients with blue or hazel eyes and fair or creamy complexions should use warm, light hair colors. Light or dark colors without red accents or overtones generally flatter persons with green eyes and florid or pinkish complexions. Brown-eyed clients with olive or yellowish complexions should use darker and ash colors.

You will quickly realize that permanent hair colors also offer cosmetologists several advantages.

1. Satisfaction of the client because complete coverage of gray hair is possible.
2. The possibility of a **permanent** return to the client's natural hair color, which requires professional services.
3. Recognition and self-satisfaction because the appearance of the client has been improved.

4. Increase in money because permanent coloring is a more expensive service than temporary and semipermanent coloring and requires regular retouches.

Don't be misled. Permanent hair coloring does have some disadvantages for the client.

1. **A patch test** is absolutely required before **each** tint. Although this test takes only a few minutes, it is slightly inconvenient.

2. Once the hair has been tinted, a **regular appointment** should be made for retouching the new growth to keep the color even. Thus, the client must spend more time in the school or salon than required by temporary or semipermanent coloring services.

3. Tinting requires **extra time** not only in terms of additional appointments for retouches but also in respect to length of time for the individual coloring sessions. The developing time (period in which the peroxide oxidizes the tint) is 20 to 40 minutes. Counting application and full processing, tinting adds 30 to 45 minutes to the time needed for a shampoo and set. Temporary and semipermanent colors can be applied much more quickly.

4. Since tints give color that cannot be shampooed out of the cortex, the **client cannot** quickly and **easily change** the hair color. It can be changed only by cutting or applying another tint.

5. The tinting service requires more supplies at a **greater cost** than do temporary or semipermanent services; therefore, the client must pay more for permanent coloring.

There also are **disadvantages** of permanent hair colors for the cosmetologist.

1. Since color selection is very important, you may spend a considerable amount of time advising the client on it. Time is money, so you must use it as efficiently and profitably as possible. Although color selection requires a lot of time in the initial service, repeat color services may make the investment of time very profitable in the long run.

2. Patch testing for possible allergies can be time consuming. You must figure the proportion of peroxide for the very small amount of color needed for the test, and you also must keep accurate records for each hair-color service. The date of the patch test, the results, the formula proportions, and the brand of product must be recorded **before each** tint.

3. Hair coloring is a complicated process that requires skill and judgment. Every product you use will react somewhat differently on each client. Colors can be mixed to achieve an endless number of choices, but skill is required to formulate just the right color for a particular client. Even an experienced cosmetologist soon realizes there is always something new, something else to learn, about hair coloring.

4. The school or salon and the individual cosmetologist must be careful in using aniline or oxidizing products because the risk of legal action in-

creases with these services. A client who has an allergic reaction to a color service can sue the cosmetologist. Much time and money can be spent in legal processes. The best way to protect yourself is by taking the following precautions:

    a. Follow label directions **exactly**.
    b. Give a predisposition test before **each** application of permanent color.
    c. Keep current, accurate, legible hair-coloring records.

    5. Tinting is a service requiring a number of supplies, such as shampooing items, many bottles or canisters of the complete range of hair colors, hydrogen peroxide, stain removers, cotton swabs, color applicator bottles, and protective gloves. Since you do not know exactly what colors your clients will select, **all** of the colors usually are stocked in the dispensary. **Fixed costs**, such as large inventories of one particular item, are always "built into" the cost of the service.

DOING SUBOBJECTIVE 3

Supplies

☐ plastic or glass dish
☐ 20-volume peroxide
☐ 28 percent ammonia water

Test hair for metallic salts.

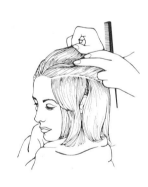

PROCEDURE

1. Analyze hair texture and condition.

2. Ask the client if any home hair-coloring products have been used in the last 12 months. If the client answers "yes" or if the hair feels harsh or coated, test for a metallic salt color.

3. Cut a small strand of hair from the bottom of the crown area of the client's head. Wind hair-setting tape around one end of the hair.

RATIONALE

1. Always check that the client's hair is in good condition before you give any chemical process.

2. Metallic salt color coatings discolor the hair when combined with professional products.

3. A strand missing from this area will be least noticeable.

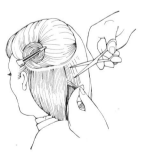

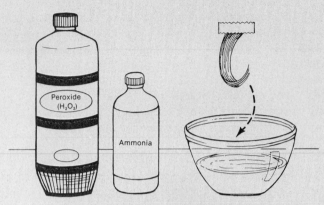

Only use **plastic** or **glass** mixing bowl

4. Mix one ounce of clear 20-volume peroxide with 20 drops of 28 percent ammonia water in a plastic or glass—not metal—dish.

5. Submerge the strand in prepared solution for 24 hours. Watch for a chemical reaction.

6. Explain to the client why the tint cannot be given.

4. This solution will detect the presence of metallic salts on the strand. Mixing peroxide and a chemical in a metal bowl can cause the peroxide to react badly.

5. If metal is present, the strand will show a reaction in 30 to 40 minutes; however, the strand should remain in the solution for 24 hours. Presence of lead will cause hair to change color almost immediately. If copper is on the hair, the solution will boil, the strand will feel hot to the touch, and the hair will easily fall apart. Also test the hair for elasticity and breakage.

6. Explain that it is for the client's protection.

DOING SUBOBJECTIVE 4

Apply a virgin tint to lighten or darken hair. (Preparation before the application)

Supplies

□ client hair-coloring record form
□ client release form
□ color-safe shampoo
□ shampoo supplies plus two laundered towels

□ sanitized plastic tint applicator bottle and top
□ 1 pair of rubber or surgical gloves
□ talcum powder
□ 20-volume peroxide

□ tint
□ color chart
□ comparison chart

□ operator apron
□ timer
□ stain remover

PROCEDURE

1. If necessary, shampoo lightly and use lukewarm dryer to remove moisture. Shampoo the hair only if it is very soiled.

2. Analyze the condition of the hair and scalp (see chapter 6) and make conditioning recommendations as needed; ask client what home or professional coloring products have been used in last 12 months.

3. Explain the cost, process, and upkeep of the tinting; answer the client's questions.

4. Use the color chart to help the client decide on a color.

RATIONALE

1. Try **not** to stimulate circulation of blood to scalp because this increases the likelihood that the client will react to the tinting material. Normally, the hair is not shampooed before a tinting service. Hair must be dry before tint is applied.

2. Hair that is very porous needs conditioning so that the tint will remain in it. If hair is extremely porous or chemically damaged, a **filler** may be needed. **Fillers** equalize the porosity of the hair shaft so that color can be spread evenly. The filler also acts as a **primer coat** on porous or damaged hair. Most fillers are ready to use and should be applied like a shampoo **only to porous** or damaged hair. **Fillers usually are left in the hair**, but follow label directions. It is important to know if other dyes are on the hair because they may interact unfavorably with the tint.

3. Some clients do not realize permanent color does **not** shampoo out of hair. They also may not realize the tint has to be retouched.

4. This helps you and your client visualize the best color. Consider the color of the client's eyes and skin tones. (Recall earlier sections on color choice.) If the hair was **not** shampooed and dried, it will appear **slightly darker**.

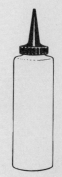
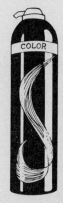
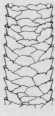
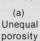
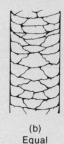

(a)
Unequal
porosity

(b)
Equal
porosity

Filler used to equalize hair porosity

5. Lift a small amount of hair on top of the client's head; look through the strand of hair. Examine the scalp for scratches, open cuts, or abrasions.

5. Lifting the hair makes it easier for you to feel its texture—fine, coarse, porous, or resilient—and helps you see if the hair has red or gold overtones, which should be considered in color selection.

6. Select the chart color that is **closest** to the client's natural color.

6. It is best to use the natural color as a guide.

7. When a client who does not have **gray hair wishes to lighten** the natural color, select a tint that is one color **lighter** than the client desires.

7. Tinting products vary in strength. It is always better to have a color lighter rather than darker than the one desired. If a color is too light, it is easy to go one or two shades darker. But it is very **difficult** to lighten a tint that is too dark (whether you do it right away or at a later appointment). If the color is too dark, the client may be very unhappy. The same probably will **not** be true if the color is a little too light.

8. When a client who has **gray hair wants a lighter** color, again select a color that is **lighter** than client's choice.

8. Remember: tints **lighten and deposit color** in hair. The lighter colors have more bleaching action than the darker ones. If the color selected by the client is very light, prebleaching and toning may be necessary. (This double application—bleaching and toning—will be discussed in the next chapter.)

9. If a client who does not have gray hair wants a darker color, use the same color that the client picks.

9. This produces the best results. As a preliminary safeguard, always strand test a color before applying a virgin tint to the entire head.

10. If a client who has gray hair wants a darker color, use a color one shade darker than the client's selection.

10. Some gray hair is resistant to color. Such hair has a resilient, "glassy" feel because the cuticle layers are closed tightly around the cortex. After some coloring experiences, you will develop a fingertip touch that identifies resistant gray hair. Because of this resistance, normally use a shade one color darker than the one desired to be sure that the gray is covered.

11. Explain to the client the need for the predisposition (patch) test and the method of application.

11. Inform the client that law requires the patch test. Describe symptoms of a positive reaction. Advise the client to phone the school or salon if these symptoms occur.

12. Give the patch test with the same tint color that will be used.

12. Be sure that the client wants the color you are testing. Only the color you test can be used in the tinting service.

13. On the client release form, record the location of the patch test and the product used. Date and initial the entry.

13. Accurate records protect you and your client. They also save you the trouble of remembering all the mixing formulas for clients.

14. Study the color comparison chart, if needed.

14. The color comparison chart is a table that lists and compares professional colors of most manufacturers. The chart shows tints that are approximately the same.

15. Schedule the tinting service for at least 24 hours after the test began. Record it in the appointment book and give this information to the client.

15. Results of the test must be negative. If the results are positive, do not give the tint.

16. Record the results of the patch test on the client release form.

16. This protects the school or salon.

(Mixing and Applying Tint)

PROCEDURE

1. Read the label directions which accompany the tint.

2. Prepare a strand test. Using the proportions in the label directions, mix a small amount of color with hydrogen peroxide in a glass or plastic container or applicator bottle. **Remember: do not mix peroxide in a metal container.** Usually, 1 ounce total material (color and hydrogen peroxide) is enough.

RATIONALE

1. Tints are always mixed with peroxide, but proportions of color to peroxide vary from one product to another.

2. Follow label directions to proportionately mix 1 ounce of tinting material. Tint bottles usually contain either 1½ or 2 ounces of coloring material. Directions usually require "double peroxide," or "equal peroxide." **Double peroxide** means twice as much peroxide as color should be used. **Equal peroxide** means that the same amount of peroxide and color should be used. For convenience in mixing a very small volume of coloring material for the strand or predisposition test, you can use milliliters (mls.) (1 ounce equals 29.573 ml., which for this purpose can be rounded to 30 ml.). To mix approximately 1 ounce of color material, use 15 ml. of color and 15 ml. of peroxide if directions call for equal peroxide; use 10 ml. of color and 20 ml. of peroxide if directions require double peroxide. All tints must be mixed in glass or plastic containers. The chemicals could react with a metal container, releasing metal particles into the tint mixture. A **hydrometer** (high-DROHM-eh-tehr) may be used to test the strength of the peroxide.

7–
6–
5–
4–
3–
2–
1–
½ color
½ peroxide

tint

peroxide

Double peroxide

tint

peroxide

Equal peroxide

PEROXIDE CONVERSION CHART
(to reduce volumes)

__When 3 ounces of peroxide used—__

Peroxide	Water	Volume	Usage
3 oz.	0	20	Resistant (normal) hair
2 ¾ oz.	¼ oz.	18.3	For color that takes too deep; or bleach to a more even color
2 ½ oz.	½ oz.	16.7	Weak limp hair; or hair that easily fades
2 ¼ oz.	¾ oz.	15	Weak limp hair; or hair that easily fades
2 oz.	1 oz.	13.2	Beige toners
1 ¾ oz.	1 ¼ oz.	11.7	Beige toners
1 ½ oz.	1 ½ oz.	10	Frosting toners
1 ¼ oz.	1 ¾ oz.	8.3	Golden blonde colors
1 oz.	2 oz.	6.6	Ash blonde tints

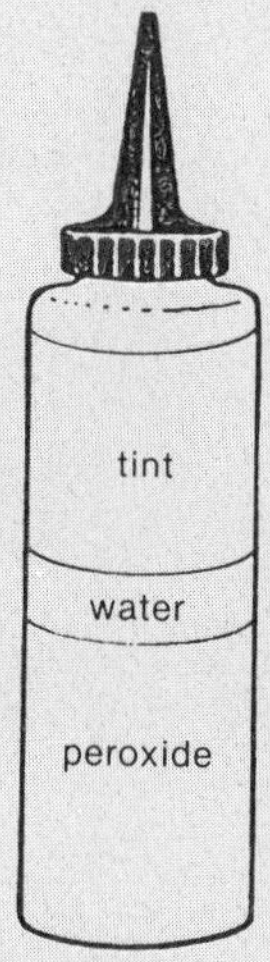

__When 2 ounces of peroxide used—__

Peroxide	Water	Volume	Usage
2 oz.	0	20	Resistant (normal hair)
1 ¾ oz.	¼ oz.	17.5	For color that takes too deep; or bleach to a more even color
1 ½ oz.	½ oz.	15	Weak limp hair; or hair that easily fades
1 ¼ oz.	¾ oz.	12.5	Beige toners
1 oz.	1 oz.	10	Frosting toners
¾ oz.	1 ¼ oz.	7.5	Ash to golden blonde tints
½ oz.	1 ½ oz.	5	Lighter than ash stain or tint
¼ oz.	1 ¾ oz.	2.5	Lighter than ash stain

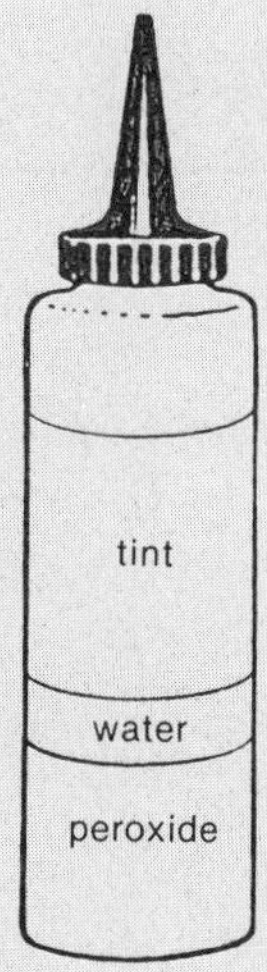

REMEMBER whenever mixing colors, contact your instructor for the best formula for you to use.

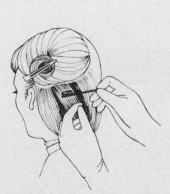

3. Explain to the client the reasons for strand testing. Since cold waving and chemical relaxing can strip the color, explain that they should be done one week before tinting.

4. Lightly powder the insides of the gloves and slip your hands into them.

5. Select a strand of hair in the lower crown area. Using the applicator bottle or brush, apply color mixture along the entire strand.

3. Make a strand test before applying peroxide to the entire head. Watch for discoloration resulting from previous chemical services, uneven coloring caused by overporous hair, and unwanted red or brassy highlights.

4. Wear gloves to protect your hands.

5. Use the lower crown area because any discoloration that might occur will be covered by the hair above it.

Strand test

6. Set the timer for 15 minutes and dispose of any remaining tint. Wash any color residue from the inside of the bottle.

6. Color usually takes 20 to 40 minutes to oxidize completely, but after the first test, you should check the strand at 10-minute intervals. Except to obtain supplies, never leave client unattended during a chemical service. Accurate measurements for the next mixture cannot be made when color residue is clinging to the inside of the bottle.

7. When the timer rings, check the test strand for discoloration.

7. Consult the instructor or manager for assistance. Usually, the color will not be fully developed after only 15 minutes. If the hair had a prior application of metallic color or is in need of conditioning, uneven or unnatural color will result.

8. Reset timer to allow color to oxidize completely according to label directions.

8. Clockwatching is a bother when you are concentrating on the right order of doing things. It is much easier to depend on a timer to indicate the proper amount of time.

9. When the timer rings, saturate the corner of a towel with water and then shampoo to remove coloring material from the strand. Thoroughly towel-dry the strand.

9. The ideal way to see exactly what color has developed is to remove the coloring material and thoroughly dry the hair. Wet hair will always appear darker than it really is.

10. Discuss the color with client and agree on the color to be applied.

10. If the color is all right except for too much red highlight, adjust it by adding small amount of drabber. A **drabber** is concentrated color that has a blue or violet base that neutralizes red or gold overtones in the hair.

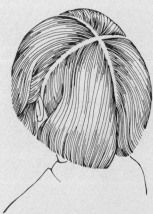

Part the hair in four quadrants (sections)

11. Using the comb, part the hair into four equal sections.

11. This step is a standard way to begin a virgin permanent hair color.

NATURAL COLOR LEVELS

Blonde

Light

Medium

Dark

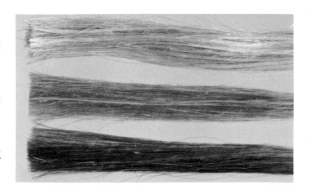

Light

Medium   **Brown**

Dark

Black

Light

Medium

Dark

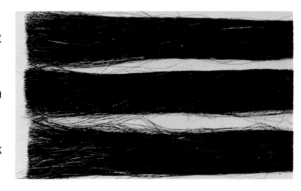

TONE EXAMPLES

COOL (DRAB) TONES	WARM TONES
1. Pale Ash-Platinum, 2. Medium Ash,	1. Yellow Gold, 2. Red Gold
3. Dark Ash	3. Red

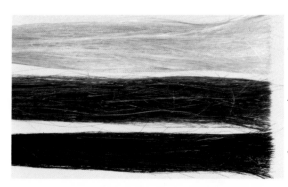

–1.–

–2.–

–3.–

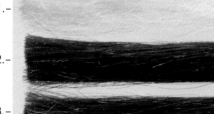

Plate 5

PERMANENT HAIR COLOR

	BLACK		RED			AUBURN		GOLDEN BROWN	

The printed colors on this chart are not exact matches . . . to ascertain exact color a preliminary hair strand test should be given first.

LAMAUR (Precision™ Hair Color)	D1.1* Black	D1.2 Black Brown	R2.1 Dark Red	R2.2 Medium Red	R2.3 Light Red	R3.1 Dark Auburn	R3.3 Light Auburn	G4.1 Dark Golden Brown	G4.2 Medium Golden Brown
CLAIROL	51™ Black Velvet			44™ Coppertone	33™ Flame	47™ Red Ginger	45™ Sparkling Sherry		
HELENE CURTIS (COLORESSENCE)	20 Deep Black			46 Red Blonde	49 Brilliant Red	42 Dark Auburn	44 Light Auburn		
ROUX® (FANCI·TONE®)	12 Black Rage			34 Strawberry Blush	33 Wild Fire	31 Dark Blaze	32 Lucky Copper		
WELLA® (COLOR CHARM®)	051 Black			544 Light Copper	633 Red Blaze	347 Dark Auburn	445 Light Auburn		
L'OREAL (PREFERENCE®)	1 Blue Black			7.4 Burnished Copper	43 Red Penny	41 Dark Auburn	66 Light Auburn		
REDKEN/LAPINAL® **AMINO COLORS**	True Black Concentrate		2FA Flame Accent	4F Med. Flame	6FA Light Flame Accent	2A Dark Auburn	3F Dark Flame		
MATRIX (SO·COLOR®)	1 Black					R-4 Mahogany			
FRAMESI (FUTURA™)	IN Black		6R Titan Red	7R Fire Red	9F Red C.				

*LAMAUR PRECISION HAIR COLOR NUMBERING SYSTEM THERE ARE 7 BASIC HAIR COLOR CATEGORIES

Designated by large number (D7.5)

1. BLACK
2. RED
3. AUBURN
4. GOLDEN BROWN
5. ASH BROWN
6. GOLDEN BLONDE
7. ASH BLONDE

D7.5

ALL BASIC COLORS AND SHADES HAVE 1 OF 3 COLOR TONES Designated by small letter (D7.5)
G. GOLD TONE
D. DRAB TONE
R. RED TONE

THE 7 BASIC HAIR COLORS ARE ORGANIZED INTO 5 SHADES Designated by small number (D7.5)
1. DARK
2. MEDIUM
3. LIGHT
4. EXTRA LIGHT
5. PALEST

Plate 6

COMPARISON CHART

	ASH BROWN			GOLDEN BLONDE		ASH BLONDE					DARK DRABBER
G4.3 Light Golden Brown	D5.1 Dark Ash Brown	D5.2 Medium Ash Brown	D5.3 Light Ash Brown	G6.2 Medium Golden Blonde	G6.3 Light Golden Blonde	D7.1 Dark Ash Blonde	D7.2 Medium Ash Blonde	D7.3 Light Ash Blonde	D7.4 Extra Light Ash Blonde	D7.5 Palest Ash Blonde	D0.1 Drabber
35™ Sunlit Brown	48™ Sable Brown	57™ Coffee Brown	46™ Chestnut Brown	43™ Sun Bronze	41™ Golden Apricot	32™ Moonhaze	42™ Moongold	40™ Topaz	30™ Flaxen Blonde		
	21 Dark Brown	31B Medium Warm Brown	33B Medium Gold Brown	47 Pale Red Blonde	36 Golden Blonde	24 Dark Ash Blonde	34 Golden Brown	37 Pale Blonde	27 Pastel Blonde		53 Dark Drabber
15 Muted Maize	13 Chocolate Kiss	21 Plush Brown			25 Gilded Lily		16 Hidden Honey	18 Spun Sand	51 Demure Mist		
555 Hazel Blonde	148 Dark Ash Brown	257 Dark Golden Brown	246 Light Ash Brown	643 Tan Blonde	841 Light Golden Blonde	1070 Honey Beige Blonde	542 Ash Blonde	940 Pale Ash Blonde	1030 Palest Ash Blonde		049 Dark Drabber
7.1 Dark Ash Blonde	4 Dark Brown	5 Medium Brown	6 Light Brown	8.4 Reddish Blonde	8.3 Golden Blonde	8.1 Ash Blonde	7.1B Medium Ash Blonde	8.1B Champagne Blonde	9 Pastel Blonde		Dark Drabber
4G Lightest Golden Brown	1N Dark Natural Ash Brown	2G Medium Golden Brown	3G Light Golden Brown	4A Light Auburn	7A Lightest Auburn		4N Lightest Natural Ash Brown	9N Extra Light Nat. Ash Blonde	9S Light Silver Blonde		Silver Blue Concentrate
	4 Dark Brown	5 Medium Brown	6 Light Brown	R-8 Medium Red Blonde	W-8 Medium Warm Blonde	A-1 Medium Ash Blonde	A-7 Dark Ash Blonde	A-8 Medium Ash Blonde	9 Light Blonde		101 Deep Ash Drabber
	3N Dark Chestnut	4N Medium Chestnut	5N Light Chestnut	7D Medium Golden Blonde	8D Light Golden Blonde	6N Dark Blonde	7C Medium Ash Blonde	8C Pale Ash Blonde	9C Very Light Ash Blonde		

Refer to plates 10 and 11 for Permanent Hair Color Results Chart.

Courtesy of LAMAUR Incorporated.

Plate 7

At 400X magnification, this series of OM color micrographs shows the formation of hair from living cells, as well as a longer section of hair.

Photo 1 shows the hair in the hair follicle. The nuclei of the cells found in large numbers around the papilla are the dark spots in the lower portion of the micrograph.

Photo 2 shows the change in shape of these cells by their elongation.

In photo 3, these cells appear only as fine reddish lines.

In photo 4, the cells have completely disappeared. The formation of keratin within the structural fibers is visible by the increasing appearance of yellow color.

(Courtesy of the Wella Corporation.)

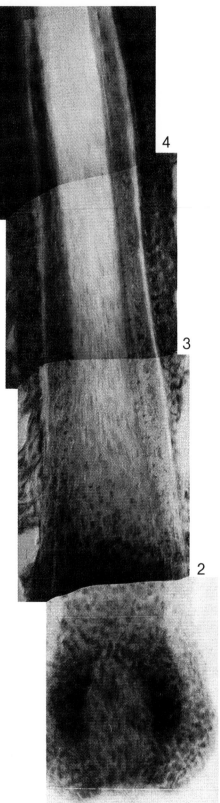

Plate 8

PERMANENT HAIR COLOR

RESULTS CHART**

**Results on this chart were
obtained by using LAMAUR
Precision™ Hair Color only.

Strand test for exact
results.
Refer to Plates 6 and 7 for
color samples.

Plate 9

PERMANENT HAIR COLOR

**Results on this chart were obtained by using LAMAUR Precision™ Hair Color only.

Strand test for exact results.

Refer to Plates 6 and 7 for color samples.

TO OBTAIN DESIRED SHADE:**

1) Locate on the chart the column heading describing the client's natural hair shade. Under this heading are listed the different results obtained with various shades of Precision Hair Color.

CLIENT'S NATURAL HAIR COLOR IS

NO.	NAME	LIFTING ACTION	BLACK Results obtained	GRAY Results obtained
D1.1	Black	0 shades	Truer, richer black	True black
D1.2	Black Brown	0 shades	Natural black	Natural black
R2.1	Dark Red	4 shades	Dark brown with red highlights	Dark red
R2.2	Medium Red	4½ shades	Brown with copper red highlights	Bright, light copper red
R2.3	Light Red	6 shades	Brown with bright red highlights	Light bright red
R3.1	Dark Auburn	3 shades	Dark red brown	Dark brown
R3.3	Light Auburn	3½ shades	Brown with red highlights	Medium auburn
G4.1	Dark Golden Brown	1 shade	Dark brown with warm highlights	Dark golden brown
G4.2	Medium Golden Brown	2 shades	Medium brown with warm highlights	Medium golden brown
G4.3	Light Golden Brown	3 shades	Brown with warm highlights	Light golden brown
D5.1	Dark Ash Brown	1 shade	Very dark brown	Dark ash brown
D5.2	Medium Ash Brown	2 shades	Medium dark brown	Medium ash brown
D5.3	Light Ash Brown	3 shades	Medium brown	Light ash brown
G6.2	Medium Golden Blonde	4 shades	Brown with reddish highlights	Medium golden blonde
G6.3	Light Golden Blonde	7 shades	Brown with very gold highlights	Light golden blonde with dark hair lightened to blend in
D7.1	Dark Ash Blonde	3½ shades	Brown with subtle highlights	Very drab ash blonde
D7.2	Medium Ash Blonde	3½ shades	Brown with gold highlights	Ash blonde
D7.3	Light Ash Blonde	7 shades	Bright warm brown	Light ash blonde with darker hair lightened to blend in
D7.4	Extra Light Ash Blonde	9 shades	Lighter, bright warm brown	Light drab blonde with darker hair lightened and toned
D7.5	Palest Ash Blonde	9 shades	Brown with bright golden highlights	Lightest drab blonde with darker hair lightened and toned

*LAMAUR PRECISION HAIR COLOR NUMBERING SYSTEM
THERE ARE 7 BASIC HAIR COLOR CATEGORIES

Designated by large number (D7.5)

1. BLACK
2. RED
3. AUBURN
4. GOLDEN BROWN
5. ASH BROWN
6. GOLDEN BLONDE
7. ASH BLONDE

D7.5

ALL BASIC COLORS AND SHADES HAVE 1 OF 3 COLOR TONES
Designated by small letter (D7.5)
G. GOLD TONE
D. DRAB TONE
R. RED TONE

THE 7 BASIC HAIR COLORS ARE ORGANIZED INTO 5 SHADES
Designated by small number (D7.5)
1. DARK
2. MEDIUM
3. LIGHT
4. EXTRA LIGHT
5. PALEST

Plate 10

RESULTS CHART**

2) Under the column that best describes the patron's natural hair, locate the shade Precision Hair Color desired. Refer to the column in line with this shade on the far left, which is the number and name of the Precision Hair Color to be applied.

No. D0.1 Drabber is not used alone, but in conjunction with the other Precision Hair Color colors to minimize undesirable red tones.

BROWN	RED	BLONDE
Results obtained	Results obtained	Results obtained
True black	True black	True black
Natural black	Natural black	Natural black
Dark red brown	Deep bright red	Deep red
Medium red brown with coppery highlights	Red with copper highlights	Medium red
Light red brown	Light bright red	Light bright red
Reddish brown	Bright red auburn	Reddish brown
Medium auburn	Light bright auburn	Medium auburn
Dark golden brown	Dark red brown	Dark golden brown
Medium golden brown	Medium red brown	Medium golden brown
Light golden brown	Warm golden brown	Light golden brown
Dark ash brown	Dark brown with red highlights	Dark ash brown
Medium ash brown	Medium brown with red highlights	Medium ash brown
Light ash brown	Light warm brown	Light ash brown
Brown with gold tones	Red with gold highlights	Medium golden blonde
Lighter shade with golden blonde highlights	Slightly lighter red	Light golden blonde
Lighter brown with ash tones	Drabber red	Dark ash blonde
Lighter brown with slight ash tone	Medium blonde with red highlights	Medium ash blonde
Lighter, with decided gold highlights	Light red blonde	Light ash blonde
Lighter shade with blonde highlights	Lightest red blonde	Light pale blonde
Lightest shade of brown with slight blonde highlights	Lighter subdued red	Pale ash blonde

Courtesy of LAMAUR Incorporated.

Plate 11

METRIC MEASURES IMPORTANT TO COSMETOLOGY

How to make conversions to metric scales:

	Symbol	Unit	Multiply by	Metric Unit	Metric Symbol
LENGTH	in.	1 Inch	2.5	Centimeters	cm
	ft.	1 Foot	30	Centimeters	cm
VOLUME	tsp.	1 Teaspoon	5	Milliliters	ml
	tbsp.	1 Tablespoon	15	Milliliters	ml
	fl. oz.	1 Fluid Ounce	30	Milliliters	ml
	pt.	1 Pint	0.47	Liters	l
	qt.	1 Quart	0.95	Liters	l
	gal.	1 Gallon	3.8	Liters	l

CONVERSIONS

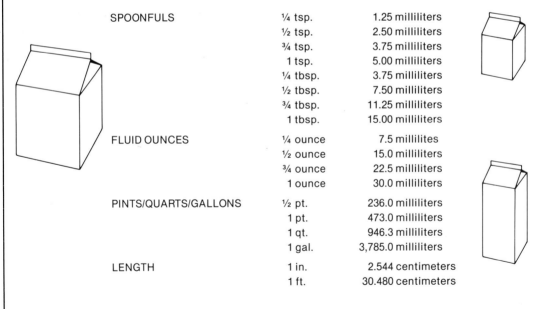

SPOONFULS	¼ tsp.	1.25 milliliters
	½ tsp.	2.50 milliliters
	¾ tsp.	3.75 milliliters
	1 tsp.	5.00 milliliters
	¼ tbsp.	3.75 milliliters
	½ tbsp.	7.50 milliliters
	¾ tbsp.	11.25 milliliters
	1 tbsp.	15.00 milliliters
FLUID OUNCES	¼ ounce	7.5 millilites
	½ ounce	15.0 milliliters
	¾ ounce	22.5 milliliters
	1 ounce	30.0 milliliters
PINTS/QUARTS/GALLONS	½ pt.	236.0 milliliters
	1 pt.	473.0 milliliters
	1 qt.	946.3 milliliters
	1 gal.	3,785.0 milliliters
LENGTH	1 in.	2.544 centimeters
	1 ft.	30.480 centimeters

Plate 12

12. Following label directions, pour clear, 20-volume peroxide into a clean applicator bottle. (Creme developers also are used.)

12. Never mix a tint until you are ready to immediately apply it. It is much easier to measure the correct proportions if you add the peroxide first! When the color is poured first, it stains the inside of the bottle and makes it difficult to see how many ounces of either liquid are in it.

13. Pour the correct amount of tint into the bottle. Check the total ounces of material in the bottle against the directions.

13. If the directions for 1½ ounces of color call for double peroxide (3 ounces), the applicator bottle should have 4½ ounces of ready-to-use material after the color and peroxide are mixed. Always recheck measurements of coloring material!

14. Secure the nozzle firmly on the applicator bottle and shake (gently or vigorously according to directions for different products).

14. Some manufacturers advise to gently shake the bottle, since heavier shaking causes the combination to thicken too much. On the other hand, some color and peroxide combinations are applied in a gel form, which requires vigorous shaking for 10 to 15 seconds.

Apply a Virgin Tint to Lighten the Natural Hair Color

PROCEDURE

1. If the color selected is several shades lighter than the client's natural color, begin to apply it one inch away from scalp area.

RATIONALE

1. When coloring lighter, body heat causes the color to develop faster at the scalp than toward the ends of hair. If you apply the color on the scalp first, the color will be uneven, lighter at the scalp and slightly darker toward middle and end of hair shaft.

2. Use the nozzle of the applicator to part off horizontal ¼-inch strands of hair in the right crown area.

2. These partings insure complete saturation of all hair within the strand.

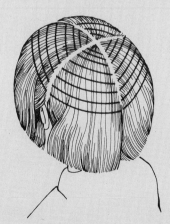

Part off horizontal ¼ inch subsections

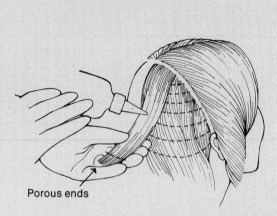

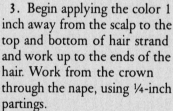

Porous ends

Apply tint only up to porous ends

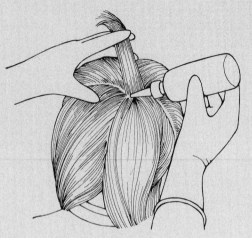

Apply color to scalp hair

3. Begin applying the color 1 inch away from the scalp to the top and bottom of hair strand and work up to the ends of the hair. Work from the crown through the nape, using ¼-inch partings.

4. After you have finished the right crown, go to the top left crown. Repeat application from the top crown through the nape.

5. Use the applicator nozzle to part off ¼-inch strands on the left front top. Apply the color 1 inch from the scalp through the ends of each strand. Work from the top to the bottom of the section.

6. Apply the color according to directions to the top right front section.

7. Set the timer for 15 minutes.

3. Apply the color in the crown first. Hair around the front hairline is usually fine-textured and less resistant than hair in the crown and nape.

4. **Do not allow coloring material to run into client's eyes or onto clothing.**

5. Since you have just completed left nape, it is convenient to continue on the left front top.

6. This will complete application of color to all the hair except the scalp hair.

7. This allows the middle and ends of the hair shaft to start developing before you apply the color to the scalp hair. Body heat will cause this hair to oxidize the color faster.

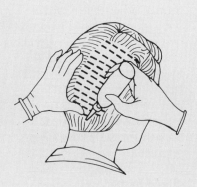
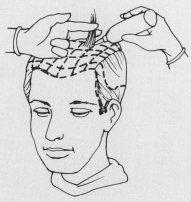
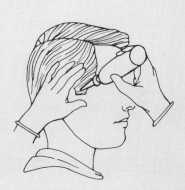
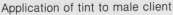
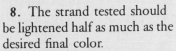

Application of tint to male client

8. When the timer rings, make a strand test.

9. Beginning in the right crown, apply color to the scalp hair in ¼-inch horizontal partings.

10. Proceed to left crown. Apply color in ¼-inch horizontal partings. Work from crown through nape to color hair.

11. Go to the left top front and continue to apply color to all of the scalp hair.

12. Apply the color to the right top front section in ¼-inch partings.

13. Set the timer for 10 minutes; strand test when the timer rings and carefully check to be certain that all of the hair has color.

14. Lightly spray lukewarm water around hairline. Use your thumbs to work the water into the color around the hairline.

8. The strand tested should be lightened half as much as the desired final color.

9. These partings help you color all of the hair.

10. This is a good systematic way to apply the color.

11. This is standard procedure.

12. This is standard procedure.

13. When color on ends of hair matches that on hair next to scalp, the color is even. It is easy to miss a small piece of hair, so check and apply color as needed.

14. This will begin the process of removing stain from hairline.

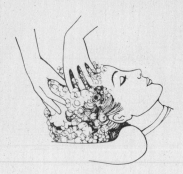

Shampoo gently, as scalp may be sensitive

15. Use circular thumb movements to work water and color into a lather. (Add shampoo as necessary.) Remove all color stains from the hairline.

15. Warm water and the tint form a lather that removes stains along hairline. This is the best way to remove it. Quickly rinsing or shampooing color from hair without using this lathering process will not remove hairline stains. Lukewarm water is used because the scalp may be sensitive.

16. Rinse the remaining color from the hairline, and shampoo the hair twice with a color-safe product.

16. All coloring material should be removed from the scalp and hair. Dark colors may require more than two shampoos.

17. Apply normalizing conditioner and discuss the results with the client.

17. Since tints have a pH of between 9.5 and 10.5, it is necessary to neutralize traces of alkali.

18. Record formula and results on the client's permanent hair-coloring card.

18. Be sure to record date, formula, result, and remarks.

Apply a Virgin Tint to Darken the Natural Hair Color

The steps and safety procedures for darkening the hair are basically the same as for previous services. The basic difference is that the tint is applied to the scalp hair **first**.

DOING SUBOBJECTIVE 5

Apply a tint retouch.

PROCEDURE

1. Prepare the client for a basic tinting service. Use the same procedures for applying a tint to new growth.

2. Apply the tint to outline partings, which divide the hair into 4 equal sections. Apply tint only to the new growth of hair. Stay 1/16-inch from the previously tinted hair.

RATIONALE

1. Procedures and safety precautions are the same as for previously described services.

2. Do not overlap tint onto hair that has already been tinted. **A line of demarcation** will result from overlapping. If color is applied on tinted hair next to new growth, the color will build up on this part and cause a line of darker (or lighter) color. (It will look like marked hair caused by improper cutting.)

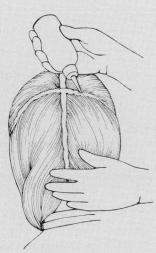

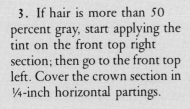

Always wear protective gloves. To begin, apply tint to outline of sections

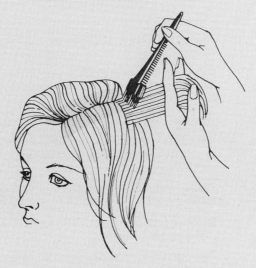

Apply tint to new growth

3. If hair is more than 50 percent gray, start applying the tint on the front top right section; then go to the front top left. Cover the crown section in ¼-inch horizontal partings.

4. After you have retouched all new growth, carefully inspect the areas in which you have applied the tint. Apply in any area missed. Gently lift the ends of the hair away from the head.
5. Develop color as usual. Shampoo and set the hair.

3. When hair is more than 50 percent gray, it is more resistant to coloring, so many cosmetologists begin applying color along the front rather than the crown. This gives better coverage of gray. If the hair is less than 50 percent gray, most cosmetologists begin applying in the right crown and work in ¼-inch horizontal partings toward the nape.
4. The tint oxidizes better if air is allowed to circulate through the hair. Do not mat the hair ends close to the head.

5. This procedure is the same as previously described services.

GLOSSARY

Aniline (AN-ehl-ehn) derivative   A substance used in tints. It comes from coal tar.

Bleaching and toning   A double-application method of coloring hair using two different products, one to take color from the hair and another to add the new color.

Coal tar   An organic substance used to make synthetic hair dyes.

Developer   A chemical that provides the oxygen to fix the color during a permanent hair coloring process. Most modern products use 20-volume hydrogen peroxide for the developer.

Double peroxide   Mixing twice as much peroxide as color in the permanent hair-coloring service.

Drabber   Concentrated color that has a blue or violet base that neutralizes red or gold overtones in the hair.

Equal peroxide   Mixing equal amounts of peroxide and color in the permanent hair-coloring service.

Hydrogen peroxide   An acid used to provide oxygen in chemical hair coloring. In this process it is called the developer.

Hydrometer (high-DROHM-eh-tehr)   An instrument used to determine the strength of the peroxide or other chemical in a mixture.

Hypersensitive (high-per-SEN-seh-tiv)   Allergic.

Line of demarcation   A line of darker or lighter color in the hair caused by overlapping the application of a tint onto hair that has already been tinted.

Oxidation   The process of combining oxygen with other substances.

Oxidation tint   A permanent hair coloring that deposits the color into the hair shaft through a chemical process. Also called penetrating tint.

Oxidizer   Any substance that gives up oxygen during the process of oxidation.

Para-phenylene-diamine (PA-rah-FEN-l-een-DIGH-eh-meen)   A synthetic organic compound that is derived from coal tar used to give color to hair dye.

Patch test   See **Predisposition test**.

Penetrating tint   Hair coloring that permanently penetrates the cuticle and deposits color in the cortex of the hair shaft. Also called oxidation tint.

Peroxide   See **Hydrogen peroxide**.

Predisposition (pree-dis-peh-ZISH-shun) test   The process of applying a small amount of hair color to the client's skin at least 24 hours before the service to determine if the client is allergic to the product.

Retouch tint   Coloring a new growth of hair that has already been permanently colored.

Single-application coloring service   Hair coloring done in one application, such as to darken the hair.

Soap cap   A service that highlights or slightly changes hair color by combining permanent hair color with shampoo and applying it like shampoo to dry hair.

Virgin hair   Hair that has not been overexposed to the sun or treated by tints, chemical straighteners, cold-waving solutions, or other chemical services.

Virgin tint   The process of using a permanent hair color on virgin hair.

QUESTIONS

1. What is virgin hair?
2. What are the three main parts of a soap cap?
3. Can you write the chemical abbreviation for hydrogen peroxide?
4. Write a definition for "double process."
5. Is hair tint ever used to color eyelashes or eyebrows?
6. In your own words, write a paragraph(s) explaining the reasons a client might want a tint.
7. Does permanent color penetrate the hair shaft?
8. What layer(s) of the hair is (are) penetrated with a permanent hair color?
9. Write another name for an oxidation tint.
10. Give the name for hair that has not been previously treated with chemicals, such as a cold wave or hair bleach.
11. When the client's tinted hair grows out, what is the name given to the service he/she will need?
12. If you are using an oxidizing tint, what is the activating chemical that makes it work?
13. What is the name for the developer used in a tint?
14. What is the main ingredient in an aniline tint?
15. What is the pH range of hydrogen peroxide?
16. What name is given to an aniline derivative color that permanently colors the hair?
17. Can a single-process tint be used to lighten the hair?
18. Does an aniline tint completely cover gray hair?
19. If the client wants to change his/her hair color, will the tint shampoo out of the hair?
20. Is it necessary to wear protective gloves when tinting the hair?
21. Is it all right to mix tint in a metal bowl?
22. How can you determine beforehand how a color will turn out on a particular natural hair color?
23. In order to dilute the volume of the peroxide 50%, how much water would you add to the following formula: 2 ounces tint and 2 ounces peroxide?
24. When applying a virgin tint, should you begin by applying the color through the porous ends?
25. If you were doing a tint retouch, would you apply the tint to the new growth first?
26. Following a tint, would the scalp be sensitive?
27. Should you keep a record of all tint clients, their formulas, and predisposition tests?
28. When applying a tint retouch, how far away from the previously tinted hair should the application be?
29. What device is used to measure the volume of peroxide?

ANSWERS

1. Hair not previously exposed to chemicals used to permanently curl, straighten, or color the hair 2. Shampoo, tint and peroxide 3. H_2O_2 4. Bleaching the hair, then applying a pastel tint (a toner) to it 5. No—never 6. (Students' own comments) 7. Yes 8. Cuticle and cortex 9. Penetrating tint 10. Virgin hair 11. Tint retouch 12. Hydrogen peroxide 13. Hydrogen peroxide 14. Para-phenylene-diamine 15. 3.5–4.0 16. Tint 17. Yes 18. Yes 19. No 20. Yes 21. No; use glass or plastic 22. Give a strand test 23. Add 1 ounce hydrogen peroxide (H_2O_2) and 1 ounce water (H_2O), then 2 ounces tint (1 oz. H_2O_2 + 1 oz. H_2O + 2 oz. tint) 24. No 25. Yes 26. Yes 27. Yes 28. 1/16 inch 29. Hydrometer

Lightening and Toning the Hair 16

You may remember from chapter 15 that the other way to permanently color the hair is by lightening and toning it. This process, called a **double-application** service, has some of the basic steps that you used to tint the hair. The double application will be explained in detail in this chapter.

Purpose

Provided with lightening and toning supplies, follow the proper steps to lighten and tone the client's hair.

Major Objective

Using the proper safety precautions and following label directions, apply a virgin bleach and retouch bleach in 30 to 45 minutes for each. Score 75 percent or better on a multiple-choice exam on the information in this chapter.

Level of Acceptability

1. Define hair lightening and toning, describe their chemical effects on the hair, and identify the 7 lightening stages of hair.
2. Identify types of bleaches and services for lightening and toning and identify the toning colors.

Knowing Subobjectives

3. Apply a virgin bleach.
4. Apply a bleach retouch.

Doing Subobjectives

241

KNOWING SUBOBJECTIVE 1

Define hair lightening and toning, describe their chemical effects on the hair, and identify the 7 lightening stages of hair.

In chapter 15 the term double-application service was used. The double-application service involves two separate services that use different products. When you lighten the hair, you apply a **bleaching agent**. After the bleaching agent has lightened the hair, it is shampooed from the hair.

Toning the hair involves applying a special pastel coloring product on hair that has been bleached. These pastel colors, called **toners**, contain molecules of color that are so large that they can only penetrate the cuticle of bleached hair. Some toners are aniline derivatives. Hydrogen peroxide must be used with them. Other toners are semipermanent colors that do not need peroxide.

Bleaches have complicated chemical formulas. Like most products they vary from one brand to the next; they generally contain ammonium, potassium, and sodium persulfates, plus water, fatty acid soaps, alcohols, and a small amount of color (usually blue or white).

You probably are especially interested in the effects these chemicals have on the hair (for safety's sake, keep their general chemical makeup in mind).

Before these bleaching chemicals are applied to the hair, they are mixed with 20-volume peroxide, which is the **catalyst*** (KAT-el-est). This mixture has a pH of about 8 to 9.5. It takes the brown, red, and yellow color out (decolorizes) of the cortex of the hair by oxidizing (adding oxygen to) the coloring pigment. The pigment actually vaporizes (evaporates) in the natural hair color. If you had a very powerful microscope, you could see that, after a hair has been bleached, the melanin is no longer in the cortex. You could see spots in the hair shaft where the molecules of melanin, or pigment, once were. The toner fills these spots with new molecules of color. Many toners in a wide variety of strengths are available. The one you choose will, of course, depend on how light a color you want. Very light toners can be used only when the natural color has been completely lightened or "lifted."

Bleaching is an **oxidizing process**, which brings hair color to different stages of lightening. Counting black hair as the starting point, there are 7 stages of lightening: **black, brown, red, red-gold, gold, yellow, and pale yellow**.

Hair must be porous enough as well as light enough to accept a toner; even hair that is naturally very light is not porous enough. All hair needs to be bleached before a toner can be applied.

Occasionally you will be bleaching a client's hair and planning to apply a toner. Suddenly the client looks up and says, "That's it! That's the color I want." You can simply shampoo the bleach from the hair—you saved your client some money and saved yourself some time.

The bleach may be shampooed from the hair at any time during the bleaching process. Bleach can be applied to the hair to prepare it for a toner, or it can sometimes be used to lighten the hair to a desirable color without applying a toner.

*The agent that starts a chemical reaction.

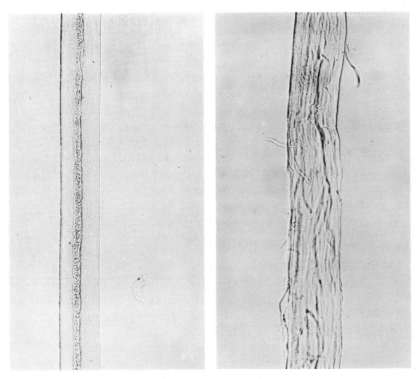

Two bleached hairs as seen under a light microscope. Note absence of pigment in cortex of each hair. Hair on right has been over-bleached (Courtesy of 3M Company)

KNOWING SUBOBJECTIVE 2

Identify types of bleaches and services used for lightening and toning and identify the toning colors.

Bleaches (lighteners) are made in 3 basic forms—creme, powder, and oil.

The best way to select a bleach is in terms of its use: how and where are you going to use it. For example, both a virgin bleach and a bleach retouch require direct contact between the scalp and the bleach, so a creme bleach, which is milder than other forms, would be the best choice.

Packages of **creme bleach** usually have one 4-ounce bottle of bleach and 4 packets of activators, also called protinators or energizers. Half of the bleach base and 2 activator packets are used per application, so a package should be good for 2 applications. When you mix the bleach, put peroxide in the bottle first. Then add the activators and shake the bottle. Finally, add the creme bleach base and mix by shaking. Now the bleach is ready to apply.

The creme base contains a very small amount of white or blue color to slightly neutralize unwanted red or brassy gold tones that are brought out during bleaching. Creme bleaches also contain buffering, or conditioning, agents, which keep the hair and scalp in better condition during the bleaching process than powder bleaches do.

When creme bleaches are mixed, they have a creamy consistency, like a gel. Their consistency makes them easy to apply. The bleach remains where it is applied; it does not dry out, drip, or run onto the forehead and neck.

Powder bleaches usually come in 3-pound cans and need only hydrogen peroxide. Since they contain few buffers or conditioners, powder bleaches may irritate the scalp. Therefore, they are used primarily for streaking, framing,* frosting, and painting (tipping), since the bleach does not come in direct contact with the scalp in these services. Hair is **streaked by using foil** to lighten large sections **around the face**. Hair is **frosted by using a cap** to lighten or darken small strands of hair **throughout the head**. Once the hair has been frosted with light strands of hair, it may be given **reverse frosting**. A **reverse frosting darkens lightened strands** of hair for the client that has been given too many lightened strands of hair. Hair is **painted** by **tipping** small strands toward the front of the head. These strands can be either lightened or darkened. Powder bleaches are faster and stronger than creme or oil bleaches, but they have a tendency to dry out when they are being used.

Oil bleaches decolorize the natural pigment, and they also add a slight amount of certified color to the hair during the process. Oil bleaches come in the following colors: neutral, which sometimes is added in small amounts to regular tints to make the tint lighter; silver, which neutralizes red or brassy gold tones; gold, which adds golden highlights to otherwise drab hair; and red, which adds reddish highlights to the hair. Remember: all oil bleaches deposit a small amount of color and lighten the hair so a toner may not be needed.

Creme, powder, and oil bleaches do not require a patch test, but the test must be given if you are going to apply a toner after the bleach.

Many manufacturers use one of the following terms to identify the color that their toner will leave on bleached hair: gold, yellow-gold-orange, red, platinum, silver, or ash.

Warm hair colors are yellow, gold, orange, red, and brown. **Cool** (drab) hair colors are ash, silver, platinum, smoke, and steel gray.

Recognizing the manufacturer's terms for toning colors will help you use the color chart to select a toning color for the client. For example, after you have studied the toning chart, you should know that a silver tone has a blue base, which would be used to neutralize bleached hair that is a little too yellow.

DOING SUBOBJECTIVE 3

Apply a virgin bleach.

Supplies

- □ client release form
- □ client permanent record form
- □ 20-volume peroxide
- □ creme bleach
- □ timer
- □ shampoo supplies, including non-color-stripping shampoo
- □ clean plastic bleach applicator bottle with nozzle
- □ protective gloves

*Framing is making a continuously lighter band around the hairline. Although a separate bleach application is not required, the tints that are used do contain bleach and the process is therefore covered in this unit.

PROCEDURE

1. Record results of the patch test.

2. Do not shampoo or brush hair.

3. Thoroughly examine the scalp and the texture and condition of the client's hair.

4. If a toner is going to be applied, use the color chart to help the client make a selection. See the chart for footnotes on lightening stages.

RATIONALE

1. You must give a patch test if an aniline toner will be used.

2. Bleach can produce small or large red blisters on the scalp if hair is vigorously brushed or shampooed before it is lightened.

3. If cuts, scratches, or abrasions are present, **do not apply** bleach. Condition hair that is very porous, fragile, or chemically damaged before you bleach it. There should not be any other coloring products on the hair. If there are, do not proceed to bleach.

4. You will not be able to get light, delicate toning colors if the natural (virgin) hair color is very red. Do not tell a client who has dark red hair that the color selected will be the one he or she will get. Consult your instructor or manager for assistance. At the bottom of the color chart, there are descriptions of the stages to which the hair must be bleached for a particular toner to give a particular color. Compare the stage needed to the condition of the client's hair. If the toner requires bleaching to pale yellow and the client's hair is fine in texture and naturally black, the hair would probably break before it reached the pale yellow (seventh) stage. Ask your instructor for help and advise the client accordingly.

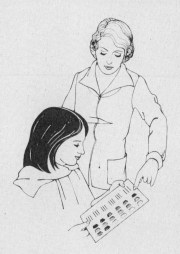

5. Part the hair into sections; then mix bleach according to label directions.

5. Creme bleaches usually have to be mixed in the following sequence. Put 4 ounces of clear 20-volume hydrogen peroxide in a bottle; add 2 activators (the protinators or energizers), cover, and **shake well**. (Activators are really alkalizers. They speed up the bleaching process by increasing the alkalinity of the product.) Then add 2 ounces of bleach base, cover, and shake thoroughly. Mixing most creme bleaches any other way causes them to be "sandy" and unusable.

6. Lightly powder the insides of surgical gloves and put them on.

6. **Always wear gloves** to protect your hands during bleaching or toning.

7. Apply bleach in the same way that you would a virgin tint to **lighten** the hair—**away** from the scalp first.

7. The principles for lightening are the same for both tinting and bleaching, but bleach lightens the hair more. This is standard procedure.

8. Begin applying the bleach in the right crown section. Apply the bleach ½-**inch away from** the scalp. Use ⅛-**inch** horizontal partings. Apply the bleach in a bead across the strand. Following the proper steps, apply bleach carefully and quickly to all the hair.

8. These partings are needed to insure that **all** hair will have enough bleach for even lightening. Apply the bleach **generously** so that it rests on and through the hair. Keep all bleach on hair strands moist. Allow air to circulate through the hair to oxidize the bleach. Apply bleach quickly so it will lighten the hair evenly.

9. Carefully examine the hair where the bleach has been applied.

9. There must be a generous amount of **moist** bleach **on** and **through** each strand.

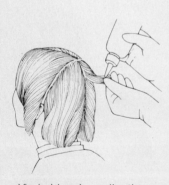

Virgin bleach application

10. Check the bleach application for dripping or running. Be sure that bleach has not dripped onto the hair next to the scalp.

11. Take a strand test after 30 minutes have passed.

12. Carefully apply bleach to the hair next to the scalp. Meet bleach that has already been applied to the hair. Apply the bleach in the same order you applied bleach to the middle and ends of the hair strands. Remove bleach by rinsing and shampooing when the hair has lightened to the correct stage.

13. Towel- or dryer-dry hair according to label directions of toner; mix **toner** and **peroxide** as directed. Apply according to directions.

14. Apply normalizing creme or conditioner.

10. Use the corner of a towel saturated with **cold** water to remove bleach that is running down the hair shaft to the scalp. Bleach should not reach hair next to the scalp because body heat will cause the hair to bleach faster and make that portion lighter than the area farther down the shaft.

11. When the hair is about half as light as you want it, you should apply bleach to the hair next to the scalp. Use horizontal partings ⅛ inch apart. If the hair is **not** ready, reapply bleach to the strand used for the test. Strand test frequently as desired.

12. Apply the bleach generously across the hair strands. Do not spread the bleach thinly across the strand. If it is spread too thinly, the hair will not be evenly lightened.

13. Carefully read label directions because they vary from product to product. **Wear protective gloves** when applying toner.

14. Use a conditioner or normalizing creme to neutralize the alkalinity of the toner.

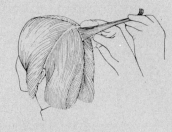

Strand testing hair

DOING SUBOBJECTIVE 4

Apply a bleach retouch.

Supplies

- □ client release form
- □ client permanent record form
- □ 20-volume peroxide
- □ creme bleach
- □ protective gloves

- □ shampoo supplies, including non-color-stripping shampoo
- □ timer
- □ clean plastic bleach applicator bottle with nozzle

Use the same steps that you used for a tint retouch. As you probably remember, bleaching is a double-application process, while tinting is a single-application process. So you have one additional step. After you have removed the bleach and shampooed the hair, apply a toner to the hair. If bleach is **overlapped** onto previously bleached hair, **breakage may result**.

GLOSSARY

Catalyst (KAT-el-est)   An agent that starts a chemical reaction.

Cool (drab) hair colors   Hair-color products that correspond to the cool secondary colors on the color chart. There are ash, silver, platinum, smoke, and steel gray.

Creme bleach   A hair-bleaching product having a gel-like consistency that makes it easy to apply.

Drab hair colors   See **Cool hair colors**.

Framing   A continuously lighter band of hair around the hairline.

Frosting   Lightening or darkening small strands of hair throughout the head by using a cap.

Painting   Lightening or darkening small strands of hair toward the face. Also called **Tipping**.

Powder bleaches   Hair-bleaching products that come in powder form and are mixed with peroxide for use. Because they contain few buffers or conditioners, they can irritate the scalp and are used primarily for applications where they will not come in contact with the scalp.

Streaking   Lightening large sections of hair around the face by using foil.

Tipping   Bleaching or coloring small strands of hair toward the front of the head. Also called **Painting**.

Toners   Pastel colors used to color bleached hair.

Toning   Applying a special pastel coloring product to hair that has been bleached.

Warm hair colors   Hair color products with bases that correspond to the warm colors on the color chart. These are yellow, gold, orange, red, and brown.

QUESTIONS

1. Using a dictionary, write a definition for the term catalyst.
2. What would be an example of a catalyst used in bleaching the hair?
3. Generally, what kind of bleach is used to streak the hair?
4. Which colors are classified as "warm hair colors"?
5. What general term is used to describe the process of bleaching and toning the hair?
6. What is the pH range of a bleach mixture?
7. Does bleach remove color pigment from the hair?
8. From which layer of the hair does bleach remove pigment?
9. Is bleaching of the hair an oxidizing process?

10. Using your own words, write a description of the process for reverse frosting the hair.
11. What are the three basic forms of bleach used in the salon?
12. Write definitions for frosting, streaking, and tipping; then compare them to the textbook.
13. Is it necessary to give a patch test before the application of a bleach?
14. Should you shampoo the hair before the application of a bleach?
15. Should you give a patch test before the application of an aniline toner?
16. When applying a virgin bleach, how far from the scalp should it be applied?
17. What size horizontal subsections should be used?
18. Is strand testing ever done before bleaching the hair?
19. Is it necessary to wear gloves when applying bleach?
20. What is "overlapping"?
21. Can overlapping cause breakage?

ANSWERS

1. (Students' dictionary) 2. Hydrogen peroxide 3. Powder bleach 4. Yellow, gold, orange, red and brown 5. Double-application service 6. 8-9.5 7. Yes 8. Cortex 9. Yes 10. (Students' comments) 11. Cream (creme), powder, and oil 12. (Students' comments) 13. No 14. No 15. Yes 16. ½ inch 17. ⅛ inch 18. Yes 19. Yes 20. Applying bleach on previously bleached hair when giving a bleach retouch 21. yes

Creative Lightening and Toning Techniques 17

Chapter 16 involved the basic principles and uses of lightening and toning. In this chapter you will learn how to apply those principles to get special effects.

Purpose

Provided with the necessary supplies, follow the proper steps to achieve special lightening and toning effects—streaking, framing, frosting, and painting the hair and tinting it back to its original color.

Major Objective

Follow the proper steps to achieve special lightening effects. Score 75 percent or better on a multiple-choice exam on the information in this chapter.

Level of Acceptability

1. Streak the hair.
2. Frame the hair.
3. Frost the hair.
4. Paint the hair.
5. Tint the hair back to its original color, either lighter or darker.

Doing Subobjectives

DOING SUBOBJECTIVE 1

Supplies

Streak the hair.

- □ client release form
- □ client permanent hair-coloring form
- □ aluminum foil
- □ powder bleach
- □ 20-volume hydrogen peroxide

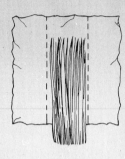

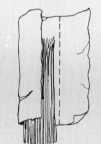

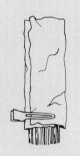

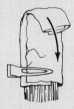

Carefully wrap foil around each strand of hair with bleach

□ shampoo supplies
□ protective gloves
□ 4–8 clips

□ color chart
□ operator apron

PROCEDURE

1. Review the client's permanent hair-coloring form and ask the client if any other products have been used.
2. Brush the hair according to its style.
3. Cut pieces of foil, place them at the base of the strands, and clip them into place.

4. Mix powder bleach with peroxide in **plastic or glass** containers according to label directions.
5. Apply the bleach to one strand and fold and clip the strand.

6. Apply bleach to the rest of these strands from the scalp through the ends of the hair. Then wrap the foil around them again and clip the foil. Leave the bleach on the hair until it is as light as you want it to be.

RATIONALE

1. Always know what other services or chemicals have been applied to the hair.

2. This helps you locate the streak(s).
3. Fit the foil to the hair's length. The longer the hair, the larger the pieces of foil should be. This helps you apply the bleach to the strand and immediately fold the foil around it.
4. Peroxide, ammonia, or other sulfonated bleaching chemicals should **not be mixed in metal containers**.
5. Enough bleach should be used to lighten the strand thoroughly. Do not allow bleach to seep outside of the foil.
6. Since foil is used on each strand, the hair will decolorize evenly.

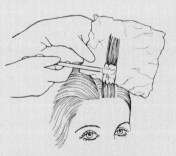

Bleach must be kept moist in order to lighten hair

7. Remove all foil when the hair has lightened. Thoroughly rinse bleach from the hair and shampoo it twice with color-safe (nonstripping) shampoo and apply normalizing creme if necessary.

8. Towel-dry the hair and apply temporary, semipermanent, or toning color, if necessary, to achieve a more becoming color.

7. A nonstripping shampoo is milder for bleached hair. Bleach should be neutralized.

8. Temporary colors are often applied to streaks to neutralize unnatural gold or brassy tones.

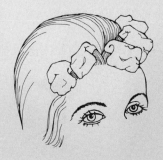

DOING SUBOBJECTIVE 2

Frame the hair.

Supplies

- client permanent hair-coloring form
- cholesterol creme
- aluminum foil
- permanent hair colors
- 20-volume hydrogen peroxide
- applicator bottle with nozzle
- protective surgical gloves
- talcum powder
- shampoo supplies
- color chart
- operator apron
- dispensary scissors

PROCEDURE

1. Apply cholesterol creme around the entire front hairline.

2. Put enough aluminum foil around the hairline to extend from the left sideburn through the top center forehead and down to the right sideburn.

3. Use the tail comb to weave a ½-inch section of hair around the entire foil line. Clip the hair if necessary.

4. Mix enough of the **lightest** tint to cover the hair you have sectioned.

RATIONALE

1. The cholesterol creme acts like an adhesive or paste to keep the aluminum foil in position at all times.

2. The foil protects the client's face (eyes, nose, mouth).

3. This is the first section that will be tinted. The lightest tint color will be applied around the hairline. Colors then will get progressively darker.

4. Mix just enough color to cover this section.

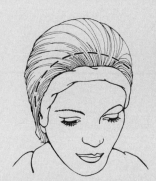

Protective cream around hairline

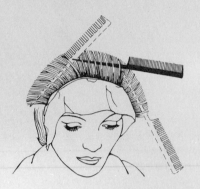 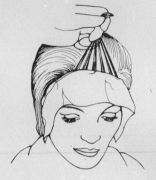 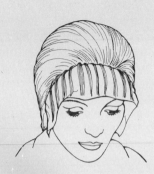

Weave comb through hair

5. Lay the tinted section on top of the foil and put another length of foil on top.

6. Weave another ½-inch to 1-inch section of hair around the front of the hairline. Mix another tint preparation slightly darker than the first.

7. Apply tint to the strand; place tinted strand along new foil toward the face.

8. Apply foil and tint to the desired color.

5. The tinted strand is placed forward toward the face on the foil so that it will be out of the way of the next strand to be tinted.

6. The change from one tint to another must be gradual.

7. The foil separates the individually tinted strands so that tints do not come in contact with other tints or with hair not to be colored.

8. The darkest tint should not be darker than the client's natural hair color.

DOING SUBOBJECTIVE 3

Frost the hair.

Supplies

- ☐ powder bleach
- ☐ plastic under-cap
- ☐ frosting cap
- ☐ plastic over-cap
- ☐ bleach applicator bottle and nozzle cap
- ☐ 20-volume peroxide
- ☐ crochet hook

- ☐ toner color chart
- ☐ talcum powder
- ☐ protective gloves
- ☐ shampoo supplies
- ☐ client release form
- ☐ client permanent hair-coloring form
- ☐ operator apron

PROCEDURE

1. Remove tangles from the hair, and comb the hair straight back and close to the head. Precondition if necessary.

2. Place the under-cap and frosting cap on the client's head. If the hair is quite long, lightly apply creme rinse before putting on the under-cap.

3. Using a fine crochet hook, begin pulling strands of hair through the holes in the top section.

4. Begin just **behind** the front hairline. Pull 8 to 12 strands through the holes in the top of the cap. Pull 4 to 8 strands through the holes on **each side** of the cap, but **avoid pulling strands that are on the hairline**.

5. Pull 4 to 8 strands through the holes in the crown of the cap.

6. Finish by pulling 8 to 14 strands in the nape section.

7. If the client complains of too much frosting, reverse frost the hair.

8. Mix the powder bleach with hydrogen peroxide according to label directions and generously apply it from the cap through the ends of the hair.

9. Put the over cap on over the frosting cap.

RATIONALE

1. Preconditioning may be necessary. Frosting is not recommended for hair having a very dark tint because brassy streaks will result.

2. The under-cap will prevent bleach from seeping through a cap that may have holes that are too large. A creme rinse makes long hair easier to pull through the frosting cap.

3. A fine crochet hook is the best implement to use. **Do not pierce the scalp with the tip of the hook.** Pull the hair **slowly**.

4. Begin behind the front hairline. Otherwise, an outgrowth of new hair will be visible in 4 to 6 weeks. The number of strands will vary with the amount of frosting desired.

5. Same as step 4.

6. This procedure completes the process for an even, attractive frosting.

7. Contact your instructor.

8. Powder bleaches, which are stronger than creme forms, can be used in frosting because the frosting cap protects the scalp from the bleach. **Each** strand must have enough bleach to evenly remove color pigment from strands.

9. Natural body heat captured in the over-cap accelerates bleaching action.

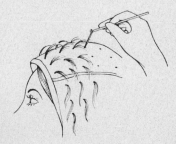

Frosting the hair

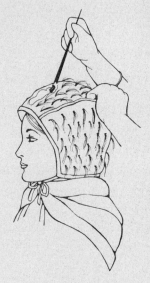

Apply bleach generously

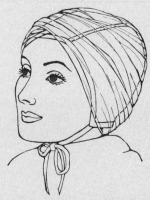

Cover with plastic cap

10. Optional step: seat the client under a warm dryer for 15 minutes or until the hair is light enough.

11. After the hair has become light and porous enough, rinse the bleach from the hair and shampoo once. **Do not remove the under-cap**.

12. Dry hair under the dryer. Mix and apply toner. Allow toner to develop. Then rinse it out and shampoo the hair.

10. Some schools and salons use heat from the dryer to speed up the bleaching action; others do not.

11. Bleach must be removed from the cap as well as from the hair, or the toner will not color the hair. Two shampoos may be necessary. If the cap is removed, you will not be able to apply the toner.

12. Toners are usually applied to dry hair. This is standard procedure.

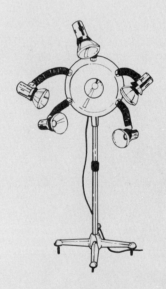

DOING SUBOBJECTIVE 4

Paint the hair.

Supplies

- powder bleach and applicator bottle
- orangewood stick
- cotton
- shampoo supplies
- 20-volume peroxide
- cellophane
- hair-setting tape
- cholesterol creme
- 4 clips
- operator apron

PROCEDURE

1. Carefully part off the top section of the hairstyle and apply cholesterol creme to the hair just **below** the top section. Apply sparingly from the hairline across the upper crown to the opposite side of the head.

2. Place the cellophane across the creme application and keep it in place on the forehead with hair-set tape.

3. Bring the top section into its regular styling position and spray **lightly** with a protein conditioner.

4. Wet the top of an orangewood stick with water; roll a bit of cotton around the point of the stick and about ½ inch of it onto the stick.

5. Mix a frosting or powder bleach according to label directions. But add ½ to 1 ounce **more** peroxide.

6. Apply the bleach on the right or left side to accent the natural movement of the hairstyle.

7. When applying bleach along the top hairline for a half-bang, paint **very thinly** on very few strands.

8. If the top section is styled to one side of the head, begin painting a fine line of bleach; then branch off one line into several others.

9. When you have finished, remove hair-setting tape and cellophane.

RATIONALE

1. Painting will be more difficult if you disturb the hairstyling lines. The creme will keep the cellophane in place.

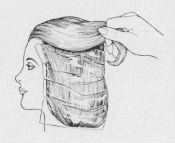

2. Be very careful. If the cellophane falls from the head, it will be very difficult to paint the hair.

3. This is the section that will be painted. The conditioner will help keep the hair from moving while you paint it.

4. The orangewood stick tipped with cotton makes an excellent, inexpensive applicator.

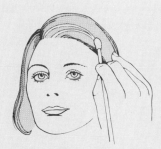

5. More hydrogen peroxide is used to make the bleach thinner and easier to apply (paint) on the hair.

6. The hairstyle will determine where you will begin painting.

7. If large strands are painted, the outgrowth of new hair will become obvious and unattractive.

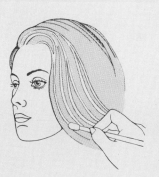

8. Branching accents the hairstyle better than many individually painted streaks.

9. When you stop depends on your judgment and artistic sense.

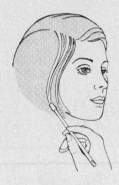

10. Rinse the bleach from the hair. Shampoo twice. Condition the hair as needed and apply normalizing creme or acid rinse.

10. The bleaching material must be removed. Some hair needs conditioning after bleaching. Alkalinity from bleach should be neutralized by normalizing creme or acid rinse.

11. Air wave or set the hair.

11. This is standard procedure.

DOING SUBOBJECTIVE 5

Tint hair back to its original color, either lighter or darker.

Supplies

- ☐ client permanent hair-color form
- ☐ oil bleach
- ☐ color fillers
- ☐ dye solvent
- ☐ filler color chart
- ☐ 20-volume peroxide

- ☐ permanent hair-color chart
- ☐ color applicator bottle
- ☐ protective gloves
- ☐ operator apron
- ☐ shampoo supplies
- ☐ tint

Lightening the Hair to Its Natural Color

PROCEDURE

1. Analyze the hair's texture, elasticity, and porosity.

2. Use a **dye solvent** or oil bleach to lighten the tinted color.

RATIONALE

1. The hair should always be in good condition before any chemical service. This service is called a **tint-back**.

2. A **dye solvent** removes artificial and natural color. Neutral oil bleaches also remove both artificial and natural color from the hair. Dye solvents are milder for hair, but they take longer to remove color. Dye solvents may require more than one application. Do not begin the tint until at least 24 hours after you have used the dye solvent. If the client does not want a temporary color between applications, you may decide to use an oil bleach.

3. Following the label directions, mix the dye solvent in a glass or plastic container.

4. Apply the dye solvent along ¾ of the strand (all except ends).

5. Strand test for desired color.

6. If dark streaks appear, rinse, shampoo lightly, and dry with a dryer.

7. Apply the solvent to the dark spots (streaks) and leave only until desired lightening results.

8. Rinse and dry when the desired color is achieved. Analyze the hair to determine if a color filler is needed, and apply if necessary.

9. Apply the selected tint to the center of the strand.

10. Strand test until half the color is achieved; then apply tint to the hair next to the scalp.

11. Work the tint through the ends with your hands.

12. Strand test until the color is even.

13. Dilute slightly with warm water and remove hairline stains.

14. Thoroughly rinse the tint from the scalp and hair. Shampoo twice.

3. For best results, dye solvents must be mixed and applied **exactly** according to label directions.

4. Since ends are more porous, the solvent removes color faster there than on the rest of the hair shaft.

5. Always strand test.

6. Dark streaks can be removed on dry hair by **spot lightening** or **spot bleaching**.

7. Apply solvent or bleach only to dark spots. Removing a dark tint from hair by using a shampoo, dye solvent, bleach, or tint is called **stripping** the hair.

8. A **color filler** is often needed before hair is tinted to equalize hair porosity, even out the color, or intensify the tint to be applied.

9. Leave the scalp and ends until later. Color will develop more quickly at the scalp because of body heat and on ends because of greater porosity. Start these areas later to get even coloring.

10. Finish applying tint to the remainder of the hair.

11. This spreads the color more evenly and does not irritate the scalp as much as combing does.

12. This is standard procedure.

13. This is the best way to remove hairline stains from the scalp.

14. The hair will be gummy and sticky if you do not remove all tint from the scalp and hair.

15. Apply normalizing cream or conditioner. Record coloring results on client's form.	15. The alkalinity from the tint must be neutralized.

Darkening the Hair to Its Natural Color

PROCEDURE	**RATIONALE**
1. Analyze the condition of client's scalp and hair and review the hair-coloring form.	1. The hair must be in good condition. This is a different procedure.
2. Explain the need for a filler, and use the color chart to select the proper color. Select and apply a gold or red filler according to label directions.	2. Fillers equalize porosity. They are made in ready-to-use form. The tint usually is applied **over** the filler. Thus, fillers are **not** usually rinsed before a tint.
3. Towel-dry the hair, or do as otherwise directed.	3. Filler applications vary, so apply according to label directions.
4. Strand test with tint selected.	4. When applying dark tint to the hair, there is a tendency for the tint to "grab," resulting in a color that is too dark. Always strand test a tint before applying it all over the hair. Select a lighter color if test strand indicates that the color is too dark.
5. Apply the tint, following the procedure for a retouch; blend immediately through the entire hair shaft.	5. Since the hair is being colored darker, the tint may be applied to the scalp hair first.
6. Allow the color to develop for 20 to 40 minutes.	6. Hair porosity will determine developing time. Strand test frequently.
7. Lightly rinse and remove stains from the client's hairline.	7. Darker colors have a tendency to stain the scalp more than light ones do.
8. Thoroughly rinse the tint from the hair. Shampoo twice.	8. Remove all traces of color and cleanse the scalp.
9. Record results and product formulas on client's permanent hair-coloring form.	9. This is standard procedure.
10. Recondition if necessary.	10. This is standard procedure.

Color filler   A product used to equalize hair porosity, even the color, or intensify the tint to be applied.

Dye solvent   A product that removes artificial and natural color from the hair.

Spot bleaching or spot lightening   Removing dark streaks from dry hair by applying a dye solvent or bleach.

Stripping   Applying solvent or bleach only to dark spots to remove them from the hair.

Tint-back   Lightening or darkening the hair to its natural color.

QUESTIONS

1. Using the facts in chapters 16 and 17, write a definition for each of the following terms: a. streak; b. painting; and c. stripping.
2. Can you explain what basic steps might be done during a tint-back?
3. During a tintback, at what stage would you use a color filler?
4. Should a filler be shampooed from the hair before tinting?
5. Would you recommend mixing bleach in a metal mixing bowl?
6. Is it important to keep bleach moist when it is lightening the hair?
7. Should a protective cream be applied around the hairline to protect the skin?
8. If a client with medium brown hair complains that the frosting has lightened the hair too much, what would you advise?
9. True or false. Bleach should be applied as sparingly as possible.
10. Is heat from a hair dryer ever used to speed-up frosting bleach?
11. When painting the hair, should you apply the bleach in thin strips or in heavy strips?
12. If a client with lightened hair wants to return the hair to its natural color, what is this service called?
13. When coloring bleached hair, what product is used to equalize the porosity of the hair?
14. What is it called when you lighten random dark spots of hair after lifting the hair close to the client's natural hair color?
15. What is the term given to the product that removes artificial color from the hair?

ANSWERS

1. a. Using foil and bleach to lighten large sections of hair around the face; b. lightening or darkening small strands of hair around the face; c. applying a solvent or bleach to lighten certain dark spots on the hair 2. (Students' explanation) 3. Before the tint application 4. No 5. No 6. Yes 7. Yes 8. A reverse frosting 9. False 10. Yes 11. Thin strips 12. A tint-back 13. A filler 14. Spot bleaching or spot lightening 15. Dye solvent

Permanent Waving (Chemical Waving) the Hair

18

Purpose

Are you one of those fortunate few whose hair falls exactly into place, has just the right amount of curl, not too much, not too little? No one has hair that is "just right" for every style. Many people have hair that is too straight. It needs a little—or maybe a lot—more curl. Others have hair that has too much curl.

Putting permanent curl into the hair is called **permanent waving**, or **chemical waving**. This is also called cold waving, acid waving, or neutral waving. Taking curl out of the hair is called chemical relaxing. (Permanent waving is used sometimes to rearrange very curly hair into a different pattern.)

All of these services are very popular and financially rewarding. In this chapter you will learn about them.

Major Objective

Using professional permanent waving chemicals and implements, permanently curl the client's hair to make it more manageable and durable from one styling to the next.

Level of Acceptability

Using safety precautions and following label directions, use the proper steps to curl the hair. Use water to wrap the client's hair on permanent-wave rods in 25–45 minutes. Score 75 percent or better on a multiple-choice exam on the information in this chapter.

Knowing Subobjectives

1. Describe three historical permanent-waving methods and list the advantages of the permanent cold-waving services used now.
2. Describe the difference between acid waves and neutral waves.
3. Describe the effects of cold-waving, the basic cold-waving chemicals, and compare the pH, cost, and methods of giving the acid wave and the regular thio wave.
4. List other services included in cold waving.

Doing Subobjectives

5. Analyze the hair and select the proper cold-wave lotion and rods.
6. Section (block) and subsection the client's hair and wrap it on cold-waving rods.
7. Process and neutralize the cold wave.
8. Subsection, wrap, process, and neutralize a ponytail cold wave on long hair.
9. Relaxing an overcurly permanent, or naturally wavy hair.

KNOWING SUBOBJECTIVE 1

Describe three historical permanent-waving methods and list the advantages of the permanent cold-waving services used now.

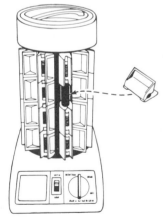

Permanent wave machine. If you are using a modern machine, it may be necessary to put cotton between clamp and scalp to prevent a heat-type burn

People have been attempting to put a permanent curl in their hair since the time of the ancient Egyptians and Romans, but these early attempts were not very successful. It was not until this century, within about a thirty-year period beginning in 1905, that the three professional permanent-wave methods introduced a new art and science in cosmetology. **Cold waving** has almost become a specialty service because of the technical knowledge and practice it demands.

The **machine permanent** method (1905) required electricity to heat large metal clamps that were placed **over** the client's hair. The hair was wound on the rods from the ends to the head. The machine had long, flexible wires that were attached directly to the large clamps, which were clipped over the rod wound on the client's head. This was called **croquignole** (KROH-kehn-ohl) wrapping (waving). When a **spiral** wrap was used, the hair was wound from the scalp to the ends. The croquignole wrap was used mainly to wave **short** hair. The machine permanent was not a very efficient way to curl hair because it required so much equipment: the machine, rubber scalp pads, small clamps, wool wave crepe, rods, and large clamps.

The **preheat permanent** wave (1931) was a "spin-off" from the machine permanent. This method was an improvement over the machine permanent because it eliminated the long electrical wires between the machine and the client. The large clamps were heated on a machine **before** they were placed on the rod wound on the client's head. Electricity did not come close to the client's head.

The **machineless permanent** wave removed the use of electricity from the waving process. The machineless wave used **chemical pads** that heated when moistened with water. After the pad was moistened, it was placed over the rod and held there by a large clamp. This method produced a curl pattern that was "pressed into the hair" by steam heat from the chemical pads. This method also required the use of protective rubber pads, small clamps, rods, and large clamps, so the procedures were basically the same, except for the use of electricity.

All three methods used two main **physical** principles to curl the hair: winding the hair **tightly** around a rod and applying **extreme** heat. Some disadvantages of all three methods were: (1) the large amount of equipment required. (2) considerable expense for the client, (3) discomfort for the client, (4) considerable time spent by the client and cosmetologist, and (5) frequent damage to the hair and scalp.

The **cold wave** was accepted for professional use in 1940. It was called "cold" because it did not require heat. The croquignole wrapping system was still used, but chemicals, instead of heat, were used to curl the hair. This is the method used today.

Cold waving uses a waving solution with a pH of 9.5, a neutralizer, rods, and end wraps. The physical effects of wrapping the hair on rods and the chemical changes produced by the waving solution and neutralizer give the hair its curl.

The liquid that causes the hair shaft to **soften** and **swell** (expand) is called the **waving lotion. End wraps** or end papers are placed on the ends of the hair strand to protect and control it as it is being wound around the **cold-wave rod.** After all the hair strands have been wrapped and the waving lotion has been applied or reapplied, the hair begins to **process.** When the hair has softened enough to make the same size circle as the rod being used, the hair must be **fixed** in this form. This is done by the **neutralizer** (or fixative). The neutralizer **hardens** and **shrinks** the hair shaft and **stops** the action of the waving lotion.

The main advantages of the cold wave over other permanent wave methods are: (1) less expense for both the client and cosmetologist, (2) less equipment and fewer supplies required, (3) faster procedure for wrapping, (4) more comfort for the client, and (5) less time required for service. The modern cold-waving service is also called chemical waving.

KNOWING SUBOBJECTIVE 2

Recently, neutral and acid permanent waves have been introduced by the various manufacturers. The **acid wave** has been the more popular of the two waves. **Acid waves** generally have a pH in the range of 5.8–6.8 (some are a little higher–7.9). Although they are milder for the hair, sometimes they can be harsher on the skin. Because of this, special care must be taken when applying the wave solution. It must be applied only to the hair, and not allowed to drip onto a towel and/or cotton, then left on the skin, which would cause a **chemical burn**.

Describe the difference between acid waves and neutral waves.

 Safety Tip

Neutral waves have a pH in the range of 4.5–5.7, and not many of them have been very successful. All neutral waves and acid waves need heat in order to curl the hair wound around the permanent wave rods. The heat tends to be of two types: heat from a hair dryer and chemical heat. In order for the hair shaft to be "opened" so that the waving solution can penetrate the hair, a plastic cap is placed over the permanent wave rods; then, the client is placed under a hot dryer. Processing is determined by the manufacturer, but "test curls" may be taken as advised by your instructor.

Chemical heat is made by adding an activator chemical to the waving solution just before the application of the waving solution to the rods. This causes the waving lotion to physically "heat-up." A plastic cap is secured around the wound permanent wave rods, and processing is usually determined by the manufacturer's directions. When the manufacturer's directions state that the particular permanent should be processed for 10 minutes, 15 minutes, or 20 minutes etc., this permanent wave is also called a self-timing permanent wave. It is self-timing in the sense that the manufacturer doesn't recommend test curls. The manufacturer feels that the best curl will be achieved on the type of hair indicated in the directions when the product is left on the hair a set period of time. Your instructor will advise you whether test curls should be taken on the particular permanent wave you are using.

Neutral waves and acid waves make up a large part of the permanent waving done today. Together, the pH range of these products is in the range of 4.5 on the low side, and 7.8 on the high side. Remember that some form of heat is necessary for them to effectively curl the hair. It is also necessary to wrap the hair with even, moderate-firm tension in order to break down the hydrogen bonds of the hair to give the final curl the strength and firmness needed to hold the hairstyle in place.

KNOWING SUBOBJECTIVE 3

Describe the effects of cold waving, the basic cold-waving chemicals, and compare the pH, cost, and methods of giving the acid wave and the regular thio cold wave.

Cold waving involves 3 steps that produce physical and chemical effects on the hair:

1. wrapping or winding strands on cold-waving rods (physical effects)
2. processing with waving lotion (chemical effects)
3. neutralizing with a separate solution (chemical effects)

Wrapping the hair on the rods physically breaks the hydrogen cross-bonds that help give the hair its form or shape.

In processing, the waving lotion softens and swells (expands) the hair. It also breaks the cystine (SIS-teen) disulfide (sulfur) bonds that help to maintain the shape of the hair. These bonds are re-formed around the rod. This means that the strand takes the shape, or diameter, of the rod. Thus the hair becomes curly. In the breaking down and re-forming actions on the cystine disulfide bonds, the amino acid **cystine** is changed to a slightly different amino acid, **cysteine**.

When the hair is as curly as you want it to be, apply neutralizer to stop the action of the waving lotion and to change the cysteine back to cystine. The neutralizer **oxidizes** as well as neutralizes. It hardens the disulfide bonds in their new curly formation and shrinks the hair shaft. The hydrogen and salt bonds also are changed, but the change in the cystine disulfide bonds is more important than those in the other bonds.

Cold waves are available in two types: thio and acid. Both have complex formulas that include chemicals to hide unpleasant odors, to buffer harsh ingredients, and to add protein to the lotion.

The most important basic chemical in the thio waving lotion is **thioglycolic acid** (thio). Ammonia is added to the acid to help the lotion penetrate, soften, and swell the hair shaft. With the addition of ammonia, the compound **ammonium thioglycolate** (thio) is formed. The ammonia makes the lotion **alkaline**, with a pH range of 8.5 to 9.5.

Acid waves are made from the same thioglycolate base as thio waves, but acid waves fall in a **lower** pH range of 5.8 to 6.8. They are called acid waves because their pH is closer to acid than regular thio waves. They are also called **ester waves** because of their chemical content. (Esters are formed by the interaction of an alcohol and an acid.)

You may want to try a few acid waves to see their advantages and disadvantages for yourself. They do have a lower pH than thio waves.

The thio wave is basically a **cold** type of wave, although a little body heat is necessary for processing. The acid wave, however, must have much more heat in a more reliable form. The heated clamps used in one method of acid waving remind the experienced cosmetologist of the preheat wave of the 1930s. There is one outstanding advantage of products using this acid-clamp waving method: they cannot be sold over the counter and used at home! (See figure on p. 264.)

At the proper time the action of the waving lotion is stopped by the **neutralizer**, or **fixative**. The basic chemical in most neutralizers is either sodium bromate or 2 percent hydrogen peroxide, though peroxide seems to be preferred by many cosmetologists and manufacturers. Peroxide neutralizers contain water and animal, vegetable, or mineral proteins with the peroxide in 2 percent strength. This preparation oxidizes the waving lotion. **Sodium bromate** is also used as a neutralizer, but its fumes can be combustable. The combustion can occur when soiled neutralizer towels are stored with soiled tint towels. The ammonia fumes from the tint mix with the sodium bromate fumes and combine to make **bromine gas, which can cause a fire**

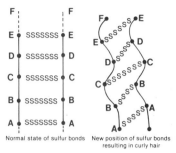

Normal state of sulfur bonds   New position of sulfur bonds resulting in curly hair

Amino acids form proteins, and peptide linkages strengthened by cross bonds

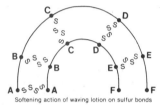

Softening action of waving lotion on sulfur bonds

Cross bonds are broken when hair is stretched on rollers

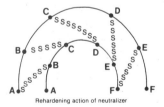

Rehardening action of neutralizer

The bonds are re-formed as hair dries on rollers

KNOWING SUBOBJECTIVE 4

For many years there has been confusion over the terms cold-waving **process** and cold-waving **service**. The process is included in the service. The price quoted for the service usually **includes**: (1) shampoo service, (2) cold-

List other services included in cold waving.

wave wrap, (3) cold-wave process, (4) cold-wave neutralizer, and (5) hair-styling service (setting and combining or air waving, etc.). You would charge extra for a conditioner.

Charges generally are made for conditioning or shaping (cutting). The cost of the cold wave does **not** include hair cutting or conditioning, but it does include services other than the cold wave **process**. Many states have laws that prohibit advertising a cold-wave price that includes the hair shaping. It must be a separate charge; for example, if the cold wave costs $50.00 and the client requests shaping, which costs another $8.00, the total charge would have to be $58.00. Your instructor will tell you what to charge in your particular school.

DOING SUBOBJECTIVE 5

Analyze the hair, and select the proper cold-wave lotion and rods.

Supplies

□ client release form
□ client permanent service form
□ shampoo supplies
□ shampoo cape
□ protein conditioner
□ styling comb
□ 2 extra laundered towels

□ operator apron
□ cold-waving rods
□ cold-waving lotion and neutralizer
□ hair-cutting implements
□ protective garment for client

PROCEDURE

1. Review the client's permanent waving form, noting chemical services that have been received in the past. **Do not brush**, but lightly **shampoo the hair once** after you have analyzed it.

⚡ **Safety Tip**

2. Analyze the porosity and elasticity of the client's hair.

RATIONALE

1. Always review the client's form so that you will know if the hair has been tinted, frosted, or when the last cold wave was given. Brushing and **excessive** shampooing may irritate the client's scalp and may cause a cold-wave (chemical) burn.

2. This is standard procedure.

3. Carefully **inspect** the condition of the client's **scalp**. Ask the client what, if any, home and professional chemical services he or she has used in the past 12 months.

4. Consider the **texture** and **color** of the client's hair. Determine if the hair is fine, medium, or coarse. Natural red and coarse gray hair will be more difficult to wave than other types and colors.

5. Assess the density and length of the client's hair.

6. Comb through the hair to determine whether it was **cut** with a **razor** or **scissors**. Ask the client if you are uncertain.

3. Cold waving is **not** permitted if **cuts, abrasions**, or **red irritation** appear on the scalp. Consult your instructor if necessary. Discoloration and breakage can result if a professional cold wave is given to hair dyed with home products containing a metallic salt tint. Some discoloration (color removal) will occur even if professional products were used in tinting.

4. Fine hair is fragile and may require a milder strength lotion than medium or coarse hair. If the hair has been tinted or frosted, use a lotion that is milder than one for medium or coarse hair, although coarse hair also may be very porous.

5. If the hair per square inch is very dense, smaller partings and larger rods seem to wave best. **Very sparse (thin) hair waves best when small partings and small rods are used.** If the hair is quite long (over 6 inches), you may wish to use the procedure for cold waving long hair.

6. Razor cuts **may** have removed too much bulk from the ends of the hair strand. In this case the end has less resistance to cold-waving lotion and becomes frizzy or fuzzy. To avoid this, blunt cut the hair (with scissors) prior to waving and wrap it properly.

Safety Tip

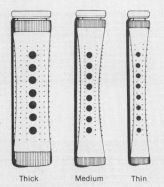
Thick   Medium   Thin

The size of the rod determines the degree of curliness

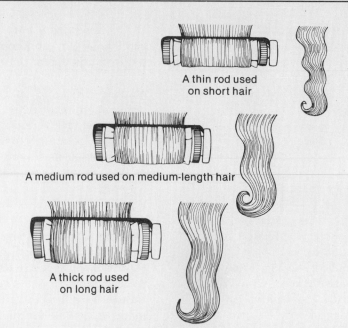

A thin rod used
on short hair

A medium rod used on medium-length hair

A thick rod used
on long hair

7. Ask the client the amount of curl desired—body, soft, or firm wave. Request picture(s) of the desired hairstyle and consider the length of the style shown.

8. Ask the client how often he or she gets a professional cold wave.

7. The **diameter** of the cold-wave rods and the **number** of rods used will determine the degree of which the hair will wave or curl. Large, straight rods or concave rods can be used for a body wave. As noted in the chapter on sculpture curling, the hair **must** rotate 1½ to 2½ turns to **wave**. A **soft** to **medium** curl will result from 2½ to 3½ turns. A **firm** cold wave formation will be produced by 3¾ or more turns. For hair that is **not** very porous, add 1 additional turn (rotation) to the above numbers. The size of the parting (blocking) also determines the size of the curl pattern.

8. The client who schedules a cold wave **once** or **twice** per year probably is accustomed to a **firm** curl. On the other hand, one who gets a cold wave 3 or 4 times per year may need only a soft or body wave.

9. Recommend a particular wave to the client, stating the reason for the choice. If you make more than one recommendation, explain the differences.

9. Always explain the reason(s) for particular recommendations. If different waves may be used, explain the differences of their effects on the hair. Similarly, if 3 prices are discussed, explain their advantages.

10. Lightly shampoo the hair once with a mild acid-balanced product.

10. Cleanse the hair and scalp, but do not manipulate the scalp to the extent that scalp circulation is increased. Mild, **good** cleansing and acid-balanced shampoos are preferred, unless an acid wave is to be used. If an acid wave is to be used, an alkaline shampoo gives better results.

11. Observe whether the hair absorbs water easily.

11. This will help you determine the porosity of the hair.

12. Shape the hair if necessary.

12. The client's hair may need blunt scissor cutting to eliminate the possibility of frizzy or fuzzy ends.

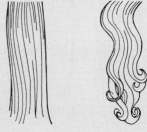

Tapered cut

13. Condition the hair if necessary.

13. Preconditioning may be necessary to equalize the hair's porosity. **If the hair is conditioned too much, the hair shaft may not have room for the waving solution.** Thus, the waving solution may not penetrate the hair shaft. Be guided by your instructor when selecting a conditioner to be used **before** cold waving.

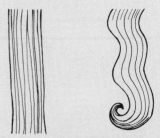

Blunt cut

14. Dry the hair according to manufacturer's directions.

14. Label directions vary from brand to brand, so it is necessary to read directions carefully.

15. If you must leave the client to get supplies, let the client know.

15. Once a chemical process has actually been started, **never** leave a client unattended without letting him or her know where you are going!

16. Select a waving lotion, neutralizer, and additives.

16. Waving lotions come in different strengths for hair that is: (1) overporous—bleached (lightened)—mildest lotion; (2) a little overporous—tinted—mild lotion; (3) slightly overporous—fine or medium—mild lotion; (4) not very porous—normal—medium lotion; and (5) slightly porous or resistant—coarse—strong lotion. Most cosmetologists who are concerned that a solution may be **too strong** for the client's hair use the next milder lotion. For example, if the client has frosted hair, the strength for tinted or bleached hair is used. If that strength does not produce a curl, the hair is towel-blotted and the next strongest solution is used. Certain systems for cold waving the hair require the addition of protein to the waving lotion and vitamins to the neutralizer, etc. Follow the advice of your instructor.

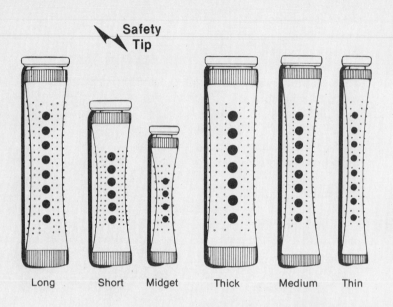

Safety Tip

Long   Short   Midget   Thick   Medium   Thin

17. Select cold-wave rods that are appropriate for the length of the client's hair and the amount of curl desired.

17. Cold-wave rods are concave, round, or oval. They are wood, plastic, or nylon. They are long, short, or very short (midget). The hair must be wound around the rod two complete turns in order to achieve a wave pattern.

DOING SUBOBJECTIVE 6

Section (block) and subsection the client's hair and wrap it on cold-waving rods.

Supplies

☐ timer
☐ end wraps
☐ rat-tail comb or styling comb
☐ one dozen double-prong clips

☐ surgical or rubber gloves
☐ cold-wave processing overcap
☐ protective cream
☐ cotton coil
☐ plastic applicator bottle

PROCEDURE

1. Test curl 2 or 3 strands of hair in the lower crown. Using the length of the rods selected, section (block) off the hair and secure with double-prong clips.

RATIONALE

1. Whenever in doubt, use test curls to determine the curlability of the hair. Use waving lotion and neutralize according to directions. The length of each section (strand of hair) can be measured by the length of the rods selected. Although there are 5 generally accepted sectioning (blocking) patterns, preference of one pattern over another will **not** make much difference in the finished hairstyle. The size of the client's head seems to determine which pattern should be selected and the outcome of the hairstyle. Commonly used patterns follow:

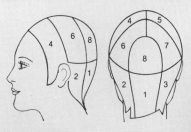

Wrapping order

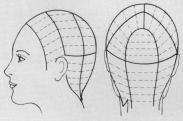

Wrapping pattern

(a) **Double horseshoe (halo)** for larger head sizes.

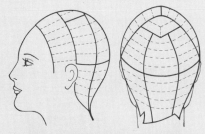

(b) **Single horseshoe (halo)** for small-to-average head sizes.

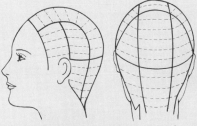

(c) **Straight-away (back)** for bouffant, off-the-face hairstyles.

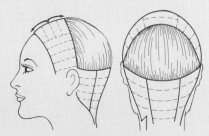

(d) **Modified straight-away** for 6- to 8-inch hair, where the hair in the crown will be combed flat or close to the head. This may also be called a dropped-crown wrapping pattern.

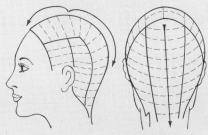

(e) **Forward wrap** for larger than average head sizes. Consult the instructor for assistance as needed.

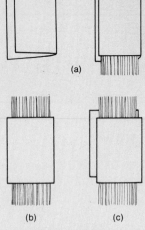

(a) Bookend fold; (b) single-end straight (c) double-end straight

2. Put on surgical gloves or apply protective cream to your hands. Select the appropriate wrapping method for end papers and begin wrapping the middle nape section.

3. Use a rat-tail comb (or styling comb) to part the strand and horizontally wind it on the rod. The size of the rod will determine the size of the subsection.

4. Check waving-lotion label and cap seal. Pour 1 ounce of lotion into the applicator bottle. Cap the lotion and screw the applicator nozzle on the bottle after adjusting lotion.

2. Waving lotion may irritate your hands. End papers serve to protect porous ends of the hair, thus minimizing the possibility of "fishhook" ends. Papers also allow you to smooth the hair evenly across the rod, which makes the hair more controllable. There are 3 basic wrapping methods:

(a) **Book-end fold**
(b) **Single-end straight**
(c) **Double-end straight**

3. Either comb may be used, depending on advice from your instructor. Rectangular subsections should be slightly **less** than the **length** of the rod but the **same** diameter.

4. Check the seal to be sure that the lotion is active. The **seal should not** be broken. Always double-check the label to make sure that the lotion, **not** the neutralizer, is used to wrap hair. The formula of the lotion may be adjusted by the instructor to improve the product's performance. Tell your instructor if the seal is broken.

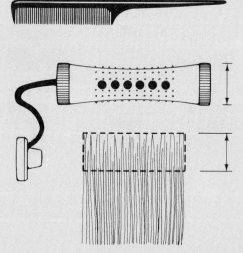

5. Apply waving lotion ½–1 inch from the scalp before wrapping **each** strand. Another method is to apply waving solution or water to the entire section to be wrapped, then reapply only if the hair becomes too dry to wrap. The hair may also be wrapped in water. Secure each rod by inserting the button attached to the elastic in the opposite end of the rod. The elastic should **not** "bind" the hair next to the scalp.

6. Using horizontal partings, complete wrapping in the center nape section.

7. Wrap the other sections, following the numbered sequence [see double horseshoe (a)] you used to wrap the nape sections. Carefully consider the length of the hair in each section before you wrap. **Do not apply excessive tension** to the hair. Apply moderate, even tension.

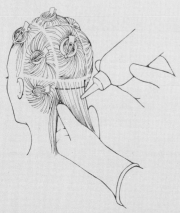

5. A **small** amount of waving lotion will run along the strand toward the scalp, and **natural body heat** will process the scalp hair quickly when the lotion is **reapplied** after the entire head has been wound. When practicing wrapping on a mannequin, or just beginning in a clinical experience center, you may be advised to wrap by moistening (not saturating) the hair with water. **Binding scalp hair with the elastic band will cause the hair to break!**

6. Because the nape hair is thought to be more resistant, requiring more processing time, schools usually advocate beginning in this section, although advanced students may use other methods. Moistening the hair only with water will soften the hydrogen bonds of the hair. They are softened further when the hair is wound around the rod.

7. Wrapping the hair in sections that are too large will result in incomplete penetration of lotion. As the length of hair **increases**, a larger (diameter) rod must be used because a small rod will require too many rotations for long hair. Hair should be wrapped **firmly** and evenly across the rod. (Do not forget, though, that the **chemical** action of the thio causes the hair to curl.) **If too much tension** (stretching) is used on the hair, the hair will break! A combination of overstretching and overprocessing also can cause the hair to appear frizzy when wet and too straight when dry. This is called **overprocessing**.

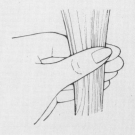

 Safety Tip

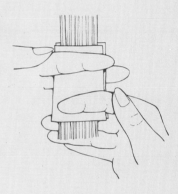

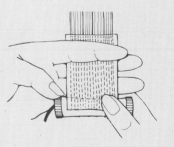

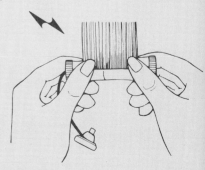

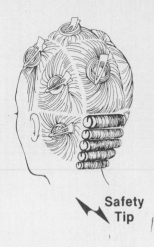

Safety Tip

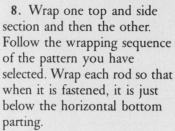

8. Wrap one top and side section and then the other. Follow the wrapping sequence of the pattern you have selected. Wrap each rod so that when it is fastened, it is just below the horizontal bottom parting.

8. Wrapping the hair this way will give maximum curl.

9. Wrap the crown sections smoothly and without too much tension to complete the wrapping procedure.

9. The hair is saturated more thoroughly when it is not wound too tightly. The hair must have room to **swell** when the lotion is applied. If wound too tightly, the hair cannot swell and may **break**.

10. Check the width of **each** subsection and compare it to the diameter of the rod that you are using.

10. To achieve uniform curl, wrap the hair according to the rod's length and diameter. Consult the instructor for an evaluation.

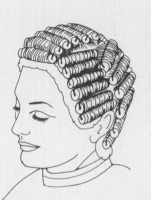

11. Check the length of each subsection and compare it to the rod used.

11. Same as step 10.

12. Check the elastic band of each rod to insure that none is binding the scalp hair. Adjust the bands if necessary. Unwind two or three rods immediately to test the curl.

12. If you used waving lotion to wrap the hair, it is fragile because of the softening effect of thio. Improperly placed elastic bands can therefore cause the hair to break. Whether you use water or lotion for wrapping, always test the curl immediately.

Safety Tip

13. Apply a piece of cotton coil around the hairline.

13. Cotton prevents the lotion from running into the client's eyes or ears and onto the face.

Application of Waving Solution

PROCEDURE

1. Prepare waving solution according to manufacturer's direction.

RATIONALE

1. Since some solutions are activated by adding two or more chemicals together, it is necessary to read the directions of each manufacturer.

2. Take special note that the waving solution you are about to use is waving solution.

2. If you are not careful, you may be applying the neutralizer in place of the waving solution.

3. Hand the client a clean, dry towel.

3. Should any waving solution drip into the client's eye(s), ear(s), face etc., advise the client to blot, **not rub,** the solution. Should waving solution drip into the client's eye(s), **flush area with cool water,** then **apply cool water to a clean towel** and blot affected area. If eye irritation persists, consult instructor. You may have to take client to a physician.

 Safety Tip

4. Beginning in the bottom of the nape section, apply a **very small amount** of waving solution to all rods in this section. Repeat until all rods in each section have been lightly saturated. Be careful and avoid dragging the nozzle of the applicator bottle across the hair on the wound rods. Should the **solution drip purple** from the hair, continue with procedure.

5. Wait 60 seconds. Reapply waving solution to each rod. Apply only the amount of solution that the hair will accept (absorb).

4. Since the hair has probably dried out, it will not readily absorb the waving solution and may drip onto the client's face, eyes, ears, or neck. Minerals in the client's hair may cause this discoloration. The client has probably been shampooing their hair using "hard water." This will not usually affect the permanent wave.

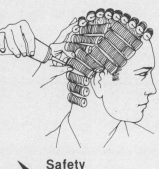

 Safety Tip

5. The 60-second wait will allow the hair to become slightly wet. The **capillary action** set up by applying a small amount of solution in the previous step will allow the hair to neatly "suck-up" the additional solution you are applying now. Slightly wet hair will absorb any solution much more readily than dry hair. This procedure will almost eliminate the need for cotton and an excessive number of towels.

6. Blot any excess waving solution that may be on the scalp between the rods. **Check neck towel for dampness. If towel is wet—change it.**

6. If waving solution is allowed to collect between the rods, or on the towel that is next to the client's neck, **a chemical burn will result!**

 Safety Tip

DOING SUBOBJECTIVE 7

Process and neutralize the cold wave.

Supplies

- ☐ timer
- ☐ end wraps
- ☐ rat-tail comb or styling comb
- ☐ one dozen double- prong clips

- ☐ surgical or rubber gloves
- ☐ cold-wave processing overcap
- ☐ protective cream
- ☐ cotton coil
- ☐ plastic applicator bottle

Safety Tip

PROCEDURE

1. Remove the saturated cotton protective strip and neck towel. Replace towel.

2. Immediately test the curl in one rod in the nape, the crown, and the front side. Unwind the rod 1¾ to 2 turns.

3. Look for a well-defined "S" formation of the depth equal to the rod diameter.

4. If very little wave appears in the test curls, touch the client's hand to see if his or her body temperature is normal or cool.

RATIONALE

1. The **cotton and the neck towel can cause a chemical burn** if they are left on the skin **after they have become saturated.**

2. Hair may be adequately curled immediately or within 12 minutes. The temperature of the client's body, the room, and the waving lotion affect the processing time of the wave.

3. When a **strong "S"** pattern is observed in each section and back-to-back "S" formations appear, the hair has processed to its maximum.

4. The client **may** be cold from the air conditioning in the building. You can place the plastic overcap on his or her head to keep what body heat there is around the waving lotion. If the hair is waving properly in one section but not in another, use the cap; then place your hand on the cap where curls are processing slowly. The heat from your hand will accelerate the chemical action of the lotion in this part of the head.

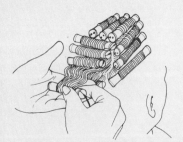

Definite "S" pattern; unwrap rod a maximum of 2 turns

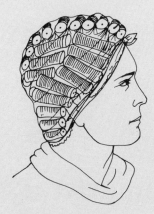

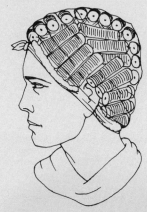

5. Using the timer, test curl **different** rods in each section of the head every 2 to 3 minutes.

6. Test curl a rod in each section of the head.

7. Hand the client a towel saturated with cold water and advise him or her to blot any solution that may drip onto the forehead or around the hairline. **If a plastic cap is used to cover rods, do not fasten it too tightly, as breakage may occur around the hairline.**

8. Test curl to the maximum processing time. Escort the client to shampoo area to neutralize the hair.

9. Using tepid to warm water, thoroughly rinse the waving lotion from the hair. Ask the client if the water temperature is too warm. Adjust temperature accordingly.

5. The hair may curl very quickly, so frequent checking is necessary to avoid overprocessing. Since hair is very fragile after waving lotion has been applied, **do not check the same rod twice.**

6. If there is no apparent curling after 10 minutes, gently blot rods with a towel saturated with warm–hot water. Apply the **next strongest** waving lotion. The first lotion may have been too weak. If the waving lotion is stored in a very cool part of the building, warm it up by placing the bottle in tepid water. Natural body heat and room temperature (72°F.) are needed for proper processing. **Ask your instructor for help in deciding the right method to use for processing the cold wave.**

7. Cold water helps neutralize the alkalinity of the waving lotion. Tell the client to **blot**, not rub, because **rubbing may irritate the skin and cause a chemical burn.**

8. Consult your instructor immediately before rinsing waving lotion.

9. Warm water not only rinses the waving lotion from the hair, but it also provides oxygen that begins to partially oxidize and neutralize the waving lotion.

Safety Tip

Plastic cap must be loose enough so fine or weak hair doesn't break! Check neck towel for wetness, and change if wet. Second coil of cotton must replace first one used for initial saturation of hair, or a chemical burn will result

10. Read the neutralizing directions that are packaged with the product.

10. Manufacturer's directions generally work best, but 2 other methods may be used. Altogether, there are 3 methods:

(a) **Instant**—Usually 5 to 10 minutes.

(b) **Splash**—A small sponge or piece of cotton is used to "splash" the neutralizer over the rods and through the hair. Neutralizer is caught in a bowl placed below the rods at the bottom of the basin; then it is poured and repoured over the rods for 10 minutes.

(c) **Self-neutralizing**—The hair is blotted, not rinsed, with a damp towel and then allowed to air dry naturally. Then, rods are removed, and the hair is rinsed thoroughly. Follow with a light shampoo to remove any excess cold-wave lotion odor; set as usual. In this case, the oxygen in the air and water oxidizes and neutralizes the hair. This method works well, but it takes a long time.

11. Obtain dispensary scissors to cut off the top of the neutralizer bottle.

11. Use an old pair of scissors to cut the top off of the neutralizer bottle. Neutralizer will corrode styling scissors, so usually there is a pair of dispensary shears used just for this purpose.

12. Mix the neutralizer and additives as needed.

12. Many schools and salons feel that since the cuticle of the hair shaft is in the open position, conditioners will penetrate better if they are mixed with the neutralizer. So, when the hair is **rehardened** and **shrunk** by the neutralizer, maximum conditioning can occur. Follow the advice of your instructor for the best results.

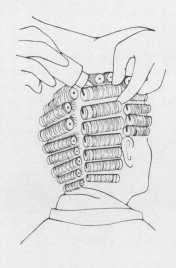

13. Gently towel-blot each rod.

13. Since the hair is soft and swollen, it is very fragile; it can break if you manipulate the towel too firmly.

14. Attach the neutralizing bib along the client's hairline and secure it at the center of the forehead.

14. The bib protects the client's ears and clothing from the neutralizer. It also catches the neutralizer in a pocket attached at the bottom so that neutralizer can be reapplied if desired. Neutralizing bibs have elastic around their perimeters, which may bind and possibly break the hair. Be careful! Bibs usually fasten with a **metal** eye hook near the center of the forehead. Cotton should be placed beneath the hook to prevent skin irritation.

Safety Tip

15. Apply neutralizer across the top and bottom of each rod; begin in the nape section and work forward. Ask the client to assume a sitting, rather than a lying, position during neutralization.

15. Applying neutralizer to the top and bottom of the rod insures thorough penetration across the hair. Neutralizer causes the **cysteine** in the hair to change **back to cystine**. (See subobjective 3.) The curl is "locked in." The weight of the client's head against the neck of the shampoo bowl could break the hair.

Safety Tip

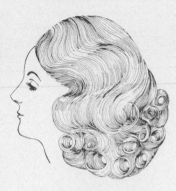

16. After 10 minutes, rinse thoroughly with tepid, then cool, water. Gently towel-blot the hair and ask your instructor if additional reconditioning is necessary.

17. Remove the rods and end papers, carefully unwinding them without pulling or stretching the hair.

18. Consult your instructor to evaluate the results of the cold wave. Record the results on the cold-wave card.

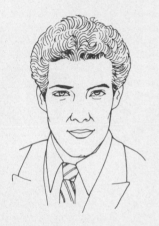

19. Discuss an appointment for the client 1 week from the date of the cold wave.

16. This removes excess neutralizer not absorbed by the hair.

17. The hair is still somewhat fragile, so you must be careful not to break the hair by stretching or pulling.

18. Your work should be evaluated continually by your instructor. **Make notes on the client's cold-wave record regarding products used, rod sizes, timing, and recommendations for future cold-waving services.** Cold-wave cards provide other useful information.

19. Always recommend the need to schedule an appointment 1 week from the date of the cold wave. This is an opportunity to determine if service was satisfactory and to correct any errors. If a couple of areas on the head are not curly enough, **pickup curls** may be used (only) for those spots.

DOING SUBOBJECTIVE 8

Subsection, wrap, process, and neutralize a ponytail cold wave on long hair.

Supplies

- client release form
- client permanent service form
- shampoo supplies
- shampoo cape
- protein conditioner
- styling comb
- 2 extra laundered towels
- operator apron

- cold-waving rods
- cold-waving lotion and neutralizer
- hair cutting implements
- protective garment for client
- 24 rubber binders (bands)
- scissors

PROCEDURE

1. Prepare client as for any cold-waving service. Discuss the advantages of the ponytail cold-waving method with the client. Also discuss the cost.

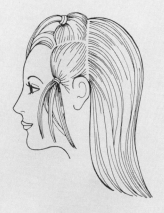

2. After you have analyzed the condition of the hair, use a brush to subsection it. Secure each subsection with a rubber binder.

3. Secure the hair in rectangular subsections until all of it is held by rubber bands in columns (or rows) of ponytails.

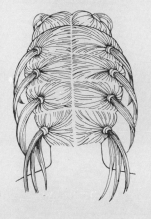

4. Select rods according to the desired curl. Spiral wrap each strand around the rod.

5. Begin wrapping at the bottom subsection of the right side, using 5 or 7 rods in each ponytail. If you use a lotion, apply it 1 inch from the elastic binder. Continue until you have wrapped all sections of hair.

6. Test the curl immediately. (If spiral rods are used, take test curl from top of rod by unwinding strand 1½ turns to check for "S" pattern.)

RATIONALE

1. The client should understand what service will be given. The advantage of the ponytail cold wave is that curl is given only on the ends; long hair does not need curl at the scalp. Placing a binder in subsections of hair and using rods only in the hair ends makes sense. The client should agree to the cost of the services.

2. A brush gives better control of long hair than a comb does. The rubber binders secure the hair next to the scalp so that only the extreme ends are curled.

3. This allows you to work in uniform, well-defined sections and makes the wrapping procedure easier. The hair is curled more evenly, too.

4. Using the guides previously discussed in this unit, select the appropriate rod sizes.

5. Since the wound rods hang down, they would be in the way if wrapping started on the top of each subsection. **If lotion is applied too close to rubber (elastic) binders, hair breakage will result from the tension of the binder.**

6. Always test the curl even if the hair is wrapped with water. Water breaks the hydrogen bonds; if a sharp wave pattern appears, the hair will quickly curl (process) when waving lotion is applied.

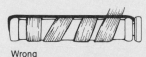

Safety Tip

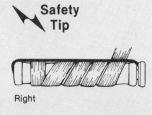

Right

Wrong

Finished "body-wave"

7. When you feel the hair has the proper curl, test the curl again in the presence of your instructor before you neutralize the hair.

8. Use a scissors to cut the elastic bands from each subsection.

9. Set or air wave the hair.

7. If the hair is neutralized before it is curly enough, the curl will be **underprocessed**. To make sure the curl is accurate, consult your instructor **before** rinsing or neutralizing the hair.

8. It is faster, easier, and safer to cut the elastic bands.

9. This is standard procedure.

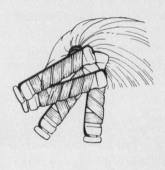

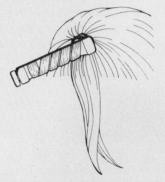

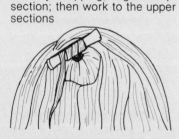

Pony-tail piggy-back wrap gives an *even* curl to long hair. When actually wrapping, begin in *nape* section; then work to the upper sections

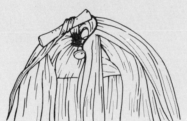

Spiral hair around rod using even tension. An end wrap is not needed for this step

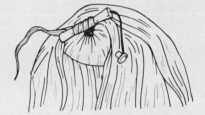

Wrap until hair covers most of permanent wave rod

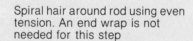

Fasten at bottom of wound rod

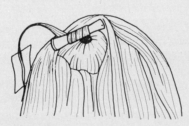

Put end wrap on the ends of the hair strand

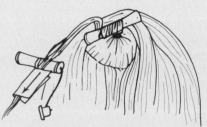

Slide end wrap down the strand, so end wrap extends beyond hair ends. Use spiral wrap and complete wrapping to other rod

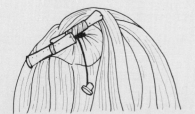

After wrapping short ends, secure
fastener at bottom of rod

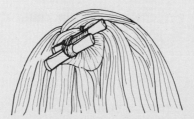

The number of sections, the
number of subsections, and
rod size will be determined by
the length and texture of the
hair and the degree of curl
desired by client

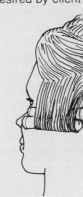

Twin wrap for longer hair lengths

DOING SUBOBJECTIVE 9

No matter how careful you are when permanent waving the client's hair, it seems that occasionally the client will complain that the permanent wave is too tight. Should this occur, you will find this doing subobjective very helpful for relaxing the client's hair to the desired degree of curliness. This procedure may also be used on naturally curly hair—provided the hair is **not** super curly. The following procedure will allow the hair to be relaxed without excessive hair damage, and the steps are relatively simple to follow. Your instructor may have a better procedure, or require you to use a particular type of cholesterol.

Relaxing an overcurly permanent, or naturally wavy hair.

Supplies

- □ towels
- □ comb (with coarse teeth)
- □ shampoo cape
- □ one tube (approximately 2 ounces) of cholesterol (check with instructor for specific brand)

- □ cold waving solution
- □ plastic or glass mixing bowl
- □ cold wave neutralizer
- □ mixing brush (and/or electric or manual mixer).

Preparation: (Drape client for a chemical service)

PROCEDURE	RATIONALE
1. Analyze the condition of the client's hair and scalp, then select waving solution. Prepare normal strength waving solution according to label directions. Do not shampoo hair.	**1.** Hair should not be dry, frizzy, or brittle, or breakage may occur. **Don't use this procedure** on hair that has been tinted or bleached as the hair will be damaged. Some waving solutions require mixing.

Safety Tip

PROCEDURE	RATIONALE
2. Squeeze an entire tube of cholesterol into the mixing bowl. Add a small amount of waving solution and blend with cholesterol using mixing brush (or electric mixer). Continue to add waving solution until your 3–4 oz. bottle is smoothly blended into a creamy mixture.	**2.** The cholesterol waters down the strength of the waving solution, and protects the hair from becoming dry. **Unless the waving solution is added slowly, it won't mix with the cholesterol**—it will separate and will not work correctly.
3. Escort client to shampoo chair.	**3.** Since dripping can become a problem, this service should be performed in the shampoo bowl area.

Application of Curl Relaxing Solution

PROCEDURE	RATIONALE
1. Begin application in the curliest section of the head first. If the hair is curly all over, begin application in the nape section of the head first. Then work your way toward the top of the head. Excess solution should be allowed to drip into the shampoo bowl.	**1.** The curliest hair will take longer to relax, so it is wise to begin applying relaxer solution in that area first. By systematically beginning in the nape first, you will be evenly applying the relaxing solution to all of the hair.
2. Continue applying solution with applicator bottle or applicator brush until all sections of the hair have been saturated with relaxing solution.	**2.** If all sections of hair are to be relaxed, it is imporant to apply solution evenly.

3. Carefully comb solution through hair using **coarse** teeth of comb. Change neck towel should it become saturated with relaxing solution. **Do not allow any solution to drip** into the client's eyes, ears, or on the client's face or clothing.

3. Combing the hair with the fine teeth of the comb, or combing the hair firmly, flat against the head may cause breakage. If solution should contact the client's skin, **flush area with tepid water**. Cool water may not rinse the cholesterol from the skin.

Safety Tip

Processing the Curl Relaxer

PROCEDURE

1. Continue to slowly comb the hair for about five minutes. Allow hair to process to the desired degree of straightness. If the hair is very resistant, you may want to place a plastic cap over the processing hair. A hot dryer is also used for 10 minutes if the hair fails to relax in 15 minutes.

2. Strand test every 3–5 minutes to check straightening action. When the hair appears shiny, feels silky, and looks straight, it probably has processed sufficiently.

RATIONALE

1. Combing the hair into a straighter position allows the curl to relax more evenly and quickly. Placing the client under the dryer to straighten resistant hair speeds up the straightening process by giving better penetration of the relaxing solution for resistant hair.

2. Check hair to insure that it is processing properly, but not overprocessing. Put client under a dryer for 10–15 minutes to achieve better penetration of the hair shaft if hair is resistant.

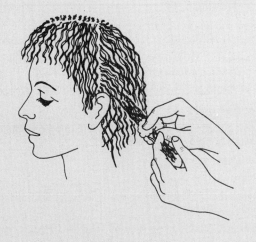

Neutralizing the Curl Relaxer

Safety Tip

PROCEDURE

1. Thoroughly rinse hair with comfortably warm water, then towel blot as much moisture as possible from hair.

2. Using the coarse teeth of your comb, begin combing in the nape section. Carefully comb the hair downward to a straight position. Air dry for 5 minutes. **Apply neutralizier** according to manufacturers' direction.

3. Condition as needed and style the hair.

RATIONALE

1. Rinsing stops the straightening action and begins the neutralizing process. **The scalp may be sensitive**, but the water must be warm enough to rinse the solution from the hair.

2. Use the coarse teeth of the comb and begin in the nape to avoid overstretching of the hair. Air assists the hair in the neutralizing process. Since almost all manufacturers "buffer" their neutralizers, there is no need to worry about lightening the hair—even with a peroxide neutralizer.

3. This is standard procedure.

GLOSSARY

Acid wave   A type of permanent wave which has a pH of 5.8–7.9; milder for the hair than the thio wave.

Capillary action   The method by which the hair "sucks up" the second application of waving solution after the small first application of it.

Chemical heat   Heat generated by adding an activator chemical to the waving solution.

Cold waving   Hair-curling method using chemicals to wave the hair.

Croquignole (KROH-kehn-ohl)   A method of wrapping hair from the ends to the scalp.

Cross-bonds   Structures that help hold the hair's internal structure together.

Cysteine (SIS-tee-ehn)   An amino acid that is formed from cystine when hair is processed with a cold-waving solution.

Cystine (SIS-teen) disulfide cross-bonds   Bonds that help give hair its shape.

End papers   See **End wraps**.

End wraps   Paper placed at the end of a hair strand to protect and control it as it is being wound around the cold-waving rod.

Ester waves   See **Acid waves**.

Fixative   See **Neutralizer**.

Machineless permanent   Hair curling that used chemical pads that heated up when moistened with water.

Machine permanent   Hair-curling method that used electrically heated clamps placed over the client's hair.

Neutralizer   A solution that stops (fixes) the action of waving lotion by hardening and shrinking the hair shaft.

Neutralizing   Stopping the activity of the waving lotion.

Neutral wave   A type of permanent wave which has a pH of 4.5–5.7.

Preheat permanent   Hair-curling method that used large heated clamps to curl hair. Unlike earlier methods it did not bring electricity close to the client's head.

Processing   The action of waving lotion on the hair.

Self-timing permanent wave   A type of permanent wave for which the manufacturer does not recommend test curls.

Spiral wrap   Method of wrapping hair from the scalp to the ends.

Thio   See **Thioglycolic acid.**

Thioglycolic (thigh-oh-gligh-KOL-ik) acid   The most important chemical in cold-waving lotion. It causes the hair to soften and swell.

Waving lotion   A liquid that causes the hair shaft to soften and swell.

Wrapping   Winding hair on rollers or cold-wave rods.

QUESTIONS

1. During cold waving, how are the physical and chemical hair bonds broken?
2. How does waving lotion affect the hair shaft?
3. In what two ways does the neutralizer affect the hair shaft?
4. What determines the degree to which the hair is curled?
5. After applying the waving lotion, why should you remove the cotton around the hairline?
6. Does cold waving solution soften or swell the hair?
7. Can the neutralizer swell the hair?
8. True or false. Neutralizer shrinks the hair.
9. Are sulfur bonds and cystine disulfide bonds the same?
10. Can the neutralizer oxidize the hair?
11. What is the basic chemical in a cold waving solution?
12. What is the pH range of a cold waving solution using ammonium thioglycolate?
13. Is hydrogen peroxide ever used as the active chemical in cold waving neutralizer?
14. Some cold wave neutralizers contain sodium _____.
15. Is cold wave neutralizer also a fixative?
16. What determines the degree of curliness when giving a permanent wave?
17. In order to achieve a wave pattern, how many turns must the hair be wound around the rod?
18. If the client is allergic to the neutralizer, how would you neutralize the hair?

ANSWERS

1. Physical—winding; chemical—waving lotion **2.** It softens and swells the hair shaft **3.** It shrinks and hardens the hair shaft **4.** The diameter (size) of the rod and the number of them used **5.** To prevent a chemical burn on the skin **6.** Both **7.** No **8.** True **9.** Yes **10.** Yes **11.** Ammonium thioglycolate **12.** 8.5-9.5 **13.** Yes **14.** Bromate **15.** Yes **16.** The size of the rods used **17.** Two and one half (2½) **18.** Blot with damp towel, and allow hair to air dry naturally

Chemically Relaxing the Hair 19

In the previous chapter, you learned about the cold-waving methods used to give hair the right amount of curl. Many people don't have to worry about putting curl in their hair. They have the opposite problem: they have more curl than they want.

Until 20 or 30 years ago, if you had very curly or **super-curly** hair, you had quite a real problem. The kinds of hairstyles you could wear were rather limited. Many people, both then and now, have liked curly hairstyles. But today people who have very curly or **super-curly** hair have an advantage. They can change easily to a style with less curl in it because the products used to relax hair have been improved greatly in recent years. Hair that is very curly or super-curly can be relaxed and styled with sculpture curls or rollers without much difficulty today.

Purpose

Using a professional hair-relaxing kit, relax the client's hair to permit setting with sculpture curls or rollers in a style for less curly hair.

Major Objective

Use the proper safety precautions, label directions, and proper steps to straighten the hair. If you use a **no-base** relaxer, apply the relaxing creme in 15 minutes. If a base relaxer is used, apply both the base and relaxing creme in 30 minutes.

Level of Acceptability

1. Describe chemical relaxing and straightening.
2. Describe the difference between a base and a no-base relaxer.
3. Identify safety precautions used in chemical relaxing and straightening services.

Knowing Subobjectives

4. Apply a base chemical relaxer to virgin hair.

Doing Subobjective

KNOWING SUBOBJECTIVE 1

Describe chemical relaxing and straightening.

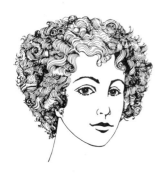

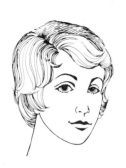

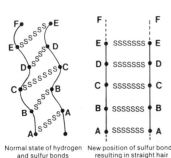

F E
E D
D C
C B
B A
A

Normal state of hydrogen and sulfur bonds

F F
E SSSSSSS E
D SSSSSSS D
C SSSSSSS C
B SSSSSSS B
A SSSSSSS A

New position of sulfur bonds resulting in straight hair

Hair bonding

Cosmetologists and their clients sometimes use the terms **chemical straightening** and **chemical relaxing** to mean the same thing. These terms actually refer to two different chemical processes. **Chemical straightening** is relaxing naturally wavy hair with products that contain ammonium thioglycolate. **Chemical relaxing** usually is used to describe relaxing super-curly hair with products that have **sodium hydroxide** (SOH-dee-uhm high-DRAHK-sighd). **Ammonium thioglycolate** (thio) and sodium hydroxide (caustic soda) produce different effects on the hair.

Thio can quickly relax naturally wavy hair without breaking it, but it is not strong enough to relax super-curly hair in a short time. If it is left on this type of hair long enough to relax it, it also may break it. Sodium hydroxide is most often used to straighten super-curly hair. It is too strong for naturally wavy hair. If you use it on naturally wavy hair, it may dissolve or break the hair.

Terms are like tools, in a way. People use what feels most comfortable and works best for them. So, you may use the terms "chemical straightening" and "chemical relaxing" interchangeably as long as you remember their different chemical effects and applications.

Even the terms "straightener" or "straightening service" are not completely accurate. Chemicals make the hair straighter, but they **should not** make the hair completely straight. If you straightened the client's hair completely, it would not have enough curl (body) to hold the hairstyle. The professional terms that more accurately describe this process are **chemical relaxing** and a **chemical relaxer**. Chemical relaxers also are called **perms**.

Hair relaxers are usually packaged in a kit that includes a variety of products.

The **base creme** is an ointment that **protects** the scalp from irritation or burns that could be caused by the relaxer creme.

The relaxer creme is a complex formula of **sodium hydroxide** or **ammonium thioglycolate**; however, most professional relaxers used today contain sodium hydroxide, which requires considerable instruction, supervision, and practice. With a pH of 11.5 to 14, a sodium hydroxide relaxer is very caustic, but it is **preferred** over ammonium thioglycolate (pH 8.5–9.5) for super-curly hair, because the thio products have a tendency to break this type of hair if they are left on long enough to relax it. Ammonium thioglycolate also tends to allow the hair to revert to its original curliness in humid climates. As in most cases, the final choice of product is yours.

Of course, hair varies from person to person, and you will need to control the relaxer. The neutralizing shampoo helps you to get just the right effect. It **stops** the softening and straightening action of the thio or sodium hydroxide relaxer. It is also called the **neutralizer, stabilizer**, or **fixative**. This shampoo is made especially for stabilizing (stopping) the strong chemical process, so this shampoo is used only in chemical relaxing. No other process in the salon uses a shampoo in this way. The neutralizing shampoo not only

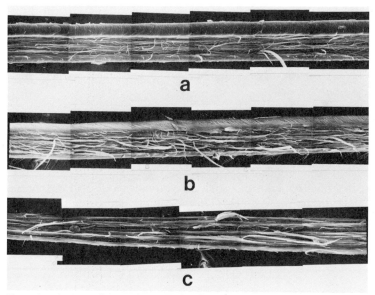

(Scanning electron micrograph supplied by Scruples)

The scan electron micrographs here show dramatically the changes which take place in the hair with the application of chemicals. Hair *a* is a normal, undamaged hair. Note the cuticle still tightly adheres, forming a protective barrier against damage. (500X)

Hair *b* shows damage by treatment with a thio permanent wave solution. Note how the cuticle has been partially eroded. This erosion allows the oozing-out of the cement-like micropolysaccharide within the cortex. The loss of this cement causes the fibers to become detached from their bundles. (600X)

Hair *c* shows treatment with a sodium hydroxide relaxer. Note the total absence of cuticle. Unprotected by the cuticle layer, the cortical fibers show excessive damage from the loss of the micropolysaccharide cement. The detaching of the fibers from the cortical bundles is even more visible here, as well as the loss of hair strength. (550X)

stops the action of the thio or sodium hydroxide, but it also cleanses the scalp.

If a neutralizing shampoo is not provided in the relaxing kit, an **acid-balanced shampoo** is used and **followed by a neutralizer or stabilizer**. In any case, the main chemical that stops the straightening action is **hydrogen peroxide** in the neutralizing shampoo form or in a separate stabilizing preparation. It should be noted that the cystine disulfide bonds broken during chemical relaxing are **not** re-formed chemically as they are in cold waving. So, while these bonds are broken by the sodium hydroxide base of the chemical relaxer, and this action is stopped by the stabilizer, it is not true that the cystine disulfide bonds reharden or re-form in a straightened position. Chemically, the bonds have been weakened too much to be re-formed.

Since chemical relaxers react strongly on the hair, many kits contain 2 conditioners to be applied after the neutralizer. One is a conditioner to normalize the hair. The other is a scalp conditioner that has an ointment-like consistency. You can apply this conditioner by parting the hair into ¾-inch sections and gently rubbing a small amount onto the scalp. It relieves excessive dryness and gives the hair luster. This type of oil conditioner usually resists moisture.

The creme rinse/setting lotion lubricates the hair, which may be in a brittle condition from the relaxing treatment. Hair can break when it is combed during setting and styling. The creme rinse keeps it from breaking.

Neutralizing Shampoo

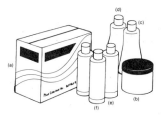

(*a*) Relaxing kit; (*b*) relaxing creme; (*c*) neutralizing shampoo; (*d*) hair conditioner; (*e*) scalp conditioner; (*f*) creme rinse and setting lotion

Creme Rinse

Thio Relaxer

When the **thio relaxer** is applied, the hair **swells** and **softens**, and the disulfide cross-bonds are broken. After you have worked the hair into a straighter position, you can neutralize it with an acid shampoo (stabilizer or neutralizer) in the straightened position. The neutralizer stops the action of the thio relaxer on the cystine disulfide bonds and hardens them in a straighter position.

Sodium Hydroxide

Sodium hydroxide actually dissolves 1 of the cystine disulfide bonds. The cystine amino acid bond has 2 sulfur bonds attached to it in the polypeptide linkage; one of these bonds is not present in the hair after it has been re-formed by the stabilizer. Like thio, sodium hydroxide **swells** and **softens** the hair, but it acts **much more quickly**. In the sodium hydroxide service, the stabilizer affects the salt bonds of the hair to a greater extent than it does in the thio relaxer.

KNOWING SUBOBJECTIVE 2

Describe the difference between a base and a no-base relaxer.

The manufacturers of professional products have research and development programs designed to improve existing products and to develop new ones. A typical example demonstrating the effectiveness of these programs was the introduction of the no-base chemical relaxer.

The **no-base** chemical relaxer has the protective base creme mixed into, or built into, the relaxing creme. This manufacturing improvement eliminates one entire step—you do not have to apply the protective creme to the scalp. If you use the no-base kit, you can apply the relaxing-protective creme directly to the hair without applying a separate protective base, but you still have to be careful. Since the no-base relaxer eliminates 1 application, you will probably find it more convenient and time-saving for both yourself and your client. Doing a process faster allows you more time for other services and, therefore, more income.

KNOWING SUBOBJECTIVE 3

Identify safety precautions used in chemical relaxing and straightening services.

Hair relaxers (straighteners) and their neutralizers are made in a very complicated way. This text could list some of the other sophisticated chemicals contained in both, but doing so might tempt some beginners to make relaxers and neutralizers themselves. This kind of experimenting is **very dangerous**. The scientific knowledge needed to make a **safe relaxer** and a **safe neutralizer** is so great that only the manufacturers of professional products should attempt to make them. Relaxing products made in the school or salon often cause hair breakage and scalp burns. Today, the makeup of the neutralizer is just as important as the makeup of the relaxer itself. Doctors do not make a list of chemicals so that just anyone can fill a prescription; in the same way professional cosmetologists should not make cosmetic hair relaxers for their clients.

Although the importance of reading and following label directions has been indicated earlier in the text, such safety measures must be **stressed** in chemical relaxing. The possibility for serious damage to the scalp and hair is great because of the strong chemicals used in this service.

Do not mix different chemical relaxing products. Mixing different products can cause serious damage to the hair and scalp. This means that you must **always** check the relaxing kit **before** you start the service to make sure that all necessary supplies (and enough of them) are available to complete the service. **Brand A cannot be used to complete a relaxing service that was started with Brand B.**

Always select a relaxer that has the proper strength for your client's hair texture. **Relaxers are made in different strengths: mild (for fine-soft hair), regular (for medium hair), and super (for coarse hair).**

Carefully read directions for each strength of relaxer. One safe way to choose the right strength is to strand test a new client's hair.

In very warm climates, you should cool the temperature of the client's scalp under a "cool" dryer before giving a relaxer!

**Safety
Tip**

DOING SUBOBJECTIVE 4

Supplies

- client chemical services record form
- shampoo cape
- 3 laundered towels
- surgical or rubber gloves
- rake comb and rat-tail comb (both hard rubber)
- timer
- base chemical relaxing kit

- label directions
- protective base creme
- chemical relaxing creme
- neutralizing (stabilizing) shampoo
- hair conditioner
- scalp conditioner
- setting lotion with creme rinse qualities

Apply a base chemical relaxer to virgin hair.

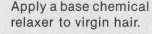

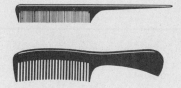

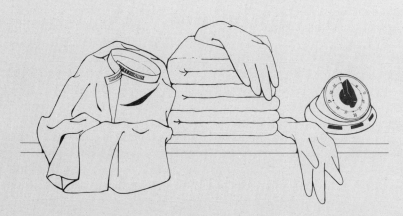

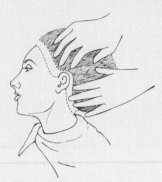

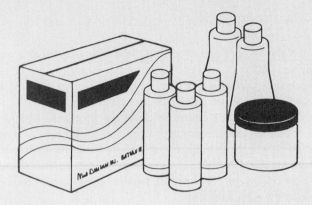

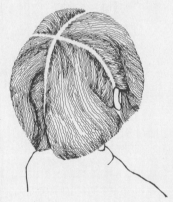

Protective base creme
around hairline

Applying base creme in
section 1

▶ Safety
  Tip

PROCEDURE

1. Using ½-inch horizontal partings, examine the entire scalp.

2. Review client's chemical record form and ask if any chemical services have been performed at home.

3. If you are unsure about which relaxing strength to use, strand test a 1-inch section of hair. Carefully read the directions on the kit you have chosen.

4. Apply protective base creme (precreme) around the front hairline and neck (nape) hairline. Cover the top and back of each ear.

5. Divide the hair in 4 equal sections. Using ¼-inch horizontal partings, begin applying the base creme in the right **nape** section. Work up to the top of the section.

RATIONALE

1. You must not use a chemical relaxer of any kind if the scalp has scratches, abrasions, or irregularities. If any of these conditions exists, the sodium hydroxide or thio will cause extreme discomfort and **possibly cause a serious scalp burn**.

2. Since chemical relaxers are applied to **dry hair**, you should know what home products, if any, may still be in the hair.

3. This is the safest way to check the condition of the hair and choose the best strength of relaxer. Different kits have different directions, so read them carefully.

4. The **protective base creme prevents** strong chemical agents in sodium hydroxide or thio **products from burning the client's scalp**.

5. These partings insure that the entire scalp area will be protected. The client's body heat will cause the base to become liquid and spread over the scalp. **Do not rub** the base creme on the scalp. **Rubbing** increases circulation, which **may cause a scalp burn**.

6. Using ¼-inch horizontal partings, apply the base creme in the left nape section. Work up to top of section. Then apply the base creme to the top left front section and work through the bottom of the section. Repeat for right front section.

7. Check the bases of strands all over the head.

8. Put protective gloves on both hands.

9. Use the handle of the rake comb or the comb part of the rat-tail comb to stir the relaxing creme gently. Apply a base and a no-base creme in the same way.

10. Apply relaxing creme in ¼-inch horizontal partings to the right nape section. Use the little finger of one hand or the rat-tail part of the comb to make partings; then with your other hand, hold the strand above where you are going to apply the relaxer.

11. Apply the relaxer ¼-inch from the scalp. Use your rat-tail comb to "set" the relaxing creme across the hair strand. **Do not use pressure**. Work in ¼-inch horizontal partings toward the top of the section.

12. Apply the relaxing creme in the same way to the left nape section. Using ¼-inch horizontal partings, set the relaxing creme ¼-inch **away** from the scalp. **Do not use pressure** when you apply creme to hair strand.

6. Same as step 5.

7. This insures that the scalp is protected well enough before the relaxing creme is applied.

8. All sensitive areas of skin must be protected from the caustic relaxing material.

9. Some of the heavier chemicals in the relaxing creme have a tendency to settle to the bottom of the container while they are sitting on the shelf. Stirring with the rake handle or a rat-tail comb blends chemicals together so they will work more effectively on hair.

10. Even distribution of creme is needed to insure uniform relaxing. Holding the strand in your opposite hand helps you see better.

11. The relaxing creme does not work until you apply **pressure** (friction) to it with your hands and the comb. The **creme should not be activated yet**.

12. This is standard procedure. Do not use pressure (friction) which would activate relaxing creme.

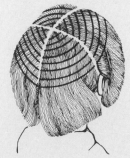

Subsectioning pattern for applying base creme

 Safety Tip

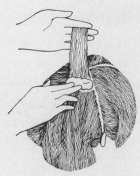

The base creme protects the scalp

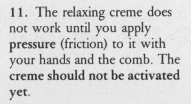

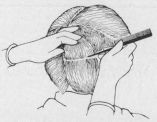

Apply relaxer using ¼ inch partings

 Safety Tip

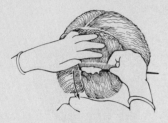

Use back of tail comb for application

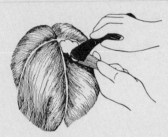

Use back of rake comb

Safety Tip

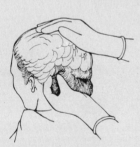

Friction (pressure) activates the relaxing creme

13. Apply relaxing creme from the left nape section through the top crown section.

14. Apply creme to the left front section. Begin application at top center and work toward the hairline around the ear. Use ¼-inch **diagonal** partings to set relaxing creme on the hair strands.

15. Go on to the right front section and apply the relaxing creme to the rest of the hair as described in the previous procedure.

16. Set timer for 15 minutes. **Spray** any irritated points on the scalp with water.

17. Using pressure (friction) with the hands and/or comb, begin in the nape section and work the relaxing creme down the hair strands **towards, but not through, the ends**.

18. Smooth the relaxing creme carefully, but quickly, through both back sections, from the nape through the crown.

19. Saturate each strand. Add creme where necessary.

13. This is standard procedure.

14. Diagonal partings make the hair lie **back** rather than toward the face. So, the chances of dripping relaxing creme into client's face or eyes are reduced.

15. This is standard procedure.

16. Once the sodium hydroxide has been activated by the pressure of the hand and comb, it straightens the hair very quickly. You may find the following timetable helpful: fine hair-3 to 6 minutes; medium hair-7 to 13 minutes; and coarse hair-8 to 15 minutes. After you have started the hair relaxer, **never** allow it to stay on the hair for more than 15 minutes. Water slows or stops action of relaxer.

17. Wait until later to work the relaxer through the ends and the hair next to the scalp. The hair will relax faster there due to porosity and body heat.

18. If you **stretch** the hair too much while you are applying, **the hair will break**. Speed is necessary so that the hair will be relaxed evenly.

19. Long or very thick hair may require additional relaxing creme to cover entire strands.

20. Activate the relaxing creme on the left and then right front sections. Smooth (spread) the creme along the strands. Work from the top of the sections through the bottom hairline over the ears.

20. This is standard procedure to activate the relaxing creme in all 4 sections of hair.

21. Work the relaxing creme through the hair. Use moderate pressure.

21. As you work the relaxer through the hair, the **"feel"** will tell you how much relaxing is taking place on the head. As the bonds within the strands are softened and broken, the hair will have a soft, mushy feel. The hair will also have a silky, shiny appearance.

22. Watch timer and compare to timetable previously discussed. (If client is **allergic to relaxer or experiences other extreme discomfort, rinse immediately with lukewarm to tepid water and neutralize according to directions.** If only a **very small area** [less than "dime" size] **stings,** spray the small area with water and continue.)

22. If you leave the relaxer on for more than 15 minutes, the hair may break. Be sure that the temperature of the water is comfortable for the client. Cool water stops the action and the stinging.

Safety Tip

23. When the hair "feels" soft enough, work the relaxing creme onto all the hair next to the scalp and through all the ends quickly and thoroughly.

23. Working the relaxer carefully but quickly avoids hair breakage or discoloration.

24. Immediately escort client to shampoo area. Using outside of gloved thumb, immediately smooth hair around the front hairline. Use firm pressure and work quickly until hairs in that area are straight.

24. Reducing the curl around the hairline without breaking the hair is a standard part of this service.

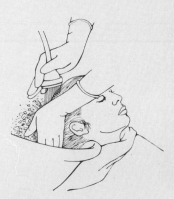

25. Use a strong spray of **tepid** water to rinse the relaxer thoroughly from hair.

25. If the water is too cool, the relaxing creme, which is heavy, will not rinse out of the hair. On the other hand, if the water is too hot, the client will be very uncomfortable.

Rinse all relaxer from hair

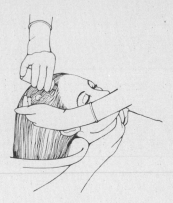

Apply neutralizing shampoo

26. Shampoo hair 2 or 3 times with the **neutralizing shampoo** and rinse until the water runs clear.

27. Inspect the scalp for protective creme or relaxing creme; shampoo again if necessary.
28. Rinse the hair thoroughly. Then apply the hair conditioner according to directions. Apply scalp conditioner if needed.

29. Allow the conditioner to remain on the hair according to label directions; then rinse the hair, towel-dry, and apply creme rinse or setting lotion.
30. Apply scalp conditioner in 1-inch partings.

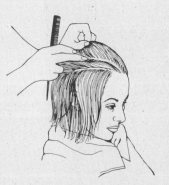

31. On client's chemical service form, record the product used, the date, timing, and recommendations for the next treatment.
32. Shape hair with scissors only.

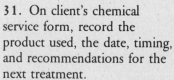

Apply scalp conditioner

26. The procedure does 5 things for hair and scalp: (1) cleanses scalp, (2) removes protective base from scalp, (3) removes the relaxing creme from the hair, (4) neutralizes (stabilizes) the sodium hydroxide or thio, and (5) hardens the hair in the straightened position (hardens the cuticle in the re-formed position). If the rinse water is milky rather than clear, chemicals are still in the hair.
27. All traces of relaxing cremes should be removed from the hair and scalp, or irritation may result.
28. The rinse water should look clear, **not milky**. Application of conditioners varies from one brand to another. **Foam will only appear if all the base or relaxer has been removed from the hair**.
29. The creme rinse or setting lotion reduces the chance of breakage from combing when the hair is brittle from the relaxing service.
30. Chemicals used in the relaxing service remove nautral oils from the scalp; conditioners replace some of these oils so that the scalp returns to a supple, good condition.
31. Accurate records should be made so that both you and the client can refer to them for dates and products used.

32. Super-curly hair that has been relaxed is very fragile; razor shaping will scrape bits of cuticle from the hair shaft because the hair possibly will be very brittle.

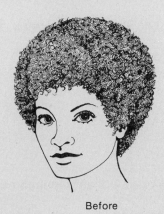

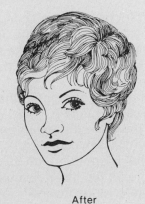

Before   After

As in a tint or bleach retouch, a relaxer retouch is applied only to the new growth. Use the base protective creme if the kit contains one. Otherwise, just apply a no-base relaxer and proceed as previously described. **Relax the new growth only.** Retouches every 3 or 4 months are recommended. The hair must **not be** thermally silked **(pressed)**, or breakage will result. The hair is either chemically relaxed or thermally silked (pressed) and curled, **but not both!**

Relaxer Retouch

Safety Tip

GLOSSARY

Base creme (Petrolatum)   An ointment that protects the scalp from irritation or burns that can be caused by relaxer cremes.

Caustic soda   Sodium hydroxide, used in some chemical relaxing products.

Chemical relaxing   Relaxing super-curly hair with products that have sodium hydroxide or ammonium thioglycolate.

Chemical straightening   Relaxing naturally wavy hair with products that contain ammonium thioglycolate.

Hair relaxers   Products that straighten curly hair by either swelling and softening or dissolving cystine disulfide bonds in the hair.

Neutralizing shampoo   A shampoo, usually containing hydrogen peroxide, that stops the softening and straightening action of thio or sodium hydroxide in hair relaxers.

No-base chemical relaxer   A hair relaxer that comes with the protective base creme mixed into the relaxing creme.

Petrolatum   See **Base creme**

Sodium hydroxide (SOH-dee-uhm high-DRAHK-sighd)   Fast-acting, caustic alkali used in chemical relaxers.

Thermal silking   Temporarily straightening the hair with pressing combs. (Also called pressing).

QUESTIONS

1. What basic chemical is used in professional chemical relaxers?
2. Name three terms for the chemicals that stop the action of the chemical relaxer.

3. After chemically relaxing the hair, would you thermally press and curl it? What if you did?
4. Is sodium hydroxide the same as sodium bromate?
5. What is the difference between a base and a no-base chemical relaxer?
6. When you straighten the hair, do you want to make it completely straight?
7. Is there any difference between sodium hydroxide and ammonium thioglycolate?
8. What is another term for chemical straightening?
9. What is the pH of sodium hydroxide and ammonium thioglycolate, respectively?
10. Why would a neutralizing shampoo be used following a chemical relaxer?
11. Does the neutralizing shampoo "fix" the hair in the straightened position?
12. Will sodium hydroxide straighten the hair faster than ammonium thioglycolate?
13. Do chemical relaxers generally come in one strength?
14. Is it necessary to wear gloves when applying a chemical relaxer?
15. True or false. If a chemical relaxer creme should drip into the client's eye(s), remove it by wiping with a towel.
16. Should a protective base be applied around the client's hairline and in back of the ears?
17. Does the application of a chemical relaxer begin in the top of the section?
18. Is the application of the relaxer done using 1½-inch subsections?
19. Does exposing the relaxing creme to air activate the straightening action?
20. What activates the straightening action once the relaxer has been applied to the hair?
21. True or false. After the application of the chemical relaxer, a plastic cap is put over the client's hair; then, the client is placed under the dryer for 15 minutes.

ANSWERS

1. Sodium hydroxide 2. Neutralizing shampoo, stabilizer, or fixative 3. No. It would most likely break. 4. No. 5. The base relaxer uses a protective scalp creme —the no-base doesn't 6. No 7. Yes 8. Chemical relaxing 9. 11.5–14; 8.5–9.5 10. To neutralize the hair in the straighter position 11. Yes 12. Yes 13. No; several 14. Yes 15. False; flush with cool water 16. Yes 17. No; in the bottom 18. No; ¼ inch subsections 19. No 20. Pressure (friction) 21. False

Silking (Pressing) and Curling the Hair 20

Previous chapters have been concerned with the methods used to chemically straighten or curl the hair. These methods involved physical means of curling the hair, too, but the main difference was the chemical treatment that was used. In this chapter you will learn about a process that physically straightens or curls the hair.

Thermal silking and curling uses a thermal comb and curling iron to silk (straighten) and then curl super-curly hair. A circular thermal curling iron (marcel iron) is used to make different kinds of curls in the hair, which can then be brushed or combed into a style. Silking normally lasts about 2 weeks. How long the style will last is determined by the amount of moisture the hair is exposed to. Moisture causes the hair to recurl.

People have their hair silked for two reasons. First, thermal curling may be used between regular appointments to correct parts of a pattern that have been disturbed by sleeping or by humid weather or to put the finishing touches on air-waved or blow-waved styles.

When **normal hair** is pressed quite straight and the pressing iron is applied once, this is called a **soft press**. Hair that is **coarse**, wiry hair with a slick "glassy" feel may need a double comb press, and this is called a **hard press**. More pressure and a hotter pressing comb may also be needed.

The second use is for hairpieces. You may use the marcel (thermal curling iron) to style hairpieces made from human hair quickly and accurately. It is a very important part of styling wigs.

Major Objective

Provided with a set of professional thermal irons and supplies, straighten the hair with the pressing comb, curl the hair with the curling iron, and comb the curls into a hairstyle.

Level of Acceptability	Use the proper steps and safety precautions to silk the hair in 30 to 45 minutes; then curl and style the hair in 45 to 60 minutes. Score 75 percent or better on a multiple-choice exam on the information in this chapter.
Knowing Subobjectives	1. Briefly describe the history of thermal irons and the kinds of thermal implements and supplies used today. 2. Describe the various techniques used to produce thermal curls.
Doing Subobjectives	3. Silk the hair with pressing combs. 4. Curl the hair with marcel irons.

KNOWING SUBOBJECTIVE 1

Briefly describe the history of thermal irons and the kinds of thermal implements and supplies used today.

Thermal curling or **waving** was originally called **marceling** or **marcel waving**. It was named after Marcel Grateau, a Frenchman who perfected the technique in 1875. The original thermal irons themselves were called **marcel irons**. These irons had to be made of very fine-quality steel so that they could be heated evenly. Various techniques were used to apply the heated iron evenly to the hair. A small gas burner was designed specifically for heating a marcel iron. Special marceling combs made of hard, non-flammable rubber were used.

Since that time, both implements and techniques have been improved. The **pressing comb** used today is made of **copper** and **brass** and has a **wooden handle**. The copper and brass comb heats and holds heat better than combs made of other metals. Pressing combs generally come in 3 sizes. The smaller, or midget, comb is used to straighten shorter hairs around the hairline; the larger combs (with wide or narrow teeth) are used to straighten hair in the crown, top, and upper side sections. Some **silking** (pressing) combs have self-contained heating units and cords, but most modern silking combs are heated inside an **electric heater**. Gas heaters were used in the past, but they are rarely used anymore.

Thermal curling irons are heated in a similar way. Some are placed into an ordinary electric heater. They are made from high-quality steel. They have a circular shape. Their handles are made of nonflammable hard plastic or rubber. They may be purchased in 3 or 4 sizes.

The comb used for thermal **silking** (temporarily straightening the hair with pressing combs) is a **nonflammable hard rubber** rake implement with wide teeth. A nonflammable hard rubber styling comb is used for thermal curling and waving the hair after it has been straightened.

Safety Tip

Special supplies are required for thermal silking and curling. Oils, cremes, brilliantines, and lusterizing sprays are applied to protect dry hair from scorching or burning. Most of these preparations have a **lanolin oil** base, which is made from sheep wool.

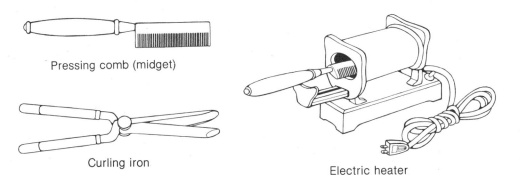

Pressing comb (midget)

Curling iron

Electric heater

Describe the various techniques used to produce thermal curls.

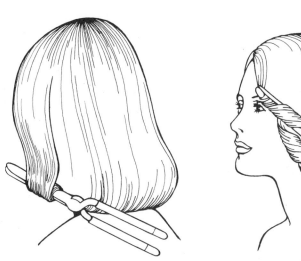

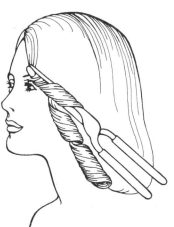

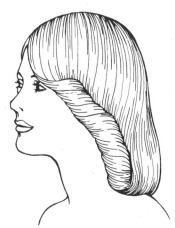

You can use three techniques to style hair with a curling iron: roller, croquignole, and spiral.

The **roller technique** (round) involves winding a short hair strand **from the end** of the strand to the scalp. Place the comb between the iron and the scalp for protection. When the heat penetrates the strand to the outside hair, slip the iron out of the curl. Then clip the curl into place and allow it to cool at room temperature.

For the **croquignole technique** (figure eight), rotate the handle and turn your wrist to wind the strand in small or large sections **from the scalp** to the ends.

The **spiral technique** (poker curling) is really a combination of the spiral and croquignole methods. Wind the strand **from the scalp** in a **spiral** fashion. The resulting curl looks like a spiral candle, and this technique is sometimes called **candlestick curling**.

DOING SUBOBJECTIVE 3

Silk the hair with
pressing combs.

Supplies

- [ ] shampoo supplies, plus chair cloth and neck strip
- [ ] hard rubber combs (rake, rat-tail, styling)
- [ ] pressing combs (regular and midget)

- [ ] pressing creme or oil
- [ ] curling wax (optional)
- [ ] hair spray
- [ ] white tissue
- [ ] electric heater for irons
- [ ] duck-bill clips

Preparation for Pressing

PROCEDURE	RATIONALE
1. Use chair cloth to drape client.	1. **A plastic shampoo cape would melt from the heat of the pressing** comb. Also, the chair cloth made of cotton, rayon etc., will not melt. It is also cooler, therefore, more comfortable for the client.

⚡ **Safety Tip**

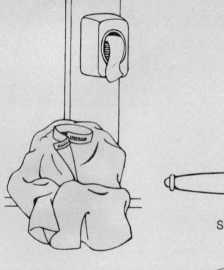

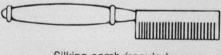

Silking comb (regular)

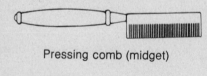

Pressing comb (midget)

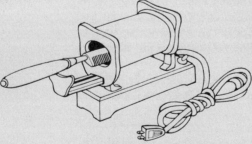

Electric heater

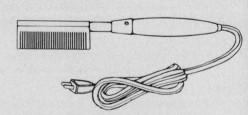

Electric pressing comb

2. Examine the scalp for possible irregularities and tightness; analyze condition and texture of hair. Rotate the scalp with the cushion of your fingertips.

3. Carefully lift dandruff flakes with your comb.

4. Ask the client if the hair has been chemically relaxed within the last 12 months.

5. Shampoo the hair thoroughly.
6. Rinse the hair thoroughly and check it for shampoo residue. Towel dry hair.
7. Apply a small amount of lanolin creme or oily-scalp conditioner to dry areas on the scalp.
8. Use your fingertips to spread the creme or oil through the strands.

9. Divide the hair into 4 equal sections and hold each in place with a duck-bill clip. Dry the hair with a dryer.

2. By rotating different areas of the scalp you will see how flexible the scalp is. A scalp that is **very flexible** and supple is hard to press because it will move as the pressing comb moves through the hair. A **normal** scalp usually moves a little, and the hair has a medium texture, elasticity, and porosity. A **tight scalp** moves very little. The hair is overporous, brittle, and dry. A tight scalp must be silked in the direction in which the hair grows.
3. This helps you see how flaky or dry the scalp is. A scalp treatment and the proper shampoo will help control this condition.
4. Hair that has been chemically relaxed within the last 12 months cannot be silked. **Silking will break hair that has been chemically relaxed recently!**
5. It is easier to silk clean, dry hair.
6. The hair should be visibly free of lather and oils.

7. This helps keep the scalp moist.

8. This lubricates brittle hair and protects it from the extreme heat and pressure of the pressing comb. The hair is easier to handle with the wide-toothed rake comb.
9. The hair is very thick next to the scalp. It is easier to section when **wet** than when dry. But the actual silking is done on dry hair.

 Safety Tip

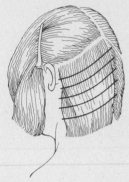

Thermal pressing
subsections

Safety Tip

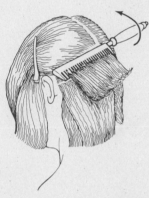

Safety Tip

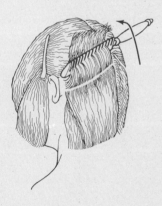

Steps for Pressing the Hair

PROCEDURE

1. Plug in or turn on the electric heater and place the pressing combs inside it.

2. Stand behind the client. Remove the clips and carefully comb tangles from the hair with the rake comb.

3. Part and secure the hair into 4 equal sections. Leave 1 crown and nape section free.

4. Remove the pressing comb from the heater and **touch it to white tissue**. Stop if the tissue discolors in a yellow or brown pattern.

5. Begin silking the **nape. From the nape hairline**, subdivide the hair into horizontal partings.

6. Secure the hair above the subsection out of the way with a duck-bill clip.

7. Insert the teeth of the pressing comb into the **top of** each ½–1 inch subsection and as close to the scalp as possible. **Do not** touch the scalp with the pressing comb. For fine hair use **large** subsections; for coarse hair use **smaller** subsections. Some subsections may be as large as 1½ inches, or as small as ½ inch.

8. Rotate the handle of the pressing comb **downward** so that the teeth of the iron are pointed directly **away** from the client. Pull the hair through the comb so the **back** of the comb presses against the hair as it is moved away from the scalp. Do not pull the comb through the hair too quickly.

RATIONALE

1. This is the best time to begin heating the combs.

2. The rake comb's **wide** teeth will make it easier to comb the hair from the ends to the scalp.

3. Start silking the section that is hanging free.

4. **Discoloration of tissue indicates** that the **comb is too hot for the hair.** Let the comb cool. Test a second time.

5. This is standard procedure. Smaller sections are easier to silk than larger ones.

6. The clip holds the hair out of the way.

7. The pressing comb is very hot; be very careful **not to burn the client's skin**.

8. Always move the **pressing comb away** from the client. The heat and pressure you put on the pressing comb straightens the hair.

9. Insert the teeth of the pressing comb into the **underside** of the **same** subsection, as close to the scalp as possible. **Do not** touch the scalp with the pressing comb.
10. Rotate the handle of the pressing comb **upward** and **away** from the client's scalp while you draw the hair against the **back** of the pressing comb.
11. Repeat this procedure for each ½–1 inch horizontal subsection of **each** large section of the head until **all** the hair has been straightened. Work sections in the same order you use for tinting.
12. Proceed to iron curling, if desired.

9. This is standard procedure. Silk **both** sides of the strand to get maximum straightening.

10. The rotation causes the hair strand to be "pressed" against the back of the comb and straightened.

11. This is standard procedure. Straightening all hair **once** is called a **soft press**. Repeating the entire procedure (straightening all hair **twice**) is called a **hard press**.

12. This is standard procedure.

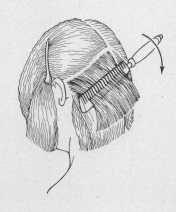

DOING SUBOBJECTIVE 4

Curl the hair with marcel irons.

Supplies

- □ curling irons of various circle sizes
- □ styling combs
- □ electric heater

- □ duck-bill clips
- □ brush
- □ white tissue paper
- □ electric curling iron

PROCEDURE

1. Heat the irons.
2. Select an iron with a large, medium, or small circumference.

RATIONALE

1. This is standard procedure.
2. The circumference of the iron must be selected according to the length and texture of the hair. Short, fine hair (especially strands around the hairline) requires an iron with smaller diameter than long, coarse hair does.

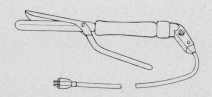

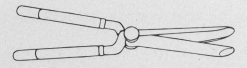

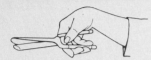

Safety Tip

Control done with ring finger and little finger

3. **Test on white tissue** for heat. Use the little and ring fingers of your right hand to control the clamp.

4. Begin curling the hair in the same sequence you used to set the hair.

5. Hold the hair strand and comb in your left hand and hold the iron in your right hand.

6. Practice holding the iron and clicking it (opening and closing the clamp) while rotating the comb. The barrel, not the clamp, of the iron curls the hair. The clamp merely holds the hair between movements.

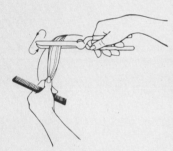

Wind the hair strand around barrel of the iron

7. Hold the strand away from scalp and put the barrel of the iron to the hair next to the scalp. Push the iron against the scalp hair and bring the end of the strand toward you. Rock the iron against the base of the strand to form the base of the curl.

8. Open the clamp and wind the strand between the barrel and then close the clamp to where it pivots next to the handle.

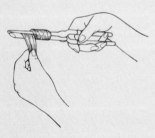

Slowly "feed" hair around iron

9. Hold the end of the strand with your left hand. Curl this part of the strand (next to the head) by rocking the iron against the strand in a movement horizontal to the head. Spiral the strand between the clamp and the barrel next to the first part of the strand; repeat until the entire length of the strand has been curled.

3. This helps you avoid applying too much heat to the hair, and helps control the iron. **Be careful not to burn client's hair or scalp!**

4. This is the easiest way to curl if a roller-type hairstyle is desired.

5. This is standard procedure.

6. Effective thermal waving takes practice. You can get practice by using a cold iron on a mannequin.

7. This directs the base of the hair strand to give it the same height and strength as a curl formed in a wet setting.

8. This is standard procedure.

9. This procedure gives an even curl to each section of the strand.

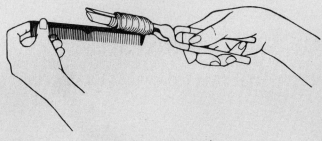

Comb protects scalp

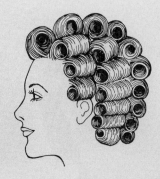

Curling pattern

10. Place the comb between the iron and the scalp. Place the fingertips of your left hand on the hair that is wound around the iron.

11. Slide the iron horizontally from one side of the curl and clip the curl to the scalp in the same way you would clip a roller. Do not allow the curl to unwind before clipping it into place. If you need assistance, consult instructor.

12. Use the curling iron on all of the hair strands.

13. Clip the curls and let them cool. All curls should be allowed to cool before the clips are removed for styling.

14. Remove the clips and arrange hair.

Wave Pattern

15. To make a wave pattern, insert the iron diagonally in the hair to the outside corner of the left eyebrow.

16. Close the clamp and rotate the iron 1 turn forward. Rest it on the comb (which is on the scalp) until the heat penetrates the hair evenly. Place your fingertips across the wound hair.

10. You must place the comb between the iron and the scalp to avoid burning the scalp.

11. The hair is quite warm when the iron is removed. A more durable curl is formed if the hair is allowed to cool in a clipped rather than an unclipped and unwound position.

12. This is standard procedure.

13. This is standard procedure.

14. This is standard procedure.

15. This is how you should begin to form the wave ridge.

16. Placing your fingertips on the hair helps you take the iron out quickly after you have finished heating the hair.

Safety Tip

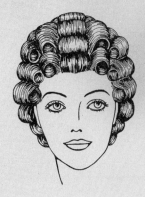

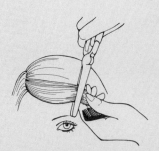

To make a soft wave, place iron diagonal to front hairline

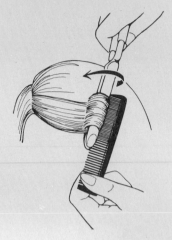

Comb protects scalp

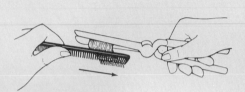

Shift hair beneath iron to form wave

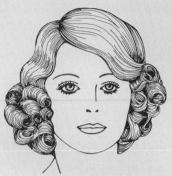

Finished thermal wave

17. Reverse the rotation of the iron, but return it to the original position.

18. Place the iron across the ridge, but do not close the clamp. Shift the hair beneath the iron with the comb to make the wave pattern.

19. Repeat steps 15, 16, and 17 until the hair on the bottom of the side hairline has been waved.

17. This gives you an even ridge.

18. This is standard procedure.

19. This is standard procedure.

GLOSSARY

Hard press   Using a thermal pressing comb throughout the hair twice.

Marcel irons   The original steel irons used in marcel waving or thermal waving.

Marcel waving (Marceling)   See **Thermal waving**.

Pressing comb   A copper and brass comb with a wooden handle; used to straighten hair.

Silking   Temporarily straightening the hair with pressing combs.

Soft press   Using a thermal pressing comb throughout the hair once.

Thermal waving (curling)   Using heated irons to curl the hair.

QUESTIONS

1. What does it mean to press the hair?
2. How long does a press last?
3. What do you use to press the hair?
4. Is a pressing comb metal or rubber?
5. How is a pressing comb heated?
6. What effect does pressing have on the hair?
7. Once the hair is pressed, what will cause it to become curly again?
8. If the hair is pressed once, but remains quite wavy, what can be done?
9. Is pressing a style by itself, or must something else be done?
10. What is another term for marceling or marcel waving?
11. Name the solution used to clean the thermal iron.
12. Is it best to use a plastic comb for marcel waving?
13. Before using the marcel iron on the hair, what safety precaution should you take?
14. Write a short definition for croquignol, spiral, and the roller technique, respectively.
15. Is it necessary to examine the scalp before pressing the hair?
16. What kind of cape should be used for the pressing service?
17. Should the hair be shampooed before the pressing service?
18. If the hair has been chemically relaxed, should you press it?
19. Is towel-dried hair pressed, or must the hair be thoroughly dried with a dryer?

ANSWERS

1. Straighten it temporarily 2. If the hair is kept dry, shampoo-to-shampoo 3. A pressing comb 4. Metal 5. In an electric heater 6. It temporarily straightens it 7. Moisture 8. A hard press 9. The hair must be thermally curled also 10. Thermal curling or thermal waving 11. Sudsy ammonia 12. No; hard rubber 13. Test the temperature of the iron 14. (Check your answers against the text) 15. Yes 16. Cloth or linen (non-meltable cape) 17. Yes 18. No 19. Dried with a dryer

Recurling the Hair 21

In earlier chapters you have learned to curl the hair by using permanent wave rods and chemicals and you have also learned to chemically relax the hair. It is important for you to have mastered those chapters before attempting this. You will find this to be true because the curl reformation service combines the knowledge and skills of permanent (cold) waving and chemical relaxing. Although the procedures are a little different, many steps of this service will be familiar to you.

Learning how to successfully give a curl reformation service will increase the number of hairstyles you can offer the client with super-curly hair. The service has two basic phases—relaxing and reforming (recurling). You have to perform each step in a quality manner—in order to end up with a quality curl reformation.

Purpose

Using professional curl reformation chemicals and implements, relax and reform (recurl) super-curly hair to make it more manageable and durable from one styling to the next.

Major Objective

Observing safety precautions and following label directions, use the proper steps to relax, then reform (recurl) the hair. Use a chemical relaxing product to relax the hair in 30-45 minutes. Then, wrap the client's hair on permanent wave rods in 45-75 minutes. Score 75 percent or better on a multiple-choice exam on the information in this chapter.

Level of Acceptability

The publisher and author of this book wish to acknowledge their debt and extend their sincere appreciation to Soft Sheen Products, Inc., who rendered its valuable service and assistance in writing this chapter.

Knowing Subobjectives	1. Define the basic curl reformation service and its advantages.
	2. Describe the chemical processes of the curl reformation service.
	3. Evaluate the condition of the hair and scalp.
	4. Identify important safety and after-care considerations for the curl reformation service.

Doing Subobjectives	5. Analyze the hair and apply the chemical curl relaxer.
	6. Section and subsection the client's hair and wrap it on cold wave rods.
	7. Process and neutralize the curl reformation.

KNOWING SUBOBJECTIVE 1

Define the basic curl reformation service and its advantages.

The **curl reformation** service is also known as a **curl rearranger** (or recurl). These terms will be used interchangeably through this chapter. A **curl reformation** is a **double-application service**, in which the hair is treated with two different chemical processes. The curl reformation service is given to a client with **super-curly hair**. The objective is to begin by straightening the hair, then to recurl the hair in a larger curl pattern.

The first stage of this process involves a chemical relaxer to **straighten** the hair. This is usually done with **ammonium thioglycolate**, also called "thio." Other chemicals are also used, but generally, most salons use the "thio"-based relaxers. The relaxer you use, however, will be determined by your school/salon manager.

 Safety Tip

Remember to read and follow manufacturer's directions for the product your are using!

During the second stage of the process the hair is wound around cold wave rods and another "thio"-based chemical is applied. The hair is processed until the desired degree of curl is achieved, and then it is neutralized. The most common type of **neutralizer** used for a curl reformation is **sodium bromate**. While a few manufacturers may use a peroxide neutralizer, the vast majority use sodium bromate. **Read product** directions **carefully**.

The basic product used to relax the hair is called the **chemical rearranger**. This is the "thio" chemical earlier mentioned. Since this product has a pH that is **alkaline, gloves** must be worn to protect the hands. Of course, prolonged contact with the client's skin and scalp may cause irritation, so care must be taken to protect them by working as rapidly as possible.

The chemical rearranger generally comes in different strengths: mild, for fine or tinted hair; regular, for average hair; super, for very curly to resistant hair. The exact description of strengths may differ from one manufacturer to another so read the directions carefully. After it has been applied, **the chemical rearranger** may be left on the hair from 17–30 minutes, depending on the resistance or texture of the client's hair. Fine, tinted hair will probably require less time; super-curly, coarse, virgin hair may take a little longer.

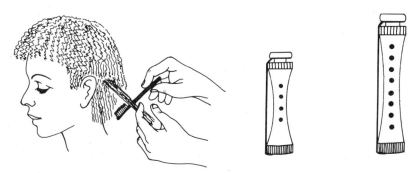

Strand test for reformation (recurl) service.   Concave, medium size short rod
Applicator bottle or brush may be used   Concave, medium size long rod

To be on the safe side, **check the rearranger every 3–5 minutes**. Unlike a hair color strand test, the curl reformation strand test is done with a strand about the size as that used for wrapping a cold wave rod.

After the chemical rearranger has been rinsed from the hair, the **curl booster** (waving solution) is applied. The **curl booster** is a "thio" chemical that is used to wrap the hair and then process it for the desired degree of curliness, based on the size of the rods used during wrapping. If the hair dries out during the wrapping process, apply only the curl booster, **not water** in most cases. Water would dilute the curl booster and may prevent the hair from curling. Although water is not used during wrapping in most cases, it can be used in some situations, according to your instructor's and the manufacturer's directions.

Rod selection tends to be **toward small sizes** for the curl reformation services. For a curly-do that can simply be "picked-out" (lifted), small diameter, yellow or blue rods achieve the results preferred by most clients. If the hair is quite coarse, blue rods are used. However, if the client wishes to blow-comb/iron curl or wet set the hair, larger pink or gray rods may be used.

Therefore, the rod used will be determined by the hair's condition, texture, and the amount of curl desired by the client for the hairstyle requested.

For several reasons, **wrapping** is somewhat different for a curl reformation service than for cold/acid waving. First, the **subsection** of hair that is wound around each rod **must be very thinly parted**. Because small subsections of hair are used, many rods are needed to wrap the entire head. For example, a typical cold wave or heat wave would most likely be wrapped in four to five dozen (48-60) rods. A curl reformation, however, will usually require ten to twelve dozen (120-144) rods.

The **tension** used in wrapping the hair for reformation is also a little different. The hair **must be wrapped with a firm degree of even tension** across each rod. Another important part of the wrapping procedure is the technique for winding the rods and positioning them in the subsection. The

**Safety
Tip**

individual strand should normally be wrapped as though you were making a **no-stem roller**. When wound, the rod should rest on the subsection of hair from which it was taken. Remember, **too much tension on the elastic rod strap will cause breakage.**

Furthermore, the best results are achieved when the right side, left side, and top sections are **wrapped forward—toward the face.**

The advantages of the curl reformation for super-curly hair are many. Some of them would be:

1. Hair is more manageable.
2. More hairstyles can be achieved.
3. Hair may be easily blow-combed/iron curled.
4. Hair may be easily wet set in rollers.

Safety Tip

KNOWING SUBOBJECTIVE 2

Describe the chemical processes of the curl reformation service.

As noted earlier, the curl reformation processes aren't really anything new to you. The "thio" found in the chemical rearranger used for relaxing the hair is **alkaline**, with a pH of 9.6. When this is applied to the hair, it **softens and swells** the **cystine disulphide bonds (sulfur bonds).** Smoothing the hair with your hands or the back of your comb causes the sulfur peptide linkages to "slip" into a straighter position. The hydrogen and salt bonds are also affected, but to a lesser extent. The action of the chemical rearranger is stopped when the hair is rinsed with **tepid water**, since water has a pH of 7.0. This is an effective way to stop the chemical action of the rearranger.

The **curl booster** is also **alkaline**, with a pH of 9.6. The curl booster continues the softening (or breaking down) process on the sulfur bonds, helping the hair to reform around the shape of the permanent wave rod. Once this new shape has been achieved, it can be said that the hair has been "reformed." You will need to take a test curl to determine how long the curl booster should be left on the rods after the hair has been completely wrapped. A **test curl** is done by unwinding a rod or two in each section of the head. Each rod should be **unwound only 1½–2 turns** to check for the

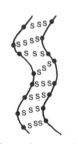

Normal state of sulfur bonds

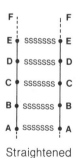

Straightened sulfur bonds

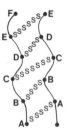

New position of sulfur bonds resulting in recurled hair

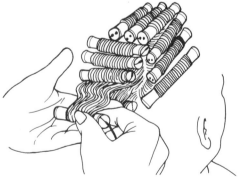

Definite "S" pattern; unwrap rod a maximum of two turns

classical "S" pattern, then refastened and another rod checked. (However, some hair may not be long enough for two complete turns.)

Heat is used to accelerate (speed up) **a chemical process.** Heat also permits better penetration into the hair of whatever chemical is used. The heat naturally generated by the client's body is used by simply placing a plastic cap over the hair to capture the heat. The artificial heat of a hair dryer or infrared light can also be used. Different manufacturers use natural and artificial heat differently. Each product's directions must be read carefully to determine when to use which source of heat with which part of a service.

Coarse hair will normally require placing the client under the dryer for **at least 5 minutes. Children under 12 years of age shouldn't** be put under the dryer at all because their bodies generate enough heat without the dryer. **As a general rule, process the rearranger without the dryer for 20 minutes on all clients before using the hair dryer for heat!**

Safety Tip

KNOWING SUBOBJECTIVES 3

Whenever you are applying chemicals that penetrate the cuticle and cortex layers of the hair, you must take **extra care before beginning** the service. This is an important step. It is your responsibility to protect the client and yourself before, during, and after the curl rearranging service.

First, ask the client if the hair has been chemically relaxed in the previous 12 months. **Hair that has been relaxed with a sodium hydroxide relaxer must not be given a curl reformation. That hair will not curl. The sodium hydroxide treated hair must be cut off to avoid straight ends.** It is necessary to explain this to the client during the evaluation process. It is all right to give a curl reformation over hair that has been treated with other ammonium thioglycolate products. Next, determine if the scalp has any open cuts, scrapes, or abrasions. If the scalp has any of these conditions, the curl reformation service will **irritate** the condition; inflammation, blisters, or open sores will result. **Do not give this service to a client with any of the foregoing condition!**

Now, you will want to determine the texture and condition of the client's hair. Coarse hair will be harder to curl than medium or fine hair. Porosity of the hair is also a factor. **Hair that is very porous will curl more easily** than hair that is not because the softening and curling chemicals penetrate (get into) the hair faster. Porous or brittle hair should be conditioned with a **polymer conditioner** or other high-quality **protein conditioner** weekly from 2 to 3 weeks **before** the curl reformation service or until the hair has regained its tensile strength. This would also apply to hair that has been tinted with permanent hair color or bleached (lightened). Bleached hair will easily break! To sum up, the curl reformation service should **only be given to strong, healthy hair.**

Finally, a personal, but brief medical history about the client may be very helpful. For example, if the client has high blood pressure (**hypertension**), or a heart condition, you may create a problem if you put the client under a

Evaluate the condition of the hair and scalp.

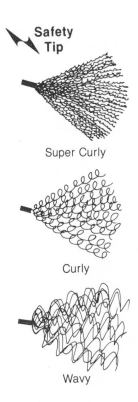
Safety Tip

Super Curly

Curly

Wavy

Safety Tip

hot dryer. **Allergies** are also an important consideration. Ask the client whether he/she is allergic or sensitive to "thio" products. Of course, **don't give this service to anyone who has had a chemical reaction as a result of this service in the past.** If there is already a record on the client, check it. Make a record for a new client.

If the client's hair has been given a curl rearranger before, simply apply the straightener to the new growth only.

KNOWING SUBOBJECTIVE 4

Identify important safety precautions and after-care considerations.

Safety Tip

Since curl reformation includes harsh chemicals, it is important to protect your client and yourself. The products in this service which are strong enough to soften and curl the hair can also soften and irritate your skin and the skin of your client. To avoid chemical burns and irritation to the skin, eyes, ears and nose, **keep all products away from these areas.** If you accidentally drop or drip a product in one of these areas, **rinse with cool water immediately.** If the irritation continues ask the client to contact a physician or dermatologist. Since you must depend on your hands in making a living, **protect them by wearing rubber or surgical gloves** during this service. Remember, failing to use the gloves on a long-term basis will result in damage to your hands. Even though you may be able to give this service today without gloves, tomorrow you may have developed an allergy, and be out of school or out of a job!

One other precaution must be observed. **Do not brush** the hair before this service. Doing so can cause the client to suffer scalp irritations or burns.

After Care

Safety Tip

Care for the hair after the curl reformation service is of the utmost importance! The hair is softened by the "thio," and the inner bonds of the hair are softened (broken), then rehardened (rebounded) during the neutralizing process. Since natural oils are also removed from the hair and scalp along with moisture, it is necessary to replace them to keep the hair looking shiny and strong. **Immediately after the hair has been neutralized, it must be conditioned** with a keratin-type protein conditioner. Then a **curl activator** should be applied to the scalp. An **instant moisturizer** should be applied after the **activator** is used. At this point in the service, the hair may be shaped (cut). If the scalp still seems to be dry, an instant curl moisturizer may be sprayed near the scalp. Now the hair is ready for styling.

The hair and scalp moisturizers may be applied every other day, or as directed. Read and follow label directions. If after-care recommendations are not followed, the client will have problems with a dry/itchy scalp and brittle hair that will have a tendency to break.

For the client who doesn't have time for or can't afford the prescribed aftercare steps, the following recommendations should be made:

1. Shampoo the hair at least weekly. Use the shampoo suggested by the curl reformation manufacturer. The shampoo must have a neutral or acid pH in order to protect the new curl formation.
2. All conditioners used should have a pH of 7.0 or less.
3. It is important to use a curl activator (oil) on the scalp.
4. Moisturizers should be sprayed on the hair before styling. If the hair is to be a "pick out," the moisturizer can be sprayed on after styling.

If care is not taken to apply the products mentioned earlier, the client will note the following change in the hair after one or two days: excessively dry scalp and hair, brittleness of the hair, and hair breakage.

The client should use a bouffant plastic cap to protect clothing after applying a moisturizer or curl activator. Of course, this also allows better penetration of the hair/scalp. However, the client must not sleep in the plastic cap because the elastic around the cap would cause breakage around the hairline.

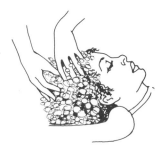

Use a neutralizing shampoo to maintain hair in good condition

DOING SUBOBJECTIVE 5

Supplies

- □ shampoo cape
- □ towels
- □ cotton coil
- □ neutralizing bib
- □ rat-tail comb
- □ rubber/surgical gloves
- □ dryer
- □ end papers
- □ large-toothed comb
- □ timer
- □ sectioning clips
- □ cold wave rods (10-12 dozen)
- □ plastic cap

- □ applicator brush (if applying to new growth)
- □ thio relaxer (chemical rearranger)
- □ waving solution (curl booster)
- □ neutralizer (sodium bromate)
- □ protein conditioner (keratin base)
- □ instant moisturizer
- □ curl activator
- □ conditioning shampoo
- □ polymer pretreatment
- □ protective base

Analyze the hair and apply the chemical relaxer.

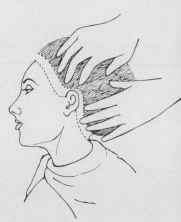

Protective petrolatum (base creme) around hairline

Safety Tip

PROCEDURE

1. Remove all neck and ear jewelry and drape client. **Apply protective base around hairline (forehead, ears, and neck). Put on protective gloves.**

RATIONALE

1. Metal and different solutions may cause a chemical burn on the skin. Draping protects the client's clothing. The base is needed to protect the client's skin. Protect your hands at all times.

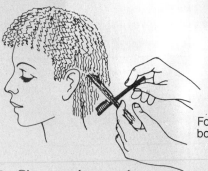

For test curls applicator brush or bottle may be used

2. Give several test curls.

2. On hair that has been curled, tinted or bleached, you will be able to determine how long it will take to curl the hair, or if the hair should be curled at all.

3. Analyze the hair for porosity, texture, and condition.

4. Part the hair into four sections and begin application of the rearranger (relaxer) in the bottom of the right nape section. Use ¼–½ inch subsections. Continue to work to the top of the section until done. Go to the bottom of the other back section and repeat application steps. Now apply rearranger to each front section, working from the bottom to the top of each section.

3. This will help you determine which strength thio relaxer to apply to the hair.

4. This is standard procedure. Small subsections are needed so that the rearranger saturates each strand (subsection) of hair.

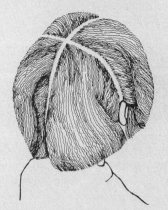

Sectioning pattern for recurl

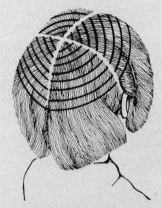

Subsectioning pattern for recurl

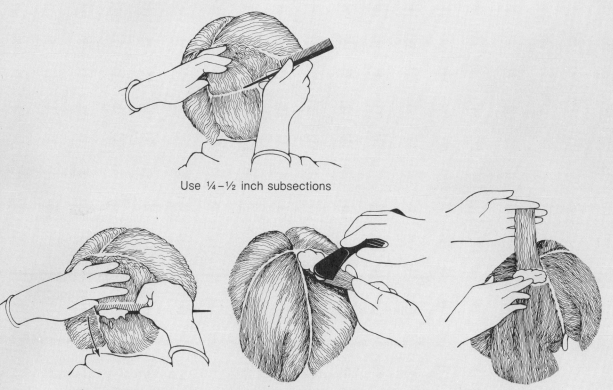

Use ¼–½ inch subsections

Begin application in *nape* subsection and work to top of section. Place plastic cap over rods

5. Begin in one nape section and work to the top of the section. Use the back of the comb or your fingers to firmly smooth the hair into a straighter position. Repeat on each section. Clients over the age of 12 may be put under a warm-hot dryer for 17–30 minutes with a plastic cap over the hair, if necessary.

6. Test rearranger for straightness every 3–5 minutes. Be careful not to overprocess. Use a timer to check processing.

5. The dryer speeds up the relaxing process by allowing for better penetration into the hair shaft.

6. Rarely will the hair process more than 30 minutes. In general, the following timetable will apply: tinted hair—15 to 20 minutes; average hair—20 to 25 minutes; coarse hair—25 to 30 minutes. A timer eliminates guessing the correct time.

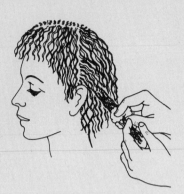

Dry strand to test for
degree of hair relaxation

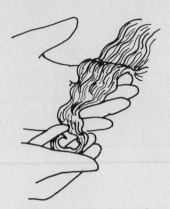

Note how second strand
test shows hair relaxing

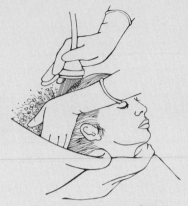

Rinse all rearranger from
hair until water runs clear

7. Strand test the rearranger.
Towel dry a strand about the
size of a cold wave rod
subsection to check for
straightness of hair.

8. Rinse the hair with tepid
(lukewarm) water for 3 to 5
minutes until all rearranger has
been rinsed from the hair.

7. This size section will give
an accurate indication of the
degree of straightness achieved.
A larger section would not. The
hair must be straight for
successful curl reformation.

8. Hot water would irritate
the scalp. Water has a pH of
7.0 so it stops the chemical
action of the relaxer.

DOING SUBOBJECTIVE 6

Section and
subsection the
client's hair and wrap
on cold wave rods.

 **Safety
Tip**

PROCEDURE

1. Select rod diameter to be
used. Now section the head for
wrapping. Put on gloves.

2. Apply waving solution
(curl booster) to the whole
section you are about to wrap.
Reapply as needed if the hair
dries out. Begin wrapping in
the top of the center crown
section (or whichever system
your instructor advises). Use
protective gloves at all times
and avoid contact with the
client's face, eyes, and ears.

RATIONALE

1. Remember, you will need
10 to 12 dozen rods. The
smaller rods will give a tighter
curling pattern than larger rods.

2. The waving solution
softens the hair so that it will
"reform" around the rod. It is
important to keep the hair wet
with the waving solution for
good penetration of the hair
shaft. **Do not use water.** Water
slows down the curling action.
**If any waving solution drips
onto the face, ear, or eye,
rinse with cold water
immediately!**

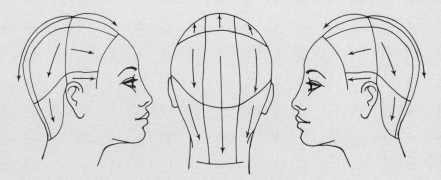

Your instructor will tell you the sectioning pattern to use. This is one

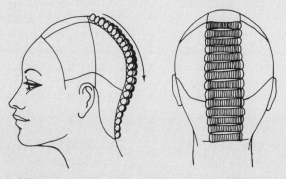

Begin in center crown section. Continue to bottom of nape. Use *small* subsections

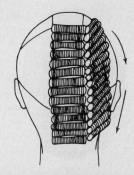

Wrap right crown section, then right nape section

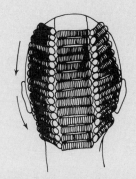

Wrap left crown, then left nape section

3. Wrap the hair, using very thin subsections (¼ to ½ the diameter of the rod used). Wrap with a firm degree of even tension.

4. Apply waving solution to each section as you wrap. Wrap the right crown section, then the left crown section, working from the top of the section to the bottom. Apply waving solution to keep the hair wet at all times. **Do not drip in client's ear or on face!**

3. If large subsections are used, the hair bonds won't be broken enough to reform around the rod you have selected. Neat rods with tension evenly applied across the rod are needed to uniformly curl the hair.

4. Dry hair won't process evenly. Precautions are needed throughout the chemical application.

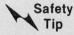 **Safety Tip**

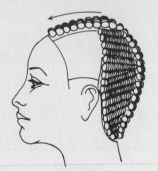

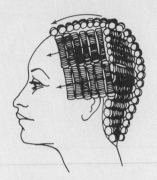

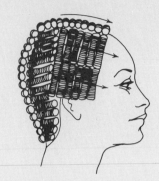

Wrap top right side sections toward the face, then wrap top left side sections, also toward the face

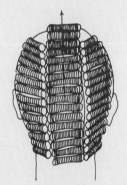

Wrap top center section forward toward the face

5. Apply waving solution to the centerfront top section. Begin wrapping from the back of the section and work toward the forehead. Rods are wrapped forward. **Do not let solution drip in client's eye, or on face!** Stand in front of client for wrapping this section.

6. Apply waving solution to right front side section and wrap **rods forward.** Begin wrapping at the back of each section and wrap the rods toward the face. **Do not drip solution on client's face!** Apply waving solution to left front side and wrap like the right side.

Safety Tip

5. It is easier to wrap the hair from the back of the section, working toward the front.

6. Since the hairs around the front hairline may be uneven, or thin amd sparse, you will find it easier to roll the rods to the face.

DOING SUBOBJECTIVE 7

Process and neutralize the curl reformation.

PROCEDURE

1. Check all rods for neat, even wrapping. Place cotton coil around entire hairline and reapply waving solution to all rods.

RATIONALE

1. Cotton stops the waving solution from dripping onto the skin, face, and ears. Resaturation with waving solution makes the hair process evenly. Some of the solution probably has evaporated from the time you started.

2. Allow cotton to become saturated for 1 or 2 minutes, then replace the cotton with a new, dry piece of cotton coil. Replace towel(s) used to drape client. Place plastic cap over rods and secure with clip or rod.

3. Place **adults (over the age of 12) under the tepid hair dryer for 10 to 30 minutes** if cap alone hasn't relaxed the hair enough. **Always process children with cap only!** After 10 minutes, **test curl** the hair by unwrapping a rod in each section **two turns**, checking for "S" pattern.

4. When "S" pattern has been achieved, remove plastic cap and rinse the hair thoroughly with tepid water for 3 to 5 minutes. Use a timer. Gently towel blot **each rod.**

2. If hair is allowed to process with the wet cotton or wet neck towel, **a chemical burn will result.** The plastic cap captures body heat and also prevents the waving solution from drying out. If the solution dries out, it won't curl the hair.

3. Normally, children have enough body heat to process the curl without the use of artificial heat. Children also have more sensitive skin than adults. Because everyone's hair is different, test curls are needed to protect against **overprocessing.** Use of the cap alone is better for the condition of the hair and scalp.

4. The water rinse removes the waving solution and stops the reformation process. Tepid water is used because hot water may irritate the scalp. Towel blotting rods removes excess water and "makes room" in the hair shaft for the neutralizer.

 Safety Tip

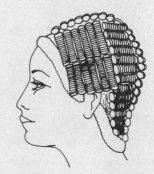

Place cotton coil around hairline. *Remove* after application of waving solution to prevent chemical burns

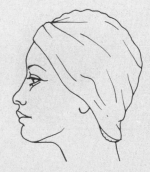

Place plastic cap over rods

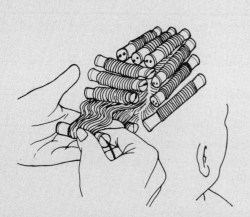

Definite "S" pattern; unwrap rod a maximum of two turns

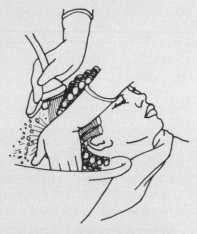

Thoroughly rinse with tepid water for 3–5 minutes

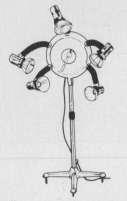

Infrared lamp for drying recurled (reformed) hair

Safety Tip

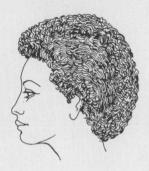

5. Attach neutralizing bib around hairline. Apply neutralizer thoroughly to each rod. Allow excess to drip into the bib.

6. Remove neutralizing bib. Place plastic cap over wound rods and secure with clip or rod. Allow hair to neutralize for at least 10 minutes or according to manufacturer's directions. **Use a dryer *only* if required by manufacturer.**

7. Rinse thoroughly with tepid water for 3 to 5 minutes. Use a timer. Gently towel blot. Apply protein conditioner and allow to remain on hair for 5 minutes. Gently unwind all rods. Next apply activator to scalp, follow with the curl moisturizer, shape, and then style the hair.

5. Neutralizing bib stops neutralizer from dripping down client's neck, ears, and forehead.

6. The plastic cap prevents the neutralizer from evaporating. **Caution**—Some manufacturers require the use of a **sodium bromate neutralizer! Do not substitute neutralizers.** Read directions carefully. **Do not drip neutralizer on client's mouth, eyes, or ears.** If you have an accidental drip, rinse immediately with cool water. A dryer **may** cause scalp burns.

7. Water rinsing removes the neutralizer from the hair. The hair should be gently unwound. Pulling may relax the curl.

GLOSSARY

Allergies   Extreme sensitivities to factors or substances in the environment.

Chemical rearranger   The basic product used to relax the hair in a curl reformation service.

Curl activator   An oily product used in the curl reformation service.

Curl booster   The thio product which is used for wrapping the hair on rods, then processing.

Curl rearranger   See **Chemical rearranger** and also **Curl reformation**.

Curl reformation   A double-application service in which super-curly hair is straightened and then recurled in a larger curl pattern.

Hypertension   High blood pressure.

Instant moisturizer   A product which puts moisture back into the hair.

Polymer conditioner   A high-quality protein conditioner.

Sodium bromate   The main ingredient used in the most common type of neutralizers in the curl reformation service.

QUESTIONS

1. What is another name for the curl reformation service?
2. Is a curl reformation a single or double-application service?
3. Is a curl reformation usually given to naturally straight hair?
4. True or false. In a curl reformation, the chemical used to relax the hair is usually sodium hydroxide.
5. Is the basic chemical used in the neutralizer for a curl reformation service generally peroxide?
6. Is it necessary to wear gloves when using the chemical rearranger?
7. Should the chemical rearranger be left on the hair more than 5 minutes?
8. Is the curl reformation service the type of service that requires a strand test?
9. Are the wrapping subsections for a curl reformation service the same as those used in wrapping a permanent wave?
10. True or false. In giving a curl reformation, it is best to use light, even tension when wrapping the hair on the rods.
11. Would the curl reformation service allow the hair to be set more easily in rollers for a bouffant hairstyle?
12. Does the curl reformation process break down the cystine disulfide bonds?
13. Would the pH of the chemical rearranger be 6.6?
14. What is the objective when using the chemical rearranger?
15. Can the processing of the chemical rearranger be speeded up by putting the client under the dryer?
16. Will porous hair take longer to process?
17. True or false. The curl reformation service obtains the best result when given immediately after a sodium hydroxide chemical relaxer.
18. Should protein conditioners be avoided when giving a curl reformation?
19. Should the chemical rearranger come in contact with the eyes or ears during the curl reformation service, would you rinse with hot water immediately?
20. Is it important to brush the hair before giving a curl reformation service?

ANSWERS

1. Curl rearranger or recurl 2. Double-application service 3. No 4. False; ammonium thioglycolate 5. No; sodium bromate 6. Yes 7. Yes 8. Yes 9. No; very thin subsections 10. False; firm, even tension 11. Yes 12. Yes 13. No; 9.6 14. To straighten the hair 15. Yes 16. No; a shorter time 17. False; hair must be cut first 18. No 19. No; cool water 20. No; do not brush the hair

Describing the Skin 22

There is a word which many of you may not be familiar with – that word is **esthetician**. The **esthetician** uses massage, skin preparations, facial devices, and the related arts and sciences to preserve and beautify the skin. Some states license estheticians separately from either cosmetologists or manicurists. On the other hand, some states include the esthetician practice as part of the basic cosmetology program. Your instructor will explain to you how your state regulates the practice of skin care.

Since the esthetician (or cosmetologist) must perform these services directly on the skin of the client, it is important that they be done safely. In order to do that, the **practitioner** (esthetician or cosmetologist) must have a thorough understanding of the **histology** (microscopic study) of the skin. This would include the structure and function of the skin.

The skin is the largest organ of the body, so it is important that you learn about it. The practitioner should know about some of the more common disorders and diseases of the skin. A doctor that specializes in disorders and diseases of the skin is called a **dermatologist**. The doctor's scientific study of the skin is called **dermatology**. Part of your job is knowing when you **cannot** safely give a service to a client and must refer the client to a physician or dermatologist. This chapter covers those disorders and diseases that you should know about.

Provided with the information in this chapter, you should be able to recognize common skin disorders that may be improved in the salon, and diseases which should be referred to a medical doctor/dermatologist.

Level of Acceptability	Score 75 percent or better on a multiple-choice exam on the information in this chapter.

Knowing Subobjectives	1. Explain the structure and function of the skin. 2. Describe the layers of the epidermis and explain their functions. 3. Classify the appendages of the skin by name and function. 4. Describe diseases of the eccrine sweat gland. 5. Explain skin pigmentation and its abnormalities. 6. Explain skin keratinization. 7. List primary and secondary lesions.

KNOWING SUBOBJECTIVE 1

Explain the structure and function of the skin.	**The skin is the largest and** one of the most efficient **organs** of the human body. It grows, reacts to sensation, and constantly renews itself. The skin is divided into three rather definite layers as follows:

1. epidermis
2. corium
3. subcutaneous tissue

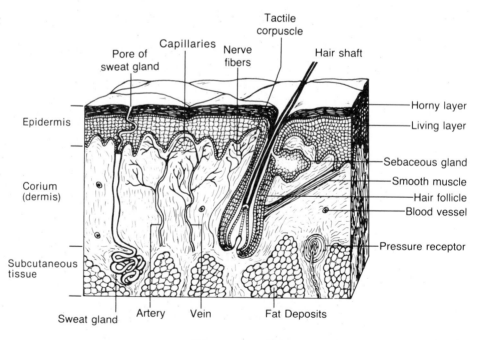

Skin cross section

The **epidermis** is the thinnest and outermost layer of skin. It is about as thick as this page. Although you can only see these skin cells through a microscope, they are very active.

The **corium** (KOHR-ee-uhm) (dermis) is the true skin. It is 20 to 30 times thicker than the epidermis and rests upon a thick pad of fatty (adipose [AD-eh-pohz]) subcutaneous tissue.

The **subcutaneous tissue** is below the corium. It acts like a shock absorber and heat insulator for the body.

Generally, the skin acts like a barrier between the organs inside the body and the rest of the world. Specifically, skin has several important functions.

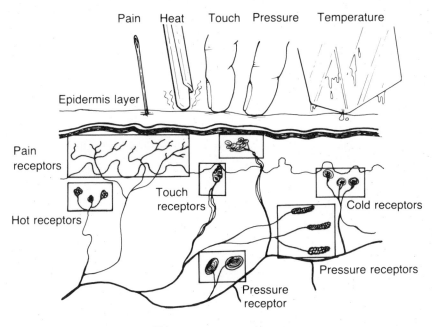

Skin sensory receptors

1. **Protection.** Healthy skin is soft and elastic. It protects the body from physical or chemical injury and from bacteria. Thus, it is both a shock absorber and barrier against bacteria and viruses.

2. **Heat regulation.** The **sudoriferous** (sweat) glands and blood vessels of the skin keep the body's internal temperature at 98.6 degrees F. Blood flows in the vessels to keep the body warm, while the sweat glands act like the cooling system. Perspiration from the sweat glands increases as the temperature outside of the body increases.

3. **Sensation.** The body feels heat, cold, pain, and touch through a network of nerve endings that are located all over the surface of the skin.

4. **Secretion.** The skin does not remove much body waste. Perspiration secreted by the sweat glands is practically the only waste removed by the skin. The kidneys are the primary excretory organs of the body.

5. **Absorption** (permeability). Many people believe that water and most others substances can go through the skin. This is not true. Most liquids will not penetrate the skin unless the layers have actually been destroyed, punctured, or penetrated. However, gases and many volatile substances easily pass through the skin. If the unbroken skin is penetrated, it occurs partly through openings of the hair follicles and sebaceous (oil) glands. Scientists do not believe that large amounts of substances enter the skin through the sweat ducts.

KNOWING SUBOBJECTIVE 2

Describe the layers of the epidermis and explain their functions.

As you learned in subobjective 1, the epidermis is the outermost layer of skin. It has five distinct layers.

1. horny layer (stratum corneum [STRAYT-uhm COR-nee-uhm])
2. lucid layer (stratum lucidum [loo-SID-uhm])
3. granular layer (stratum granulosum [gran-yoo-LOH-suhm])
4. prickle layer (stratum malpighii [mal-PIG-ee-eye])
5. basal layer (stratum germinativum [germ-in-ay-TYE-vuhm])

    1. The **horny layer** of skin is made up of several layers of dead, keratinized cells. This layer contains only 10 to 20 percent water, while the other

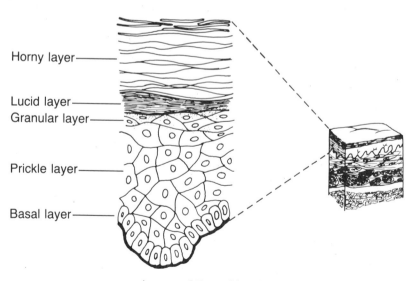

Layers of the epidermis

4 layers of the epidermis contain 70 percent water. The microscopic cells of this layer are constantly peeled or scaled off by clothing and bed linens. Surface skin is replaced completely every month. Keratin helps the skin hold water, which makes it soft and supple. It also prevents water from leaving the body and bacteria from entering the body. When the water content of the horny layer falls below 10 percent, the skin becomes chapped and visibly dry and scaly. Many people think that dry skin is due to the lack of skin oil (sebum), but it actually is caused by a lack of moisture. Humidity affects the amount of water the horny layer absorbs or loses. For example, in heated homes and offices during the winter months, dry skin is frequently a problem because the inside humidity is lowered by heating units. Installing a humidifier or using moisture lotions helps remedy this problem.

2. The **lucid layer** (clear layer) of skin is evident only in the palms of the hands and the soles of the feet where the epidermis is thick. The lucid layer lies directly above the granular layer of skin; they are the two most important barrier layers which protect the body.

3. The **granular layer** (cells look like granules) is the strongest in the areas where the lucid layer is absent. In these areas the granular layer protects the body from physical and chemical penetration.

4. The **prickle layer** is made up of several layers of epidermal cells that connect 4 or more keratin or melanin cells.

5. The **basal layer** of cells lies above the corium (dermis). Cells which are located here form **keratin** and **melanin**. The melanocytes are sandwiched between the more numerous keratin-forming basal cells. As you know, keratin is the soft cornified tissue of the skin, while melanin is the pigment which gives skin its color. In the making of pigment and skin, the basal and prickle layers work together.

KNOWING SUBOBJECTIVE 3

An **appendage** is something that is added to or extended from something else that is larger or more important. Two types of appendages are the cornified appendages (keratinized protein) of the skin–the hair and nails–and glandular appendages. The hair and nails are discussed elsewhere, so this chapter will deal only with glandular appendages of the skin.

Glands are groups of cells that take specific substances from blood, make new substances out of them, and then release the new substances which are called **secretions**.

Skin glands fall into 2 general categories–**sebaceous** and **sudoriferous.**

The **sebaceous (sih-BAY-shuhs) glands** are present all over the body except in the palms of the hands and soles of the feet. They secrete an oily fluid called sebum through a duct to a follicle that might contain a hair. The secretion of sebum is a continuous flow of material that cells have broken down. When sebum is secreted through its duct, the entire gland falls apart and is pushed out. Sebaceous glands are much larger and most numerous on the scalp and face.

Classify the appendages of the skin by name and function.

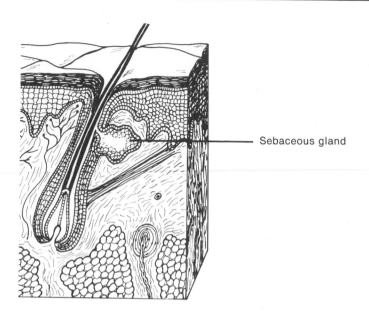

Sebaceous gland

Sebaceous gland with hair follicle and hair

The oily **sebum** covers the skin with a film that helps fight bacteria and fungus. It also slows the evaporation of moisture (water) from the skin and protects against bacteria. The amount of sebum secreted depends on several factors.

Individual differences   Some persons have small, underdeveloped sebaceous glands, while others have numerous large glands that cause greasy, oily skin.

Age   In infancy, persons produce little or no sebum, but as they grow older, activity of the sebaceous glands increases, particularly at puberty. After the age of 50, sebum production usually decreases.

Race   Black persons usually have larger and more numerous sebaceous glands.

Climate   Persons living in warm climates secrete more sebum than those living in cooler climates.

Scientists have not yet figured out how to increase or decrease the production of sebum. Drugs, hormones, and special products do not seem to affect the flow of sebum, but some prescribed drugs change the composition of the sebum to make it less irritating to the skin.

Sudoriferous (sood-ah-RIF-ah-ruhs) sweat glands are found everywhere in the human skin and are controlled by the nervous system. Sudoriferous is a general term used to describe the apocrine and eccrine sweat glands.

Apocrine (AP-ah-krehn) sweat glands are found only in the ear canal, under the arms, and in the genital region of the body. Each apocrine sweat gland opens into a hair follicle as does each sebaceous gland. Although the sweat is sterile when excreted, it becomes contaminated by bacteria on the surface of the skin. This causes "body odor." The gland secretes continuously into a reservoir beneath the skin; the sweat is excreted to the surface when the reservoir overflows (sometimes this is set off by the adrenal glands activated by emotional stress). The overall importance of these glands has not been determined. The composition of apocrine sweat is a whitish fluid containing water, salt, uric acid (found in urine), lactic acid (formed from sugar), proteins and carbohydrates. The pH of sweat is 5.4-5.6 and the body secretes 2 lbs. (2 pints) per day.

The eccrine (EK-rehn) sweat glands, by contrast, are the heat regulators for the body. Although they are much smaller than the apocrine sweat glands, there are many more of them. The eccrine sweat glands are regulated by the hypothalamus (high-poh-THAL-eh-muhs). Eccrine sweat glands are all over the surface of the skin, but they are heavily concentrated in the areas of the forehead, underarms, palms, and soles of the feet. Eccrine

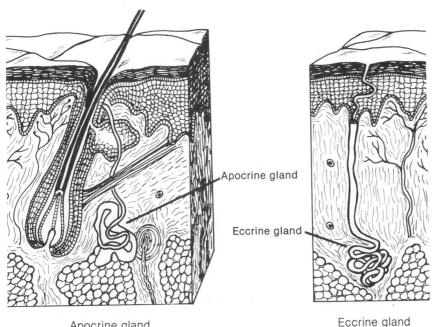

Apocrine gland

Eccrine gland

Apocrine gland

Eccrine gland

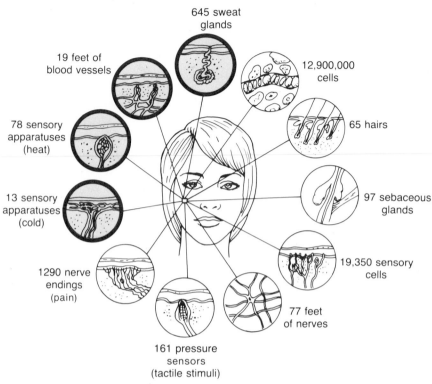

645 sweat glands

19 feet of blood vessels

12,900,000 cells

78 sensory apparatuses (heat)

65 hairs

13 sensory apparatuses (cold)

97 sebaceous glands

1290 nerve endings (pain)

19,350 sensory cells

77 feet of nerves

161 pressure sensors (tactile stimuli)

Sensor points of one square inch of skin. Screened area indicates those controlled by pituitary gland

sweat glands secrete sweat into a duct or tube from which it is excreted directly to the surface of the skin. Heat is the main activator of eccrine sweat glands.

Unlike the apocrine sweat gland the eccrine sweat gland stays inactive unless something, such as heat or emotional stress, stimulates it to cool the body. The eccrine sweat gland is not important for excreting body waste.

Cosmetic companies manufacture many products for underarm perspiration which have one common ingredient called aluminum chloride. This ingredient shrinks the openings of the sweat pores. A fragrance is often added to mask any odor that does occur.

KNOWING SUBOBJECTIVE 4

Describe diseases of the eccrine sweat gland.

Hyperhidrosis (high-per-high-DROH-siss) is an abnormal increase in the amount of sweat. It can be caused by something affecting one part of the body or the entire body.

Hot, humid weather or increased body heat caused by work or exercise can cause it. Localized sweating, such as from the palms, soles, underarms, and face, is often caused by emotional stress. It may also be caused by menopause in women, overweight, gout, alcoholic intoxication, and reaction to drugs. This condition needs a doctor's treatment.

Anhidrosis (an-high-DROH-siss) is the inability of the body to regulate its temperature. The body cannot make or send sweat to the skin's surface (sweat retention). Since the body's temperature cannot be controlled (cooled), a doctor should be consulted.

Bromhidrosis (brom-hi-DROH-siss) (also called osmidrosis [oz-mi-DROH-siss]) is abnormal, or foul-smelling, sweat. This may be caused by eating garlic or onions or taking certain drugs. Some diseases produce sweat that has a peculiar odor. They are diabetes, gout, typhoid fever, and others. Bromhidrosis is caused by surface skin bacteria coming in contact with secretions from the apocrine sweat gland. Underarm hair is the collection site for keratin, secretions, and bacteria that can cause odor on contact with sweat. Therefore, odor can be reduced by shortening or shaving hair in the area. Carefully washing underarms with an ordinary antiseptic soap in the mornings and evenings and changing clothes regularly will also help.

Miliaria rubra (mil-ee-AR-ee-ah ROOB-rah), also called prickly heat or heat rash, is caused by blockage of the sweat duct openings. It is common in very hot, humid climates. The sweat ducts rupture into the midepidermis. Itching and burning results. Mild powders and lotions will stop itching and burning, but the best treatment is an air-conditioned environment.

KNOWING SUBOBJECTIVE 5

As discussed earlier in this chapter, **melanin cells (melanocytes)** are made in the basal layer of the epidermis. The chemical that activates the production of pigment is a basic amino acid called **tyrosine (TIGH-roh-sin).** Tyrosine causes the melanocytes to make melanin. (Ultraviolet rays from the sun, for example, can cause the release of **tyrosinase (tigh-ROH-sin-ayz),**

Explain skin pigmentation and its abnormalities.

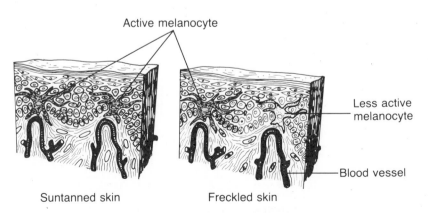

Active melanocyte

Less active melanocyte

Blood vessel

Suntanned skin   Freckled skin

During tanning, melanin moves into the corneum

an enzyme that acts on the tyrosine to start the melanin synthesis–tanning). Once the melanin is formed, it works its way through the epidermis to the horny layer. Melanin itself is colorless, but when it is exposed to oxygen, it becomes dark.

Melanin tans the skin to protect it from the sun's burning rays. It is generally accepted that overexposure to sunlight after a number of years causes thickening and wrinkling (aging) of the skin. Overexposure to the sun also causes different forms of skin cancer. Daily use of a sunscreen* (such as lotion) is advised to protect the skin. White skin and black skin do not differ in the number of melanocytes they contain. Black skin does, however, contain more pigmentation, and these pigment granules differ in size and shape and black skin can be sun burned just like white skin.

Abnormalities Involving Melanocyte Activity

The Federal Food and Drug Administration (FDA) recognizes the importance of sun tanning lotions (sun screens) as a simple way to prevent skin cancer. The FDA requires all sun tan lotion makers to label their products with a number to indicate how much of the sun's ultraviolet rays are allowed to penetrate through their product and reach the skin. The sun protection factor is important because wherever the skin is burned by the sun, the person can develop a form of **herpes simplex,** a severe, and very painful

Safety Tip

*PABA–P-Amino benzoic acid.

Examples:

SPF-15 screens out 100% of ultraviolet rays
SPF-8 screens out 50% of ultraviolet rays

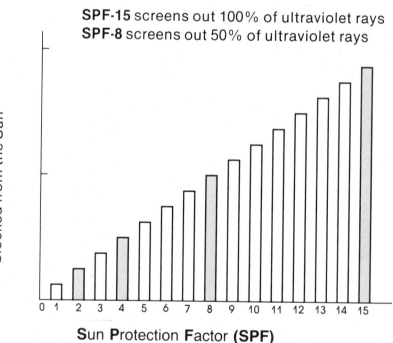

Sun Protection Factor (SPF)

skin condition. The sun triggers the herpes virus, which causes the nerve endings in the skin to become inflamed and irritated. This condition must be treated by a physician and can be difficult in some cases to clear up.

The system that is used is called the **sun protection factor** (SPF). The **SPF** is a numbering system from "1 to 15." A rating of "1" would tell you that almost all of the sun's rays are allowed to penetrate through the lotion to your skin. On the other hand, a lotion with a **SPF** of "15" would act as a "**sun block.**" A **sun block** doesn't permit any of the sun's rays to reach your skin. People with average skin color and sensitivity should use a tanning lotion with a SPF in the range of "8-10" to begin with. Individuals with a very light complexion should begin using a product with a SPF of at least "12."

Since no one wants his/her skin to prematurely wrinkle, thicken, or develop cancer, it is best to begin tanning on a gradual basis. **Avoid sun tanning** between the hours of 10:00 A.M. and 2:00 P.M. Limit exposure time at the beginning of the season to 15–20 minutes. If you live near the equator, where the sun is closer to the earth, take extra special care to use a sun screen **daily.** Individuals that live near water or snow should also be very careful because water and snow reflect the ultraviolet rays, and you will receive a double dose of sun.

Read label directions carefully because the maker will explain whether the product needs to be reapplied after the person swims or perspires heavily. Perspiration will usually water-down the sun tanning lotion 50%. A few sun tanning lotions will stain clothing, so read the label to be sure the one you are purchasing doesn't stain clothing.

There are many reasons why the pigmentation of the skin can change. A few of the more common changes in pigmentation will be discussed.

Before scientists discovered how melanocytes work, they called the overproduction of pigment melanoderma and underproduction of pigment **leukoderma (loo-koh-DER-mah).** Although more specific terms can be applied now, these terms are basically correct.

Melanoderma (mel-an-oh-DER-mah) is a term used to describe any hyperpigmentation (overactivity) caused by overactivity of the melanocytes in the epidermis. Hyperpigmentation may be triggered by four factors: overactivity of the pituitary gland, circulation of hormones, disease, and drugs.

Two common examples of melanoderma are **chloasma (klo-AZ-mah)** and **ephelides (ef-EE-li-deez).**

Chloasma is a group of brownish macules (nonelevated spots) occurring in one place. Most people call them liver spots. They often occur on the face, pubic area, or on the nipples. Chloasma is usually the result of a hormone disturbance, so it is seen in women during the use of oral contraceptives, in pregnancy, or menopause. Children usually between the ages of 2 and 5 get **ephelides (freckles).** The freckles appear more in summer than winter. Freckles are also called **lentigines,** although technically they are different from freckles. Sunlight is the most effective activator of melanocyte activity. An inflammation of the skin called **photodermatitis** is caused by

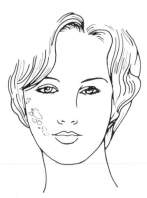

Vitiligo pigmentation

the ultraviolet light in sunlight and sun lamps, internal or external drugs, and cosmetics, shaving lotion, and perfume.

Leukoderma describes **hypopigmentation** (underpigmentation) of the skin, caused by a decrease in activity of melanocytes. It is occasionally the result of a congenital defect such as albinism; however, acquired hypopigmentation, such as vitiligo, can occur.

Albinism is a congenital failure of the skin to form melanin pigment. Persons with albinism have pink skin, white hair (sometimes it may be reddish), and pink eyes. Albinos have a marked hypersensitivity to light. Their skin ages very early, sometimes in early adulthood.

Vitiligo is characterized by oval or irregular patches of white skin that do not have normal pigment. It usually is seen on the face, hands, and neck, as patches of depigmentation. They may enlarge slowly. These patches of skin must be protected from overexposure to sun or any exposure to ultraviolet lamps. Gradual exposure of the sunlight, ultraviolet lamps or Wood's light (cold quartz light) may restore pigment, but a doctor should be consulted before these procedures are tried.

Miscellaneous Pigmentation Abnormalities

A **nevus flammeus (NEE-vuhs FLAM-ee-uhs)** is a birthmark or congenital mole. The nevus birthmark may look like a stain (port wine stain) on the face. It is a reddish purple, flat mark. The stain is caused by dilation of the small blood vessels in the skin. Cosmetic makeup is the only remedy for it. If it does not disappear shortly after birth, it is permanent.

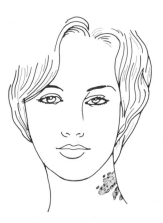

Nevus flammeus

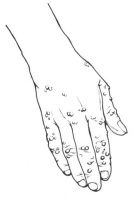

Verruca

Moles (melanocytic nevi [mel-an-oh-SIT-tik NEE-vigh]) are the most common tumors of the skin; almost everyone has one or more of them. These brown pigmented nevi first appear as macules. After a period of time they may become elevated. Hair often grows through moles, but this hair should not be removed. Any change of color in a mole should be reported to a dermatologist.

Melanotic sarcoma (fatal skin cancer) begins with a mole. The main characteristic is an overabundance of pigment.

Verruca (veh-ROO-kah) is one name assigned to a variety of warts. Warts are caused by a virus. They can be contagious and spread all over the body. Dermatologists use a variety of methods to easily remove one wart or a cluster of them.

Callus (also called hyperkeratosis [high-per-ker-eh-TOH-siss]) is a thickening of the cornified layer of the epidermis, which results from physical trauma, e.g., very heavy work involving the hands or feet. It occurs from pressure or friction applied to the skin.

Wrinkles are caused by the breaking down of the elastin and collagen fibers below the surface of the skin. The epidermis can not be supported when the fibers become broken and lumpy, causing the loss of resiliency; grooves, lines and wrinkles are the result.

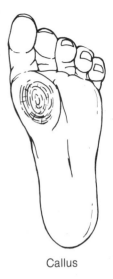

Callus

KNOWING SUBOBJECTIVE 6

Keratin is a very tough and elastic layer of protein that protects underlying skin. It is the main (not the only) ingredient in the horny layer of the epidermis. It is **not easily penetrated** or dissolved by diluted alkalis, weak acids, organic solvents, or water.

Explain skin keratinization.

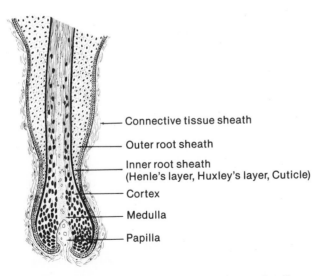

Connective tissue sheath

Outer root sheath

Inner root sheath
(Henle's layer, Huxley's layer, Cuticle)

Cortex

Medulla

Papilla

Vertical cross-section through hair and root sheath

There are two kinds of keratin. **Soft keratin** is produced by the epidermis all over the body. Soft keratin is present throughout all five layers of the epidermis, although mature hard scales (protective keratin) are found only in the horny layer of the skin.

Hard keratin is found in the nails and hair. It forms compacted and hard scales. Soft keratin is continually shed in fine loose scales.

The process of **keratinization (ker-eh-tin-eh-ZAY-shun),** formation of keratin, begins in the **basal** and **prickle** layers of the epidermis and is completed in the horny layer, where it appears as a tough elastic substance, the outer layer of skin. The elasticity of the horny layer and the chapping of the skin depend mainly on the water content of the keratin, not the amount of sebum.

KNOWING SUBOBJECTIVE 7

List primary and secondary lesions.

Since this chapter deals with the skin, you should know terms used to describe the skin. Most of the time, if you see a client who has an abnormal skin condition, tell him or her to see a dermatologist. A dermatologist is a doctor who specializes in treating diseases of the skin. The dermatologist can determine the **etiology (eet-ee-AHL-eh-jee)** (cause) of a skin disease, **diagnose** (identify) a specific skin disease, treat it, and offer a **prognosis** (prediction of the chances for improvement and the time needed for it). The dermatologist may even take a skin sample and send it to a **pathology laboratory** (a place to study the origin, nature, cause, and development of disease) for examination.

A **lesion (LEE-zhun)** is any abnormal or harmful change in the structure of an organ or tissue. Lesions are classified as primary and secondary. Twelve primary lesions are described below.

The difference between primary and secondary lesions is time. As the name implies, "primary" means first. So, primary lesions develop on the skin first. The secondary lesion is often the **result** of an untreated primary lesion. For example, you may develop a "patch" of dry skin at the corner of your mouth. This would be a primary lesion. If you didn't moisturize that area, it would become so dry that a fissure (crack) would result. The crack would be an example of a secondary lesion.

Twelve primary lesions:

1. **Macules (MAK-yoolz)** are as large as 1 centimeter. They are discolorations appearing on the skin's surface. Macules are flat and have **distinct edges (circumscribed).** Freckles and tattoos are examples.

2. **Patches** are macules that are larger than 1 centimeter. They are circumscribed, flat discolorations of the skin.

3. **Papules (PAP-yoolz)** are up to 1 centimeter. They are circumscribed, elevated, solid lesions. Warts are papules.

4. **Wheals (WEELZ),** hives, are a type of papule. Sharply circumscribed, as in an insect bite, they are solid, rising above the skin–for instance, mosquito bites.

5. **Nodules (NAHDJ-yoolz)** are also referred to as tumors, but they are smaller than true tumors. Nodules are up to 1 centimeter. They are solid lumps and may be above or beneath the skin's surface.

6. **Tumors** are larger than 1 centimeter and are deeper than nodules. They are circumscribed penetrations of skin and subcutaneous tissue. They are above and below the skin's surface.

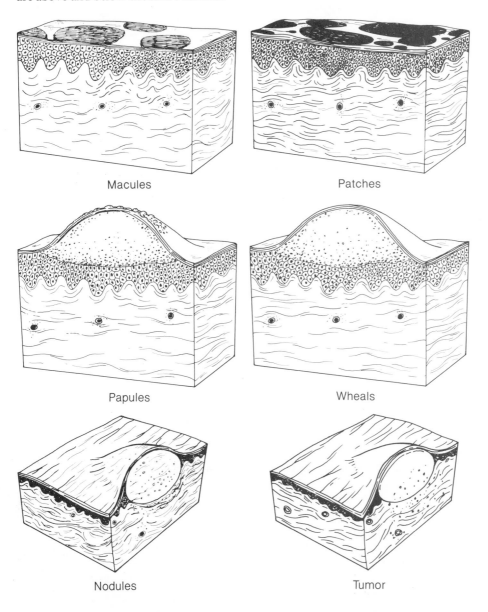

Macules

Patches

Papules

Wheals

Nodules

Tumor

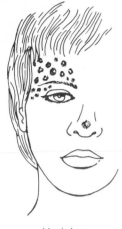

Vesicles

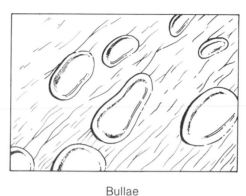

Bullae

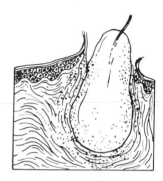

Pustule

7. **Vesicles (VES-ih-kehlz)** can be as large as 1 centimeter. They are circumscribed elevations of skin containing a clear, watery fluid. Examples are chickenpox, contact dermatitis, and blisters.

8. **Bullae (BULL-ee)** are larger than 1 centimeter. They are circumscribed lesions above and below the skin. They contain a clear watery fluid. Second-degree burns are characterized by bullae.

9. **Pustules (PUS-chyoolz)** vary in size. They are circumscribed elevations of the skin containing pus-like fluid. Acne and impetigo are examples of pustules.

10. **Cysts** are semisolid or fluid lumps above and below the skin. An example is a sebaceous cyst.

11. **Furuncles** (boils) are large localized infections of hair follicles, usually caused by staphylococci. They appear above the surface of the skin.

12. **Carbuncles** are extreme infections of several adjoining hair follicles that drain by multiple openings onto the skin's surface. They are above and below the skin.

Five secondary lesions are described below.

1. **Scales** are shedding, dead cells of the horny layer of the epidermis. The cells may be dry or greasy, as seen in dandruff or psoriasis.

2. **Crusts** (scabs) are the dried remains of an oozing sore. They may consist of dried blood, dried pus, dried sebum, or a combination of these substances.

3. **Excoriations** are abrasions of the skin, usually superficial and traumatic. They occur in scratched insect bites and scabies.

4. **Fissures** are almost straight-line breaks in the skin (cracks) that are sharply defined. They are commonly seen around the fingertips and heels.

5. **Scars**, also called **cicatrices (sik-eh-TRYE-seez),** are formations of connective tissue replacing tissue lost through injury or disease. Scars occur when the corium is damaged.

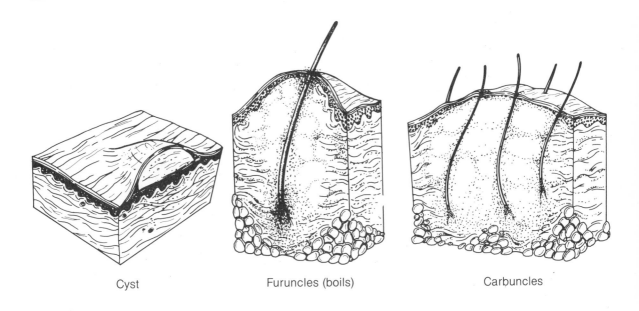

Cyst   Furuncles (boils)   Carbuncles

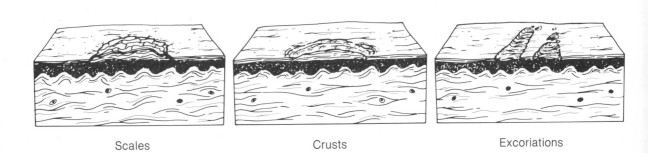

Scales   Crusts   Excoriations

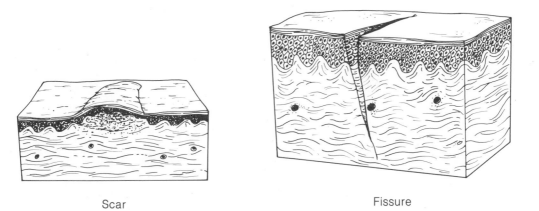

Scar   Fissure

GLOSSARY

Adipose (AD-eh-pohz) tissue Fatty tissue beneath the epidermis and the corium. See **Subcutaneous tissue.**

Albinism (AL-beh-niz-uhm) A congenital failure of the skin to form melanin pigment.

Anhidrosis (an-high-DROH-siss) The inability of the body to regulate its temperature through perspiration.

Apocrine (AP-ah-krehn) sweat glands Sweat glands in the ear canal, under the arms, and in the genital region. They open into the hair follicle.

Basal layer The layer of the epidermis where cells form keratin and melanin.

Birthmark See **Nevus flammeus.**

Boils See Furuncles.

Bromhidrosis (broh-mi-DROH-siss) Abnormal or foul-smelling sweat. Also called osmidrosis.

Bulla (BULL-ah) A circumscribed lesion such as a second degree burn, which occurs above and below the skin and contains a clear, watery fluid. See also **Vesicles.**

Callus See **Hyperkeratosis.**

Carbuncles Extreme infections of several adjoining hair follicles that drain with multiple openings onto the skin's surface.

Chloasma (klo-AZ-mah) An overpigmentation producing brownish macules (nonelevated spots) occurring in one place; caused by a hormone imbalance. Also called liver spots.

Cicatrices (SIK-eh-trigh-seez) See **Scars.**

Corium (KOHR-ee-uhm) Sometimes called the true skin, it is between the epidermis and the subcutaneous layers. It is the horny layer.

Crust The dried remains of an oozing sore on the skin, commonly called a scab.

Dermatology The science dealing with the study of the skin.

Eccrine (EK-rehn) sweat glands Heat regulators of the body.

Ephelides (ef-EE-li-deez) Freckles.

Epidermis The thinnest, outermost layer of the skin.

Esthetician The practitioner who specializes in the preservation and beautification of the face and neck.

Etiology (eet-ee-AHL-eh-jee) The cause of a disease or a disorder.

Excoriations (ek-sko-ri-AY-shunz) Abrasions of the skin.

Fissures Almost straight-line breaks (cracks) in the skin that are sharply defined and are commonly seen around the fingertips and heels.

Furuncles Large, localized infections of hair follicles caused by staphylococci; commonly called boils.

Glands Groups of cells that take specific substances from blood, make new substances out of them, and then release the new substances which are called secretions.

Granular layer The layer of the epidermis that protects the body from physical and chemical penetration.

Histology The microscopic study; histology of skin includes its functions, diseases, and disorders.

Horny layer   The outermost layer of the epidermis; it is made up of several layers of dead keratinized cells.

Hyperhidrosis (high-per-high-DROH-siss)   An abnormal increase in the amount of sweat.

Hyperkeratosis (high-per-ker-eh-TOH-siss)   A thickening of the cornified layer of the epidermis that results from pressure or friction applied to the skin; commonly called callus.

Hypothalamus (high-poh-THAL-eh-muhs)   The gland that regulates the eccrine sweat glands.

Keratin   A very tough and elastic layer of protein that protects underlying skin; found in two forms: soft keratin, present through all five layers of the epidermis, and hard keratin, found in the nails and hair.

Keratinization (ker-eh-tin-eh-ZAY-shun)   The process of forming keratin in the skin.

Lesion (LEE-zuhn)   Any abnormal or harmful change in the structure of an organ or tissue.

Leukoderma (loo-koh-DER-mah)   Underpigmentation of the skin that can either be congenital (albinism) or acquired (vitiligo).

Liver spots   See **Chloasma.**

Lucid layer   A layer of the epidermis on the palms of the hands and soles of the feet. It is directly above the granular layer.

Macule (MAK-yool)   A flat discoloration with distinct edges appearing on the skin's surface.

Melanocytic nevi (mel-an-oh-SIT-ik NEE-vigh)   Tumors of the skin that may become elevated and often have hair growing from them; commonly called moles.

Melanoderma (mel-an-oh-DER-mah)   Overactivity of the melanocytes in the epidermis caused by overactivity of the pituitary gland, circulation of hormones, disease, or drugs.

Miliaria rubra (mil-ee-AR-ee-ah ROOB-rah)   A heat rash caused by blockage of the sweat duct openings; common in hot, humid climates.

Moles   See **Melanocytic nevi.**

Nevus flameus (NEE-vuhs FLAM-ee-uhs)   A birthmark or congenital mole.

Nodules (NAHJ-yoolz)   Solid tumorlike lumps above or beneath the skin.

Osmidrosis (oz-mi-DROH-siss)   Abnormal or foul-smelling sweat. Also called bromhidrosis.

Papules (PAP-yoolz)   Circumscribed, elevated, solid lesions, such as warts.

Patches   Macules that are larger than 1 centimeter.

Photodermatitis (foh-toh-der-meh-TIGH-tis)   An inflammation of the skin caused by ultraviolet light, drugs, cosmetics, shaving lotion, or perfume.

Prickle layer   A layer of the epidermis made up of several layers of cells that connect four or more keratin or melanin cells.

Prickly heat   See **Miliaria rubra.**

Pustules (PUHS-chyoolz)   Circumscribed elevations of the skin containing a pus-like fluid; examples are acne and impetigo.

Scales   Shedding, dead cells of the horny layer of the epidermis that may be dry or greasy; occurs with dandruff or psoriasis, for example.

Scars Formations of connective tissue replacing tissue lost through injury or disease that damages the corium.

Sebaceous (si-BAY-shuhs) glands Glands located over most of the body that secrete a lubricating and bacteria-fighting substance called sebum.

Sebum (SEEB-uhm) An oily substance that helps fight bacteria and slows evaporation of moisture from the skin.

Secretions Substances made and released by glands.

Stratum corneum (STRAYT-uhm KOR-nee-uhm) See **Horny layer.**

Stratum germinativum (STRAYT-uhm germ-in-ay-TIGH-vuhm) See **Basal layer**

Stratum granulosum (STRAYT-uhm gran-yoo-LOH-suhm) See **Granular layer.**

Stratum lucidum (STRAYT-uhm loo-SID-uhm) See **Lucid layer.**

Stratum malpighii (STRAYT-uhm mal-PIG-ee-igh) See **Prickle layer.**

Subcutaneous tissue Layer of tissue beneath the epidermis and corium.

Sudoriferous (sood-ah-RIF-ah-ruhs) glands Sweat glands.

SPF See **Sun Protection Factor.**

Sun protection factor A numbering system from 1-15, indicating the level of screening from the sun's rays provided by the product.

Tumors Solid lumps, larger than nodules, which penetrate the skin and subcutaneous tissue above or below the skin's surface.

Tyrosinase (tigh-ROH-sin-ayz) An enzyme that acts on tyrosine to start the melanin synthesis called tanning.

Tyrosine (tigh-ROH-sin) An amino acid that activates the production of pigment.

Verruca (veh-ROO-kah) Warts, which are caused by a virus and may be contagious.

Vesicles (VES-ih-kehlz) Circumscribed elevations, smaller than 1 centimeter, of skin containing a clear, watery fluid; examples are chickenpox, contact dermatitis, and blisters. See also **Bulla.**

Vitiligo (vit-i-LIGH-goh) Oval or irregular patches of the skin that do not contain normal pigment. The cause is unknown, but may involve mental or physical trauma.

Wart See **Verruca.**

Wheals (WEELZ) Sharply circumscribed, solid, elevated papules. A mosquito bite is a wheal.

QUESTIONS

1. How do the following relate to skin: epidermis, dermis, adipose tissue, corium, keratin, lesion?
2. What is another name for miliaria rubra?
3. What would a break or crack in the skin be called?
4. What does the word etiology mean?
5. What does subcutaneous mean?

6. What is the technical name given to the study of the skin?
7. What is a lesion?
8. Is the epidermis the outermost layer of the skin?
9. Does perspiration (sweat) help to regulate the temperature of the body?
10. Is it true that anything you rub on the skin will penetrate into the areas below the skin?
11. How often is the outer layer of the skin replaced?
12. Does the skin act as a barrier to prevent bacteria from entering the body?
13. What is another name for the corium?
14. Do you have sebaceous glands on the palms of your hands and the soles of your feet?
15. What is the name of the substances that are released from glands?
16. Do sweat glands empty directly onto the skin, or do they empty into the hair follicle?
17. What is the technical term for excessive perspiration?
18. What does the abbreviation SPF stand for?
19. True or false. For the most beneficial type of sun tan, it is best to tan from 12:00 P.M. to 2:00 P.M.
20. True or false. If a sun tanning lotion has a rating of "10," very little protection will be given to the wearer.
21. What is the coloring substance in skin called?
22. Does over-exposure to the sun cause premature wrinkling, and may cause skin cancer?
23. What is the technical name for a mole?
24. What form of protein gives skin its soft elastic quality?

ANSWERS

1. Outermost (top) layer of skin; below the epidermis; fatty subcutaneous tissue; same as dermis; protein of the skin; any abnormal skin condition 2. Prickly heat or heat rash 3. Fissure 4. The cause of a disease or disorder 5. Below the epidermis and dermis (corium) 6. Dermatology 7. Any abnormal skin condition 8. Yes 9. Yes 10. No 11. Monthly 12. Yes 13. Dermis 14. No 15. Secretions 16. They empty in both locations 17. Hyperhidrosis 18. Sun Protection Factor 19. False 20. False; good protection 21. Melanin 22. Yes 23. Nevus or nevi 24. (Check against text*)

Giving Facial Treatments 23

The beauty industry is placing more emphasis than ever on developing two types of beauty salons—the "full-service salon," and the specialty or "esthetician salon." The full-service salon provides a complete shopping list of services from which the client can select. The esthetician salon specializes in preservation and beautification of the face and neck.

Cosmetologists of both types of salons have come to realize the importance of skin care as well as hair care. The result has been that many of them attend skin-care seminars. So, learning some of the basic procedures used for facial treatment services will allow you to enter either type of salon with the fundamental knowlege and skills to become employed.

Purpose

Use the information in this chapter and the knowledge you gain in class to give a facial massage and skin analysis.

Major Objective

Use the steps prescribed by your school or the steps in this chapter to give a facial treatment in 45 minutes. Score 75 percent or better on a multiple-choice exam on the information in this chapter.

Level of Acceptability

1. Describe the 5 basic massage movements.
2. Describe the nature and benefits of light therapy.

Knowing Subobjectives

3. Use the proper steps and safety precautions to give facial treatments to normal skin, dry skin, and oily skin.

Doing Subobjectives

KNOWING SUBOBJECTIVE 1

Describe the 5 basic massage movements.

Safety Tip

Most people want to have a good appearance, but no amount of makeup can really give the "natural look" of a **healthy skin.** Facial massages help to keep skin fresh and smooth and keep muscles firm. They are one of the best ways to enhance facial beauty.

Facial massages should **not** be performed on **diseased, broken, bruised, or scraped** skin.

Facial massages benefit the skin in several ways: stimulation of skin, which causes blood vessels to dilate and increases the blood supply to the skin; stimulation of facial muscles, which gives stronger muscle tone and fewer wrinkles; reduction of adipose (fatty) tissue in the subcutaneous layers, which gives the skin a firmer texture; relaxation and soothing of facial nerves; and normalization of the metabolism of the skin glands and the keratinization process.

There are 5 basic massage movements:

1. **Effleurage (ef-fler-AZH)** is a **light, stroking movement** applied with either the palm of the hand or the ball of the finger. It creates a soothing effect on the skin.

2. **Petrissage (peh-tri-SAHJ)** is a **kneading or rolling movement** applied with both the palm and fingers. It creates a stimulating effect on the skin.

3. **Tapotement (ta-poh-MAHN)** is a **light tapping or slapping movement** applied with the fingertips. It creates a slight stimulating effect on the skin.

4. **Friction** is a **rubbing movement** applied with either the fingertips or the flat of the hand. It creates a stimulating effect on the skin.

5. **Vibration** is a **shaking movement** done with fingertips and arm. Because it is a very stimulating, it should be used for only a few seconds in any one location.

KNOWING SUBOBJECTIVE 2

Describe the nature and benefits of light therapy.

Although you do not need a sophisticated understanding of light, you should have a basic knowledge of how light therapy is used in facial and scalp treatments.

Light is a form of energy. Its energy is related to wavelengths, which have two ranges or spectrums: visible and invisible. Ordinary light, which is visible, can be seen in a spectrum (array of different colors) when sunlight passes through a prism. This **visible light** comprises about **12 percent** of sunlight. The spectrum of visible light is also seen in a rainbow. See color plate 3 in the center of this book.

In light therapy, cosmetologists are concerned with two types of invisible light: infrared and ultraviolet.

Infrared (in-frah-RED) rays have long wavelengths capable of deep penetration. These light rays have wavelengths of 7,700 angstroms Å and longer. (An angstrom is a unit used to measure the wavelength of light.) Infrared rays comprise about 80 percent of sunlight.

Source   A therapeutic lamp specially made to produce these rays.

Distance and Time   30 inches from client for about 5 minutes; to protect the tissues from damage, make the exposure to skin intermittent by constantly turning the base of the lamp so that the pattern of the light rays is broken.

Precautions   Use of recommended distance and exposure time only; **protection of eyes by cotton** saturated with water. If used to dry the hair, **be careful not to burn the hair.**

Effects   Relief of pain by soothing heat, increase in circulation by dilation of blood vessels, increase in metabolism of skin cells and other chemical changes within tissues, stimulation of perspiration and oil production.

Ultraviolet rays (also called **actinic rays**) comprise about **8 percent** of sunlight. They have shorter wavelengths and do not penetrate as deeply as infrared. Ultraviolet light rays range from about 1850Å to 3900Å. These rays are helpful in the control of acne. **Ultraviolet can be very dangerous. Always follow directions for the specific lamp being used.**

Source   Therapeutic lamp designed to produce these rays.

Distance and Time   12 to 36 inches, depending on effects desired; initial exposure should be 1 to 2 minutes, which can be increased gradually to 8 minutes in later treatments, depending on the sensitivity of the client's skin.

Precautions   Use of recommended distance and time only; (overexposure can produce severe damage to skin); protect your eyes and your client's eyes by using cotton saturated with cool water. **The eyes must not receive any exposure to ultraviolet rays.**

Effects   Stimulation of chemical effects on the skin include an **increase in vitamin D** and an increase in blood and lymph circulation. Tanning of skin results from stimulation of the pigmentation process in the skin cells.

Infrared (Invisible Light) Used in Therapy

Safety Tip

Ultraviolet (Invisible Light) Used in Therapy

Safety Tip

DOING SUBOBJECTIVE 3

Use the proper steps and safety precautions to give facial treatments for normal skin, dry skin, and oily skin.

Give A Facial Treatment for Normal Skin

Supplies

□ cold creme
□ cleansing creme
□ cleansing lotion
□ emollient creme
□ astringent lotion

□ skin freshener
□ cotton
□ towels for head band
□ spatulas
□ cotton pledgets or tissue

Preparation

PROCEDURE

1. Check record for notes on previous services. Lower facial chair to reclining position and adjust headrest.

2. Wrap a head band around the client's head. Be sure to cover the hairline.
3. Use a sanitized spatula to remove all cremes from the jars for each client.

RATIONALE

1. A reclining position gives you easier access to the face. The client's head must be supported at all times to prevent injury.
2. This protects the client's hair from creme and other facial preparations.
3. Foreign substances can contaminate creme.

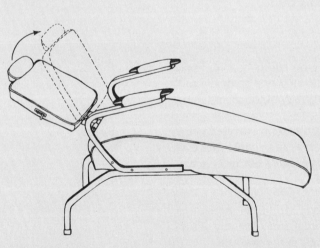

Adjustable facial chair. Head rest covering should be changed after each client

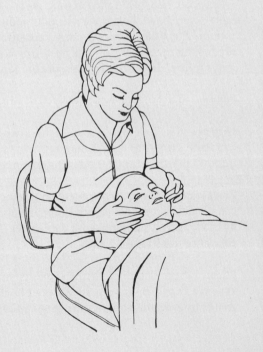

4. Apply dabs of cleansing creme to the forehead, cheeks, chin, nose, and throat and spread across the entire face. Start at the chin and work out and up toward the ears and cheeks. Continue along the eyes, nose, forehead, hairline, neck, and chest.

5. Using upward movements of both hands, remove creme with tissues folded into mittens.

Manipulations

PROCEDURE

1. Apply emollient creme in the same way that you applied cleansing creme.

2. Use the index, middle, and ring fingers of each hand to stimulate the regions described in step 4. Keep your fingers on the client's face at all times. Repeat each manipulation 5 times.

4. Massage will open the pores. Before this occurs, all impurities and makeup must be removed so that dirt cannot get into the pores to cause blackheads and milia. Use cold creme for normal skin. Use cleansing creme or cleansing lotion for oily skin.

5. All facial movements are upward to prevent dragging and sagging of muscles and wrinkling of skin.

RATIONALE

1. This is standard procedure; emollients lubricate and soften skin.

2. Stimulation is a major effect of facial massage. Using these middle fingers keeps a constant, even pressure. Keeping the fingers on the face helps you keep an even rhythm and tempo.

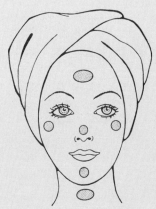

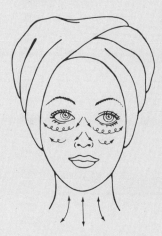

Application of cleansing cream

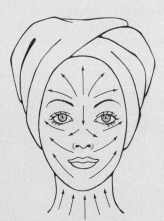

Spread cleansing cream over face and neck

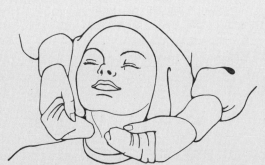

Remove cleansing cream using upward movements

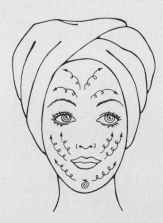

Begin at chin and go along jawline

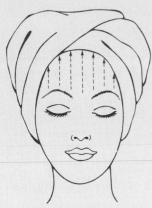

Stroking forehead to smooth wrinkles away

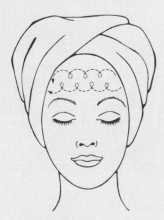

Circular etfleurage across forehead

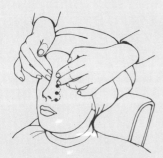

Start at inner corner of eyes, press and rotate, then slide down nose

3. Stimulate the **frontalis** (frahn-TAH-liss) by using the cushions of the middle and index fingers of both of your hands. Alternating hand positions, move hand over hand from the upper side of the nose to the hairline. Do this in short strokes without applying pressure. Move across the forehead to the left temple, then to the right temple, and back to the middle of the forehead. Complete this 5 times for each area.

4. Intensify movement 1 (used in procedure 2) by using the middle fingers of both of your hands in an effleurage (light, stroking) movement from the left to the right of the forehead that stops at the middle of the forehead. Do not take your fingers off of the face.

5. Slide your fingers to the **supratrochlear** (soo-pra-TROK-lee-ar) **nerve** (between the eyes on both sides of the upper part of the nose). Press and rotate your fingers once; then slide your fingers down the sides of the nose in a circular effleurage. Press and rotate your fingers on the tip of the nose (nasal nerve), both sides of the nose, and back to the supratrochlear nerve. Repeat 5 times.

3. Stimulating the frontalis (forehead) makes transverse wrinkles (from left to right) smooth out and relaxes the browline. Do each manipulation 5 times for maximum stimulation of muscles and nerves.

4. Greater stimulation at the browline is needed to relax and smooth the frontalis. Keeping your fingers on the face makes the movement constant.

5. The supratrochlear (branch of the trifacial nerve, which is also called the fifth cranial and trigeminal) affects the skin between the eyes and upper side of nose and eyelids. Effleurage is the most beneficial movement in this area. Do not press, pull, or stretch the skin near the eyes since the muscles, nerves, and tissues are very close to the skin's surface. Repeat for maximum benefits.

6. Slide your fingers down and take a firm grip under the chin. Hold your thumbs at the supratrochlear nerve (the inner brow area). Move your thumbs out along the rim of the browline. Press at 4 points along the brow. Rotate 5 times at the temples and slide your thumbs back lightly under the eyes to the supratrochlear nerve and rotate that area 5 times.

7. Slide your thumbs to the jawbone and separate your fingers above and below it; move to the left and right ears. Press firmly. Stroke the motor point for the facial nerve (the upper part of the cheekbone below the eye). Return around the chin with a light upward stroke, alternating between your left and right hands. Continue toward the left and right ears. Repeat stroking movement on this nerve 5 times.

8. Stimulate the muscles of the cheeks (the **zygomaticus**); slide your fingers to the right ear and separate the index and middle fingers of your left hand to hold the skin in front of the ear firmly. With the fingers of your right hand, rotate the skin 5 times on the **auriculo-temporal nerve** (located in front of the ear—it affects the external ear and the skin above the temple to the top of skull).

6. Manipulations in this area should be firm. They will affect the corrugator muscle, which draws the brows down and inward and produces wrinkles; these movements will help smooth wrinkles.

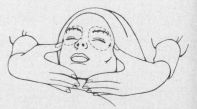

Slide thumbs around eye area

7. The **mentalis muscles** (chinline) and the zygomaticus muscles (cheekbones) often relax, become flabby, and sag. It is important that all of your movements are firm and directed up toward the ear.

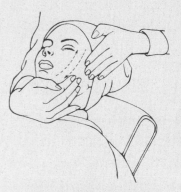

Using firm strokes, lift upward around chinline

8. Rotating and sliding movements stimulate the muscles and increase circulation.

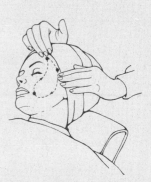

Use rotation and pressure by ear, then slide to temple

9. Hold the client's head steady with your left hand and slide your right hand under the chin. Bring your thumb and middle finger up to the corners of the mouth to do a circular effleurage (light, circular stroking) 5 times. Continue around the mouth to the side of the cleft in the upper lip. At the same time, press the side of your index finger into the cleft and pinch the 2 sides together.

9. These movements will stimulate and raise the corners of the mouth. The nerves and muscles affected include: the **mental nerve,** which serves the skin of the lower lip and chin; the **levator labii superioris** (li-VAT-ehr LAY-bee-igh soo-PIRH-ee-or-iss) which affects the upper lip; the **triangularis** (trigh-an-gyoo-LAY-riss) muscle, which stimulates the muscle that pulls down the corners of the mouth; and the **depressor labii inferioris,** (di-PRES-ehr LAY-bee-igh in-FIHR-ee-or-iss) which affects the muscle of the lower lip. The other muscles affected are the **orbicularis oris** (or-bik-yool-LAY-riss OH-riss) (the band of muscles around the upper and lower lip) and the **risorius** (ri-SAH-ri-us), which draws the corners of the mouth out and back.

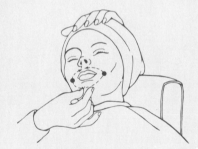

Begin at lower lip and draw fingers around mouth to upper lip

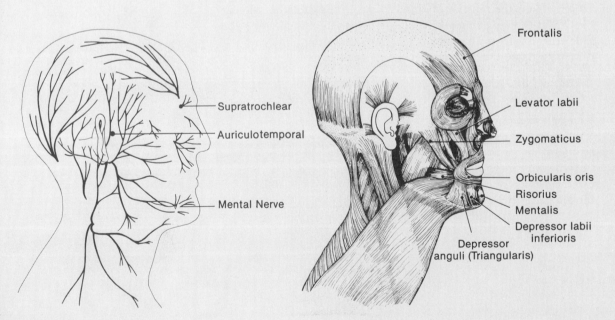

Supratrochlear

Auriculotemporal

Mental Nerve

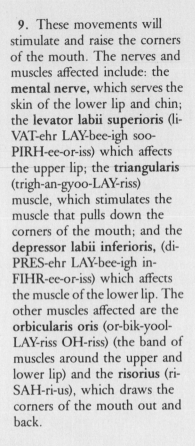

Frontalis

Levator labii

Zygomaticus

Orbicularis oris

Risorius

Mentalis

Depressor labii inferioris

Depressor anguli (Triangularis)

10. Stimulate and tighten the muscles of the cheeks. Slide the fingers of both of your hands firmly on the point of the chin and slide them with pressure toward the right and left ears. Press 4 points along the mandible (jawbone). Press your middle finger on the motor point for the facial nerve (below the ear at the end of the jawbone) and rotate twice. Return with a light stroke to the chin; slide to the corner of the mouth. Repeat pressure, pressing 4 times across the cheeks toward the ears. Press and rotate twice on the motor point for the fifth cranial nerve (in front of the ear). Return with a light stroke to the mouth; slide to the corner of the nose and repeat the pressure, pressing 4 times across the cheeks toward the temples. Press and rotate twice on the temporal nerve (at temple) and repeat 5 times.

11. Continue stimulating the cheeks, using tapotement over the same areas covered in step 10.

12. Pinch the cheeks with your thumb and index fingers; grasp the flesh at the chin between the thumb and knuckle of the index finger. Work up face with a pinching, plucking movement. Work both sides of the face from the chin to the inner corner of the eye and from the chin to the outer corner of the eye, and from the chin to the ear at the same time.

10. Upward movements help keep the muscles of the cheeks (zygomaticus muscles) from sagging. The tringularis muslces cover the tip of the chin. The zygomatic nerves affect the temple, the side of the forehead, and the upper part of the cheeks.

11. Tapotement is a light tapping movement that stimulates all the muscles and nerves of the cheeks.

12. Pinching will further stimulate the area of the cheeks and will help tighten the muscles.

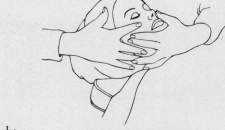

Start at the chin, then slide to upper cheek and rotate

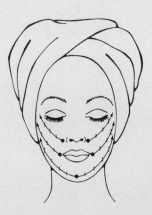

Tap entire cheek area

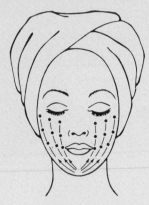

Pinching movement

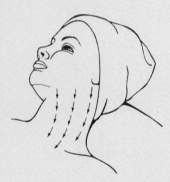

Stroking and lifting in an upward direction

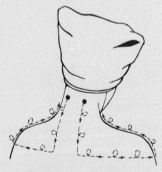

Pattern for massaging trapezius muscles

13. Place 3 fingers of both hands under the chin and "iron" a double chin by using firm friction movements under the chin and under the line of the mandible (jawbone) toward the ear. Alternate your hands, stroking from one side to the other.

14. Slide your hands completely off the face.

15. Massage the trapezius muscle.

16. Remove the emollient creme according to the procedure used for removing cleansing creme.

17. Soak 2 sterilized cotton balls in an astringent, squeeze out the excess, and dab over the entire face, chin, and eyelids with light, quick, tapping movements.

13. This strong friction movement will break up fatty deposits under the chin. The stroking movement has a relaxing effect.

14. Until this point, your hands should have been on the face for the entire time.

15. This is standard procedure.

16. It is important to remove the emollient creme thoroughly because (a) the epidermis of the skin will absorb only a small amount of it and (b) any impurities that may have surfaced during the manipulations need to be wiped away.

17. Astringent will remove any trace of emollient creme residue, close the pores, and help remove excess sebum.

Give a Facial Treatment for Dry Skin

Supplies

- cleansing lotion
- dry-skin lotion
- emollient creme
- cotton pledgets or tissue
- towels for head

- spatulas
- infrared or red dermal lamp
- high-frequency electrode (optional)

PROCEDURE

1. Follow the usual procedural steps for a plain facial.

RATIONALE

1. This is standard procedure.

2. Sponge the client's face with a cleansing lotion formulated for dry skin. Avoid using a product that has a high alcoholic content and apply the emollient creme.

3. **Cover the client's eyes** with cotton pads moistened lightly with cool water.

4. Expose the client's face to an infrared lamp for 5 minutes. Do not put the infrared lamp closer than 30 inches to the client. Cover the rays from time to time so that exposure is not constant. Do not exceed recommended time.

5. Reapply emollient creme.

6. Give manipulations. You may also use an indirect high-frequency treatment.

7. Remove the remaining emollient creme, using a tissue folded like a mitten.

8. Sponge the face with skin lotion formulated for dry skin. Pat dry.

2. Alcohol will have a drying effect on the client's skin.

3. The client's eyes must be covered before light therapy begins. If the cotton pads are moistened, they will stay in place. This a safety precaution.

4. The heat from the lamp will help skin absorb the emollient creme.

5. The skin will have absorbed some of the creme, so it is necessary to add more to allow your fingers to slide easily during the massage.

6. The manipulations help to normalize the activity of the sebaceous glands.

7. The skin will absorb only a small amount of creme, so it is necessary to remove the excess.

8. Sponging the skin will remove impurities along with excess creme.

Safety Tip

Give a Facial Treatment for Oily Skin

Supplies

- cleansing creme
- abrasive facial cleanser
- astringent
- cotton pledgets or tissue
- towels for head
- extra towels

- spatulas
- medicated soap
- antiseptic lotion
- facial steamer
- comedones extractor
- Wood's light

Note to student: Use of the Wood's light has been prohibited in some states.

Safety Tip

PROCEDURE

1. Give the client a hand mirror. Warn client **not to look into** Wood's light.

2. Turn off the light in the work area. Following manufacturer's directions, turn on the Wood's light. Allow 2 to 3 minutes for the Wood's light to warm up.

3. Show the client in the mirror the points that appear coral, orange, red.

RATIONALE

1. The mirror will allow client to see what you see during the examination. The client must never look into any ultraviolet instrument for long periods.

2. Directions may vary from one manufacturer to another. The Wood's light is always used in a darkened area for best viewing results.

3. Any of these colors identify overactivity or inflamation of the oil glands and indicate the need for corrective measures, such as medicated soap, abrasive facial cleansers, or a steamer treatment. Use of the steamer will flush the oil ducts and allow oil to flow normally.

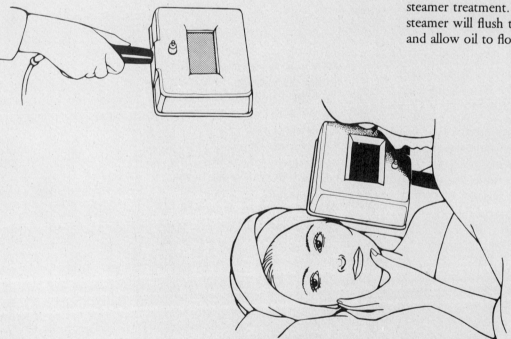

Wood's light was developed by Robert Williams Wood and is used to help determine skin conditions. Substances become luminous when exposed to the deep violet rays of the lamp. Blemishes which are not visible to the naked eye become visible. Varied shades indicate different conditions: normal healthy skin—blue to white; dehydrated skin—violet; oily areas—yellow to pink; pigmentation and dark spots—brown; the thicker the skin, the whiter the light

4. Turn on area light and turn off the Wood's light. Proceed to apply abrasive cleanser to areas identified by light. Use a facial steamer if desired, following manufacturer's directions.

4. This completes the analysis and corrective procedure.

5. Remove excess cleanser from the skin with a tissue folded like a mitten.

5. This will also remove excess oil and impurities.

6. Apply an astringent skin lotion to the skin and pat dry.

6. The astringent lotion will dry the skin and close the pores.

Treatment for Minor Problem of Oily Skin: Acne

PROCEDURE

1. Cleanse client's face with medicated soap and apply acne creme to the client's face.

RATIONALE

1. Medicated soap will help prevent the spread of infection. The creme will allow the facial electrode to glide smoothly over the skin.

2. Apply direct high-frequency current for 3 to 5 minutes. Watch the affected areas closely.

2. High-frequency current has a germicidal and drying effect on skin.

3. Remove the creme with a tissue folded like a mitten or a towel moistened with warm water.

3. This will remove excess creme and impurities.

4. Saturate cotton pads with astringent lotion and apply them to skin.

4. Astringent lotion will help the skin dry and the pores close.

5. Apply antiseptic lotion to cotton pads and place them on the affected areas.

5. Antiseptic lotion will help reduce the spread of infection.

6. Do not apply makeup unless it is medicated.

6. Makeup has a tendency to clog the pores, thus increasing the spread of the acne condition.

Treatment for Minor Problem of Oily Skin: Comedones/Milia

PROCEDURE

1. Apply the abrasive cleansing creme and remove it with a cool, moist towel.

RATIONALE

1. This is standard procedure.

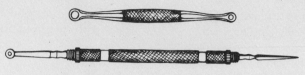

Comedones extractors

2. Apply a clay mask formula, let dry, and peel it off.

2. Comedones or milia indicate oily skin. A clay mask is made to break up and remove oil from the skin.

3. Reapply the abrasive cleansing creme and steam the face with warm towels, a facial steamer, or a direct high-frequency current for 3 to 5 minutes.

3. The warmth and moisture will open the pores.

Safety Tip

4. Remove comedones or milia with a sanitized comedones extractor.

4. Extractor must be sanitized to prevent an infection.

5. Sponge the face with an antiseptic lotion and apply towels moistened in cool water.

5. This will prevent the spread of infection and cause the skin to contract and the pores to close.

6. Apply an astringent lotion to the face, concentrating on the affected areas. Pat dry.

6. This will dry the oils and close the pores.

GLOSSARY

Absorption   The process by which one substance takes in (soaks up) another.

Auriculotemporal nerve   A nerve located in front of the ear.

Depressor labii inferioris   A muscle which affects the muscles of the lower lip.

Effleurage (ef-fler-AZH)   A light, stroking movement used in massage to soothe the skin.

Friction   A rubbing movement used in massage to stimulate the skin.

Frontalis (frahn-TAH-liss)   Part of the epicranius muscle located in the eyebrow area.

Infrared (in-frah-RED) light   Light with long wavelengths (7,700 angstroms or longer) used in light therapy on the skin.

Levator labii superioris   A muscle which affects the upper lip.

Mentalis muscle   A chin muscle that makes the lower lip protrude.

Mental nerve   A nerve serving the skin of the lower lip and chin.

Orbicularis ohriss   A circular band of muscle surrounding the mouth.

Petrissage (peh-tri-SAHJ)   A kneading or rolling movement used in massage to stimulate the skin.

Risorius   A mouth muscle used in smiling.

Supratrochlear (soo-pra-TROK-lee-ar) nerve   A subdivision of the opthalmic branch involved in facial massage.

Tapotement (ta-poh-MAHN)   A light tapping or slapping movement used in massage to stimulate the skin.

Triangularis   A muscle which stimulates the muscle that pulls down the corners of the mouth.

Ultraviolet light   Light with wavelengths of 1850 to 3900 angstroms used in light therapy on the skin. This is the type of light that causes suntan.

Vibration   A shaking movement used in massage to stimulate the skin.

Wood's light   A light with deep violet rays used to help detect various skin conditions.

Zygomaticus   A muscle in the area of the cheekbones.

QUESTIONS

1. For sanitation purposes, how often should the head rest covering for the facial chair be changed?
2. What should be used to remove facial cremes (creams) from their jars?
3. Are most facial movements upward—away from the neck, or downward toward the neck?
4. Is it necessary to give facial treatments using an even rhythm and tempo?
5. Is the frontalis muscle located in the jaw area?
6. Is the supratrochlear nerve located between the eyes on the upper part of the nose?
7. Is tapotement a facial massage movement?
8. Is the trapezius muscle located along the forehead?
9. Is the Wood's Light used to identify a scar?
10. Does high frequency have a germicidal effect on the skin?
11. Would a clay mask temporarily cleanse the face of excessive oil?

ANSWERS

1. After every client 2. Sanitized spatula 3. Upward 4. Yes 5. No; the forehead 6. Yes 7. Yes 8. No; the back of the neck and shoulder area 9. No 10. Yes 11. Yes

Applying Makeup 24

Purpose

You have already read about the "total look" that many clients want and many salons offer. Makeup is an important part of this look. As in hairstyling, makeup is applied in basic patterns and adapted to the individual's needs to accent good features and camouflage undesirable ones. Therefore, you need to know how to apply makeup techniques in the correct way for a particular client. These techniques include application, contour (corrective) styling, and color selection. Special services related to makeup are applying false and semipermanent eyelashes, tinting lashes and brows, and arching brows.

Major Objective

Using professional cosmetics and implements and using the proper principles and techniques, apply makeup to enhance your client's particular facial features and other needs.

Level of Acceptability

Use the proper steps to apply makeup on the client in 40 to 60 minutes. Score 75 percent or better on a multiple-choice exam on the information in this chapter.

Knowing Subobjectives

1. Define basic cosmetics used on the face.
2. Explain how to select an appropriate color of foundation (base).
3. Describe the cosmetics and techniques used for facial features and used to correct specific problems.
4. Describe techniques used to apply false (strip) eyelashes and semipermanent lashes (eye tabbing) and to tint lashes and brows.

KNOWING SUBOBJECTIVE 1

Define basic cosmetics used on the face.

You need to know the products used in facial care and makeup. Some of the basic types follow. Others, such as eye and night cremes, have not been included because they usually are not applied in the salon.

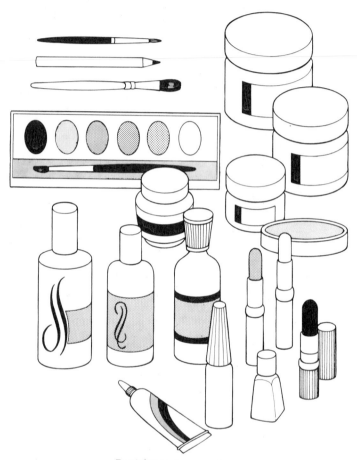

Basic facial cosmetics

    1. **Cleansers,** usually in creme or emollient forms, clean the epidermal layer of the skin. They remove makeup and unsightly matter that could cause skin eruptions and then prepare the face for a new application of makeup. Cleansing products usually come in formulas for oily and dry to normal skin.

    2. **Liquid and bar soaps** also can be used to cleanse the skin. You must consider the pH rating of a soap that you are going to use. Because alkaline products are very drying to skin, do not use soap that has a pH of more than

6.5. Doctors often suggest medicated soaps and those having a low pH rating for blemishes and acne. Superfatted soap is sometimes recommended for very dry or sensitive skin. Castile soap can be used on almost any skin.

3. **Skin fresheners (toners)** usually come in liquid form. They are used to remove traces of cleansing cremes and to close the pores of the skin. They are preferred for normal and dry skin.

4. **Astringents,** which contain alcohol, are made in liquid and creme form. They can be used on oily skin to close the skin pores and help dry excessive sebum. Because of their drying effect, however, they are not used as widely as fresheners.

5. **Moisturizers,** ususally in emulsion or a thicker creme form, are needed for all types of skin. They help retain moisture in the skin and give it a fresh appearance.

6. **Emollient cremes** contain lanolin to lubricate the skin. They are used in facial massages.

7. **Foundation** (base) comes in a variety of forms, including liquid, creme, cake, and stick. All of these forms help to cover blemishes. They also protect the skin from unsightly matter in the atmosphere. Some manufacturers have made bases especially for black skin. These or dark shades of other foundations can be employed for black clients.

8. **Corrective sticks** (both white and dark) are used to give the illusion of the oval-shaped face. White contour is used to give fullness to sunken areas, and dark contour is used on areas that need to be toned down.

9. **Blusher** is used to enhance the cheekbone area. It comes in many forms, including liquid, creme, creamy cake, and powder cake. The powder cake types can be used to add color to the forehead, cheekbone, and chin areas.

10. **Lipstick** comes in a number of forms, including gloss, liquid, creme, creamy stick, and crayon. In the salon this cosmetic must be applied with a lip brush that can be sanitized with 70 percent alcohol.

11. **Powder** is used over the foundation to set the makeup and keep it from rubbing off on clothing. Powder also provides a matte (dull rather than shiny) finish for the face.

12. **Eye shadow** is used both to highlight and shadow the area of the eyes. With eye shadow, a small eye can be made to look larger, and a large eye can be made to look smaller. It comes in powder cake, creamy cake, creme, and stick forms.

13. **Mascara** is used to make lashes darker and thicker looking. It comes in the forms of cake, creme, and liquid. (Some state boards do not allow the use of cakes in salons.)

14. **Eyeliners** are employed to outline the eyes. They come in liquid, creme, and cake forms. (Some state boards do not allow the use of cakes in salons.)

15. **Eyebrow pencils** fill in and/or darken the brows. They are pencil-like waxy products.

KNOWING SUBOBJECTIVE 2

Explain how to select an appropriate color of foundation (base).

Like many of the skills you have learned in this book, the first step, the one that no one actually sees, is the most important. This is true for foundations.

After you have prepared the skin with a cleanser, moisturizer, and freshener (or astringent), it is ready for the application of a foundation. This cosmetic will be partially absorbed into the epidermal layer, providing enhancement of an individual's skin tone.

Since you want a **natural** look rather than a painted one, select a shade that is one shade darker than the client's natural skin tone. Natural skin tones are usually classified as **pink, florid, cream white, sallow, olive** and **dark.** They can also be grouped more simply as light, medium, and dark. These names are helpful, but you can use an additional factor in choosing a color: your knowledge of pH.

The **natural pH** of **skin** ranges from 4.5 to 5.5, but agents used in cleansing, toning, etc., can alter this value. Cleansing with soap and water (and some cleansers) can change the skin's pH to about 7.

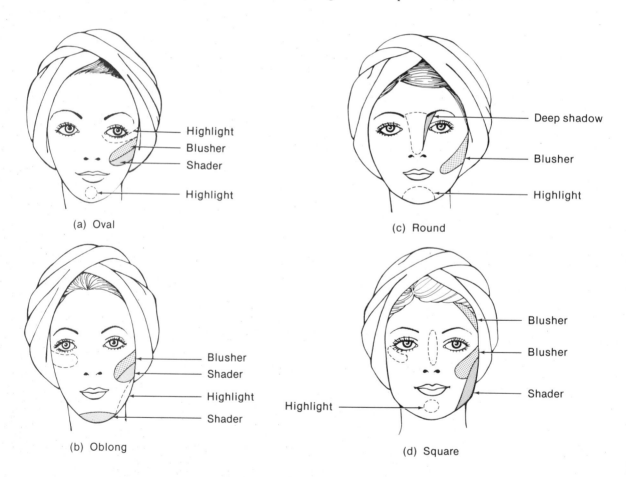

(a) Oval
— Highlight
— Blusher
— Shader
— Highlight

(c) Round
— Deep shadow
— Blusher
— Highlight

(b) Oblong
— Blusher
— Shader
— Highlight
— Shader

(d) Square
— Blusher
— Blusher
— Shader
Highlight —

If the skin has a pH of more than 7, foundation makeup tends to **stand out** from the natural skin tone. In using a line of foundation that stands out on the skin, you should select a toner that is one tone lighter than the skin tone itself. On skin that is acid, foundations have a tendency to disappear on (absorb into) the face; for this type, a darker than normal color should be used.

Although knowledge of basic skin tones and pH factors can help you choose a good color, you will still need to try one or more colors on the client before making your final decision. Apply a small amount of the foundation to the lower jawbone on the skin just in front of the ear. If the color is too light or dark, you can remove the foundation with cleansing creme, and try a different color.

KNOWING SUBOBJECTIVE 3

As you know, the **oval face** is considered to be the ideal shape. Corrective makeup techniques can be applied to other facial types to create the **illusion** of the oval shape. You must use the contour of the face to give the optical illusion of the oval shape. You can use corrective makeup to enhance an oval face, to make an oblong face look shorter, to make a round face look thinner, and to make a square face look softer.

This chapter will concentrate on 4 basic facial shapes. If you learn the principles involved in applying makeup to these shapes, you should be able to handle any problems that might arise for any shape.

You can use a simple rule when applying corrective or contour makeup: "lights in the valley—shadows on the hills." This means, for example, that **highlighting** adds width. Shadowing narrows and plays down prominent features. **Highlighting in this sense is not accenting.** For an oval face, follow the general procedures for cosmetic application. This shape is the model (standard).

The rest of this subobjectve will illustrate corrective techniques that can be used for specific facial features.

Describe the cosmetics and techniques used for facial features and used to correct specific problems.

Corrective Techniques for the Nose

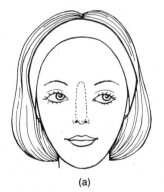 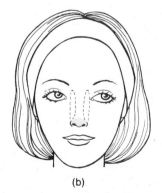

(a)   (b)

Corrective makeup for: (*a*) short nose, (*b*) protruding nose

Corrective Makeup for the Chin

You can use the same principles for applying makeup on the chin:

(a) Protruding—Apply shadow to the areas to be played down.
(b) Receding—Lighten in a shallow area.
(c) Sagging double chin—Play down the extra chin by applying darker foundation.

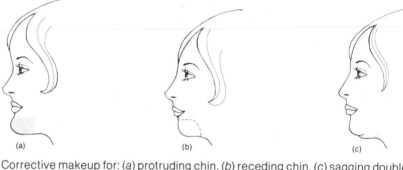

Corrective makeup for: (a) protruding chin, (b) receding chin, (c) sagging double chin

Corrective makeup can be applied to the jawline in these ways:

(a) Narrow—Lighten to give width to a narrow jawline.
(b) Broad—Shadow to play down a broad jawline.

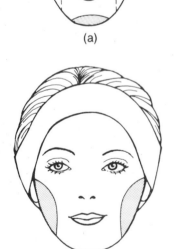

(a)

(b)

Corrective makeup for: (a) narrow jawline, (b) broad jawline

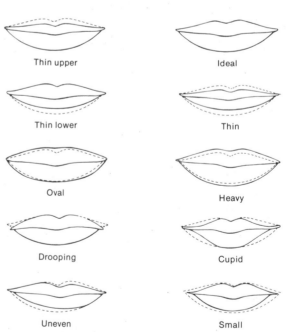

Thin upper

Ideal

Thin lower

Thin

Oval

Heavy

Drooping

Cupid

Uneven

Small

Corrective makeup for the lips

Corrective techniques for the lips are shown in the figure on page 374.

Use the following steps to shape the eyebrows (as shown below).

Eyebrows

1. Place the eyebrow pencil in a straight line at the side of the nose. Start the eyebrow at this point.
2. Measure a 45-degree angle from the outside corner of the eye to find where the eyebrow should end.
3. Hold the pencil parallel to the nose along the outside edge of the iris of the eye. This is where the arch of the eyebrow should be.
4. Hold the eyebrow pencil horizontally just above the eye. The pencil should connect the beginning and the end of the eyebrow in an evenly curved arch.

You will need a good deal of practice to shape eyebrows, but these rules will help you avoid improper shapings (see figure below right).

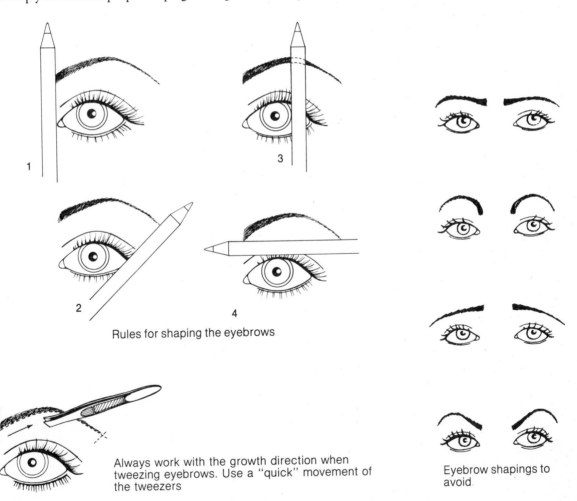

Rules for shaping the eyebrows

Always work with the growth direction when tweezing eyebrows. Use a "quick" movement of the tweezers

Eyebrow shapings to avoid.

KNOWING SUBOBJECTIVE 4

Describe techniques used to apply false (strip) eyelashes and semipermanent lashes (eye tabbing) and to tint lashes and brows.

Applying False Eyelashes

Use the following steps to apply false strip eyelashes:

1. Measure the false lash on client by placing it from the inside to the outside corner of the eye; cut off any extra lash at the outside corner.
2. Using tweezers or your fingers, put the center of the false lash directly above the center of the left eyelash.
3. Press the inside corner of the false lash with your thumb; then, press the outside corner with your index finger. Hold for 1 minute.

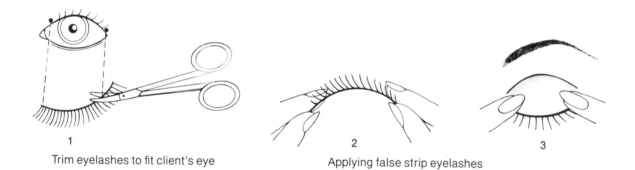

1   Trim eyelashes to fit client's eye   2   Applying false strip eyelashes   3

Use the following steps to apply semipermanent lashes (eye tabbing):

1. Use tweezers to take the lash bulb from the tray. Dip the bulb in the glue.
2. Start in the center of the lashes of the right eye. Stroke the lash bulb from the beginning (at the lid) to the end.
3. Place the semipermanent lash on the client's glued lash; continue this procedure to the inside corner and then to the outside corner of the eye.

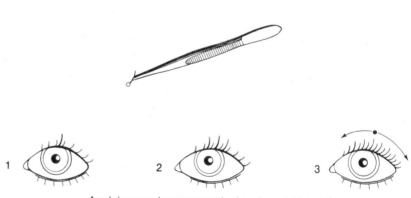

Applying semipermanent lashes (eye tabbing)

There are 4 basic steps to follow to tint lashes and brows:

1. Apply petroleum jelly around the eyes and on paper shields.
2. Apply paper shields under the bottom lashes on both eyes where skin and lashes begin.
3. Use an upward stroke to apply tinting solution on the upper lashes several times. Stroke the lower lashes of both eyes from the eyelid to the tips of the lashes.
4. Stroke the eyebrows in the direction of the growth, and then against it.

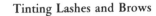
 Safety Tip

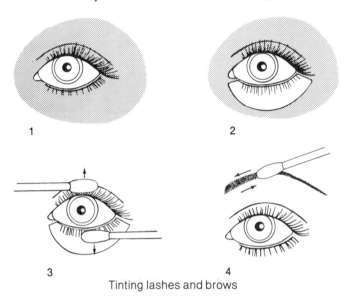

Tinting lashes and brows

GLOSSARY

Astringent   A liquid or creme containing alcohol that is used on oily skin to close skin pores and help dry excessive sebum.

Blemish sticks   See **Corrective sticks**.

Blusher   A product coming in a variety of forms used to add color to an area of the face. It may be applied to the forehead, cheekbones, and chin areas.

Cleanser   A creme or emollient to clean the epidermal layer of the skin.

Contour makeup   See **White contour makeup** and **Dark contour makeup**.

Corrective stick   A makeup stick used to help cover blemishes and scars.

Dark contour makeup   A dark stick or thick creme used to tone down areas on the face.

Emollient creme   A creme containing lanolin to lubricate the skin, used in facial massage.

Eyebrow pencil   A pencil-like, waxy product used to fill in and/or darken the eyebrows.

Eyeliner   A product coming in liquid, creme, or cake form used to outline the eyes.

Foundation   A makeup product coming in a variety of forms that helps cover blemishes and protects the skin from matter in the atmosphere.

Lipstick   A product coming in a variety of forms used to add color or gloss to the lips.

Mascara   A product coming in cake, creme, or liquid form used to make eyelashes look darker and thicker.

Moisturizer   An emulsion or creme that helps the skin retain water.

Powder   A product used over makeup foundation to keep it from rubbing off and to give a matte finish.

Skin freshener   A liquid product that removes traces of cleansing cremes and helps close the pores of the skin.

White contour makeup   A white stick or thick creme used to give the illusion of fullness in sunken areas of the face.

QUESTIONS

1. How does an astringent affect the skin pores?
2. Does an emollient lubricate the skin?
3. How is an eyeliner used?
4. What name is given to products used to remove makeup and other matter from the face?
5. What product contains alcohol and is used to remove oil from the skin, plus close the pores of the skin?
6. What product helps skin retain moisture by lubricating it?
7. What is the makeup used to enhance the eyes by highlighting them, or shading these areas?
8. What is the natural pH of the skin?
9. What facial shape is considered the "ideal" facial shape?
10. Should tweezing be done with a slow movement, or a quick movement?
11. Is tweezing normally done in the same direction of the hair growth, or opposite the direction of hair growth?
12. When applying artificial eyelashes, are the false lashes glued to the natural lashes only?
13. When tinting eyelashes, is it necessary to use protective eye shields?
14. Is eyelash tint usually applied with a cotton ball?

ANSWERS

1. It closes them 2. Yes 3. To outline the eyes 4. Cleanser 5. An astringent 6. An emollient creme 7. Eye shadow 8. 4.5–5.5 9. Oval 10. A quick movement 11. The same direction as hair growth 12. No 13. No 14. No

Describing the Principles of Electricity 25

The word electricity is very familiar to most of you because you have been using it all of your lives. It is used to run almost all of the devices found in your home; from stereos and blow dryers to air conditioners and clothes dryers. A better understanding of electricity is important to you because many of the devices you will be using in the field of skin care as well as hair care which are needed to perform beauty services are electrical. For you to perform various skin care services safely and effectively, you will need to know which form of electrical current will give the best results for the service requested by the client.

Provided with the information in this chapter and help from your instructor, define and describe professional terms used in cosmetology

Score 75 percent or better on a multiple-choice exam on the information in this chapter.

1. Define basic electrical terms.
2. Identify sources that make and control electricity.
3. Describe electro-therapy terms.
4. Define electrolysis and thermolysis (diathermy) terms.
5. Describe the benefits of a high-frequency scalp treatment.

6. Give a high-frequency scalp treatment.

The word electricity is very familiar to most of you because you have been using it all of your lives. It is used to run almost all of the devices found in your home; from stereos and blow dryers to air conditioners and clothes dryers. And yet most of us should have a better understanding of electricity.

As a licensed cosmetologist in a profession which relies heavily on the safe and effective use of electricity to serve the needs of your clientele, you will have to learn about a few basic electrical concepts. In order to do this, you will have to learn a small part of the "language of electricity."

KNOWING SUBOBJECTIVE 1

Define basic electrical terms.

This subobjective will define and describe some of the basic terms common to the theory of electricity. The terms included in this subobjective are as follows: **voltage, current, resistance** and **power**.

Volts

The word "**volt**" is used in electricity to explain **how much electrical potential is available** for you to use in the form of electricity. Volt is a unit of measure for **voltage**. Generally, the bigger the "**voltage**" is, the more it can do. For example bigger muscles can do more than smaller ones.

The two voltages found in your home or salon in North America are 120 volts and 240 volts. All small electric devices (appliances) run on 120 volts, except those that operate on batteries. On the other hand, the very largest devices, such as an electric clothes dryer, operate on 240 volts. If you were to connect a device requiring 120 volts to a 240-volt source, the appliance could be damaged, but more importantly, you or your client could receive an electrical shock. To prevent this from happening, manufacturers of electrical devices use **different plug shapes for each type of voltage**. Therefore, you will **not** be able to plug a 120-volt device into a 240-volt outlet. So, if the plug fits the socket, the voltage will be safe for you to use.

There are some basic differences between electrical power sources. The typical outlets in the salon provide 120 or 240 volts of **alternating voltage**. This means that the voltage is always changing from a positive charge to a negative charge, then repeating the process over and over again. The positive-to-negative change (or alternation) happens 60 times per second in the U.S.A. and Canada. Each change or **cycle** per second is called a **hertz**. (Hertz used to be called cycles per second.) So the change or alternation is said to occur at a **60-Hertz rate**. Another way to say this is that the frequency of the alternating voltage is 60 hertz.

Describe Voltage

Earlier voltage was compared to a muscle. Like muscle, voltage by itself is of no use. Voltage is only useful when it makes something happen. To be of any use, a muscle must move your body. For voltage to be useful, it must move electricity. You will learn how electricity is moved in the next paragraph.

Most wire used to operate electrical appliances is **made of copper**. Billions and billions of copper atoms are strung together side by side to make a copper wire. Each one of these copper atoms can be thought of as a miniature sun with planets rotating around the sun.

The name given to the center of an atom is "**nucleus**." The name for the rotating particle is "**electron**." These two particles each have a charge. The **nucleus is positively charged**, and the **electron is negatively charged**. Voltage makes electrons **move** in the wire. Copper and other metal atoms have loosely bound electrons that can easily leave the atom and move through the wire under the influence of voltage. They move because of the fundamental electric principle that two **similar charges repel**, and two **opposite charges attract**. The name for moving electrons is **current**. When specifying how much electron **current** is in the wire, the term **amperes** is used.

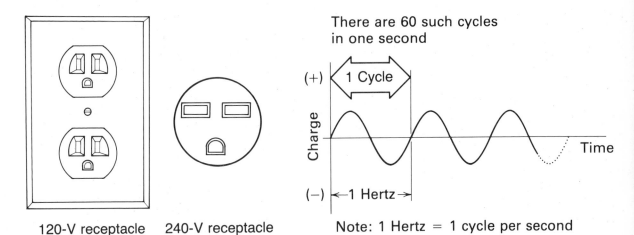

120-V receptacle   240-V receptacle

There are 60 such cycles in one second

(+) 1 Cycle

Charge

(−) ←1 Hertz→

Time

Note: 1 Hertz = 1 cycle per second

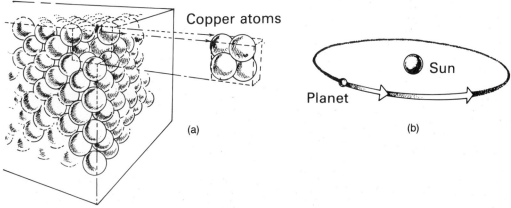

Copper atoms

(a)

Sun

Planet

(b)

(a) Crystalline structure of copper wire. (b) The structure of the copper atom is like a planet rotating around the sun

The larger the voltage, the larger the number of energy packages sent through the wire.

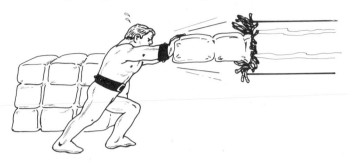

Voltage Concept

If the energy packages move rapidly, a large current results.

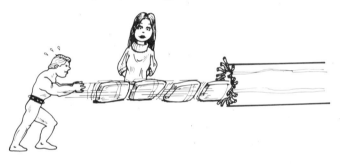

If the energy packages move slowly, a small current results.

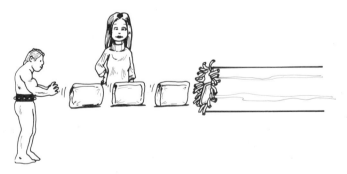

Current Concept

An easy way to imagine electron current moving through a wire is to think of it as water in a garden hose. The voltage is what makes the electrons flow. Unlike water, electricity is invisible, but that doesn't mean it is any less real. As voltage "alternates," it causes the electrons to first move in one direction and then in the other, so the current in the wire is said to be **alternating current** or simply "A.C." This is different from the current produced by a battery. A battery will cause current to go only in one direction. Because of this, it is called **direct current** or "D.C." The negative end of the battery repels electrons, and the positive side attracts electrons, so they "**flow**" from negative to positive through the wire. However, the current direction is opposite to the direction of electron flow.

Current

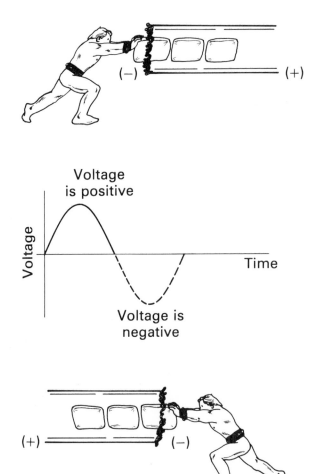

Alternating Current (AC)

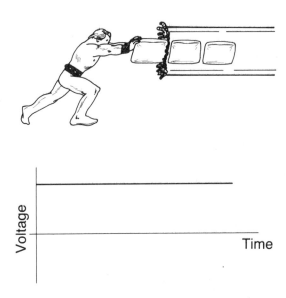

Unlike an alternating current, direct current *does not* fluctuate from negative to positive.

Direct Current (DC)

If many energy packages are consumed, we say there is a high power usage.

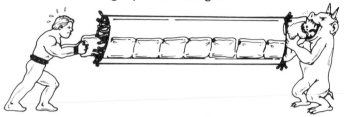

If few energy packages are consumed, we say there is a low power usage.

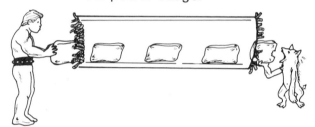

Wattage Concept

Resistance

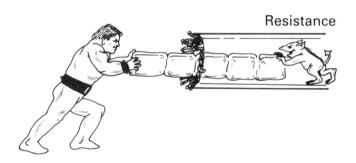

Power

You have now learned what voltage and current are. When they are both considered together, they determine power, which is measured in **watts**. The term "**wattage**" is sometimes used to refer to electrical power of appliances. A 1000-watt blow dryer works on the same A.C. voltage (120) as a

1500-watt blow dryer. It has a smaller power rating because it uses fewer amperes of current when it is turned "on." At the same time it produces **less heat**.

Current and heat are closely related. The greater the current the greater will be the amount of heat from the hair dryer. You know how current moves through wire. Any material that will normally allow electrons to move through it is called a "**conductor**." **All metals and most liquids are conductors** of electric current. But, not all conductors will allow current to move through them with the **same** ease. No conductor is perfect. Even a good conductor like copper will offer some opposition to the current. In the field of electricity the word used for opposition is "**resistance**." How much resistance is in a conductor is measured in "**ohms**." So, conductors with the most resistance (opposition) will have the highest ohms values.

This opposition can also be thought of as friction, and **friction causes heat**. So, as current flows through a blow dryer or curling iron, it causes heat to be produced because of the resistance in the wire used. The wire chosen for heat-producing devices has a high resistance. But, the wire used to plug the device into the wall receptacle should not produce heat—it should have very low resistance. A complete circuit is the route that an electrical current travels from its source of generation via conductors and back to the source.

Conductors

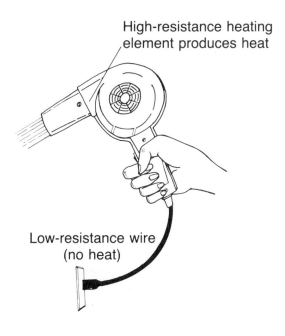

High-resistance heating element produces heat

Low-resistance wire (no heat)

Insulators

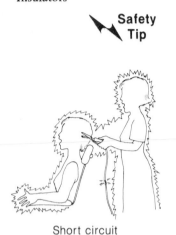

Safety Tip

Short circuit

Conductors are used to move current from one place to another, but often we want to stop current from moving someplace. To do this, insulators are used. **Current cannot pass through an insulator. Plastic, rubber, glass, and air are examples of insulators.** They are placed around all conductors of electricity for safety. If the insulation around a wire becomes damaged and exposes the inner wire, a dangerous condition exists. If any other conductor comes into contact with this uninsulated wire, current may leave the wire and flow through the conductor it contacts. This causes what is called a "**short circuit.**" If you are the conductor, current flows through you, rather than through the device it should flow through, and you would get a "shock!" **This is very dangerous, and may be deadly to you.**

KNOWING SUBOBJECTIVE 2

Identify sources that make and control electricity.

In this subobjective you will read about how electricity is produced and controlled.

Electricity can be produced in a variety of ways. In this subobjective you will read about each source of electric voltage. The first two sources of electrical volts we will describe are the most common, and the most widely used voltage sources.

D.C.

Batteries are called either "**wet cells**" or "**dry cells**." Batteries produce **direct current only**. An example of a wet cell battery that you may know about would be a 12-volt car battery. An example of a dry cell would be a 9-volt portable radio battery. Both of these sources of electricity are very similar. Each uses two metal plates, which have a nonmetallic electrical conductor between them called an "**electrolyte**." Because of a chemical action, one plate becomes charged negatively, and the other becomes charged positively. The result is either a wet or dry cell battery which is a source of voltage.

A.C.

Generators are used to produce A.C. voltage. Your local power supply company uses huge generators (as big as a semi-trailer truck) to provide your home with 120 and 240 volts of electrical power. A.C. is created by rotating conductors through a magnetic field. This action will make one end of the conductor positive, and the other end negative at the same instant in the voltage cycle. Because of the way it is rotated, the voltage of the conductor will change at 60 hertz, so it will be safe for use in all appliances.

There are devices which will change alternating current into direct current. A **converter** is a mechanical electrical device used to change direct current so it can be used to power alternating current appliances. (This term is now obsolete and has had several opposing definitions in the past.) A **rectifier** is generally an electronic device which changes alternating current into direct current.

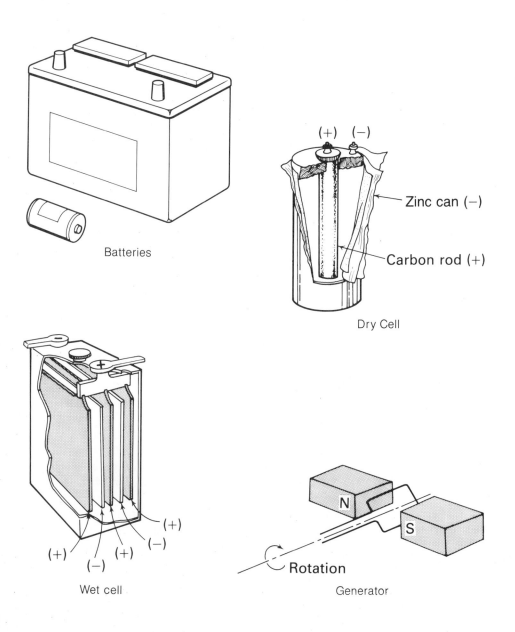

Batteries

Zinc can (−)

Carbon rod (+)

Dry Cell

Wet cell

Rotation

Generator

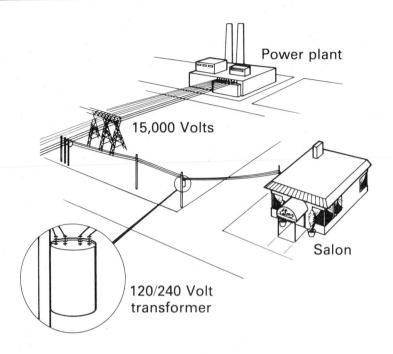

Power plant

15,000 Volts

Salon

120/240 Volt transformer

Thermocouples consist of two different metals joined together at one point. Voltage is produced between the two metals when the junction is heated. The amount of voltage depends on the metals used and the temperature where the two metals are joined. A heat device, such as a furnace is controlled by a thermocouple. It can produce only a small voltage of about one or two volts.

Photoelectric cells are made of materials which will produce a voltage when exposed to any light. The strength of the voltage depends on how strong the light is. They are used to turn street lights on at night, and off during the day.

Piezoelectric crystals will develop a voltage if pressure is applied to them in the form of twisting or bending.

You can readily see that only A.C. line voltage and D.C. battery voltage sources are strong enough for the needs of a salon. Secondly, while battery-powered devices are used in a salon, the primary power source will be the 120/240 volts of A.C. supplied by the local power company. It is not really practical for the power company to supply 120 volts all the way from a generating plant located miles away to the salon. Instead the power company generates thousands of volts at the plant and uses power lines to bring it almost into the salon. Very close to the salon the power company installs a **transformer**. This electrical device can "transform" A.C. voltages. It can raise them if desired, but usually they are made to lower the voltage down to 120 or 240 volts. Transformers only work on A.C.

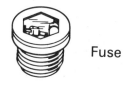

Fuse

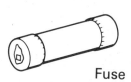

Fuse

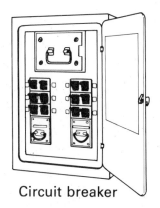

Circuit breaker

Since more than enough power is available from the power companies, safety devices have been designed and codes established to protect the consumer from drawing too much current for the salon or house wiring to handle safely. Two such protective devices are the **fuse** and the **circuit breaker**. **Fuses** are designed to **stop the flow** of current to an electric device if more is being used than is safe. Fuses should never be by-passed. You should **never install a larger fuse than the one you take out**. For example, if a 15-ampere fuse "blows," it must be replaced only with a 15-ampere fuse! Their purpose is to eliminate the chances of property damage or personal injury which could occur through overheating an electrical device.

Another similar protection device is a **circuit breaker**. These devices are **not replaceable** like a fuse. Instead, they operate something like a light switch to shut off power. To reactivate the electrical device, you simply slip the breaker lever back on.

It is possible to determine how much current (amperes) a piece of equipment will draw in one of two ways. Most equipment will include the rating on the label. Another way is to calculate the amperage of the device by simply dividing the wattage of the device by its operating voltage (120 or 240). So, a 1000-watt blow dryer operating on 120 volts will use just over 8 amperes.

Because many salon and home power lines are fused at 15 amps, you could **not use** two 1000-watt blow dryers on the same line without the fuse stopping the current.

Another safety feature widely required is **grounding**. In simple terms, this means that a third wire is used in the cord which connects the electrical appliance to the electrical plug in. One end of the third wire is connected to all exposed metal parts of the device. The other end is connected to ground through the salon wiring in such a way that minimizes the danger for shock.

It is becoming much more common to see what is often called **double-insulated** appliances instead of grounded appliances. The wide use of plastics has made it possible to eliminate all exposed metal parts from most electrical devices.

Fuses and Circuit Breakers

 Safety Tip

 Safety Tip

KNOWING SUBOBJECTIVE 3

Describe electro-
therapy terms.

The use of electricity to stimulate the body is called **electro-therapy**. Electro-therapy uses current to stimulate the muscles under the skin. This makes the muscles move and flex. There are presently three types of electro-therapy. They are called **faradic therapy, galvanic therapy,** and **sinusoidal therapy**.

Introduction to Electro-
Therapy

Safety
Tip

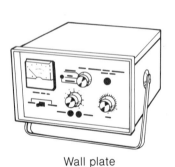

Wall plate

Galvanic electro-therapy uses D.C. current. The other two types use A.C. current. Each type of therapy produces a different result. And each type is believed to have its own advantages and disadvantages. All three types are given to the client for somewhat different reasons. These differences will be explained.

First of all, it is important for you to know that the current that comes from your wall outlet is **never** applied directly to the client's skin. Since there are 120 volts as it comes from the city power plant, if applied directly to the skin, you would **kill your client**. Instead, the 120 volts is reduced (or changed) to a level the human body can safely tolerate. The name for the appliance that does this is the **wall plate** (not to be confused with the wall plate around an outlet). This name is interesting because this device isn't actually attached to the wall, and it is portable. The wall plate is plugged into the wall outlet. The wall plate comes in different sizes and styles.

Galvanic electro-therapy is the oldest and most common type of electro-therapy. It is believed that galvanic electro-therapy causes a **chemical reaction on the skin,** for the purpose of promoting **beautiful, healthy** and **youthful** looking skin.

Galvanic electro-therapy causes the muscles to contract and relax. It **produces heat** because current flows through the client's skin, and skin offers some **resistance** to the flow of the current. The D.C. current causes a **chemical reaction** on the skin. This is said to be a **chemical current.** Current can be used to force chemicals through unbroken skin. This process is known as **phoresis**.

All electro-therapy devices have two poles. One is positively charged, and the other is negatively charged. The positive electrode of a device is called the **anode**. It is usually marked either with the word "**positive**," a large "P," color-coded "red," or marked with a plus ("+") sign. The negative electrode of a device is called the **cathode (kath-oh-d)**. It is marked with the word "**negative**," a large "N," color-coded black, or marked with a negative ("-") sign. The positive and negative electrodes can look different. It depends on which company manufactured the device.

Some of the older machines required the client to hold one of the electrodes. Some newer machines attach the electrode to the client using a moistened pad held in place with elastic tape or strap. In galvanic electro-therapy, **the client holds** (or is attached to) the **inactive electrode**. The **active electrode** is held by the cosmetologist and applied to the client's skin. When using galvanic therapy, **never use the indirect method** in which a

Safety
Tip

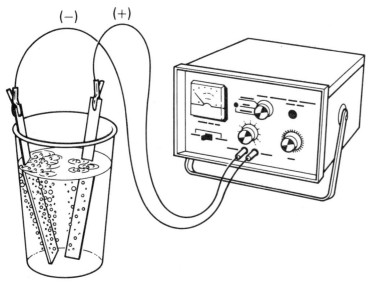

Determining which electrode is negative (−)

part of your body is between the client and the active electrode. Be sure that you **always read and follow the directions in the operating manual very carefully!** If the manual is not available, have your instructor present when you use the device. This is important for your safety and that of your client.

Safety Tip

Sometimes the electrodes aren't marked in any way. If this is the case, a simple test can be done to determine which is the negative electrode and which is the positive electrode. Place **just the tips** of the two electrodes in a glass of tap water **without touching** them together. Should they touch each other—you will probably blow a fuse, or trip a circuit breaker in the machine. Gradually turn up the current on the machine. The water will "bubble." This is caused by the current flowing between the electrodes. The flow of current makes the water break down into gases which produce the bubbles. Although there will be bubbles on both electrodes, **the negative (-) electrode will have more bubbles, and they will be smaller bubbles.** The positive electrode will have the larger bubbles.

Identifying the Negative or Positive Charge of the Electrode

It is believed that **the positive electrode** produces an **acidic reaction** on the skin. It is used by the cosmetologist to **close the pores, firm up skin tissue**. The positive electrode is said to be a **vaso-constrictor** (reducing the flow of blood in blood vessels). This means that the blood vessels get smaller and limit the flow of blood through them. This will also slow down glandular activity, and this has a sedative effect on the skin. Galvanic electro-therapy can be used even on red irritated skin, and it will have a soothing effect. You will also note that the positive electrode is said to have an **astringent effect**, which tends to firm and harden skin tissue.

Using the Positive Electrode for Galvanic Electro-Therapy

Using the Negative
Electrode for Galvanic
Electro-Therapy

When the client is in contact with the positive electrode and the cosmetologist touches the negative electrode to the skin, it is said that an **alkaline reaction is produced.** This has the opposite effect of the positive electrode. It is believed that the **negative electrode softens the skin and increases glandular activity.** It acts as a **vaso-dilator** (increasing the flow of blood in blood vessels). This means the blood vessels get larger. This is irritating to the skin. **Never** apply the negative electrode to red, irritated skin! You would probably use this type of therapy to relax the skin before a facial treatment.

Caution

 Safety Tip

Regardless of the type of therapy you use on your client, **never allow the current to go above 1 milliampere!!** You can determine the amount of current by looking at the current meter on the machine. **Larger amounts will cause pain and discomfort to your client.** The current is easy to regulate if you start at "0," then gradually increase the current to a comfortable level for your client. Remember, the "comfort level" will vary from client-to-client, so **begin at "0" each time you use this therapy.**

Different Treatments
Using Galvanic Electro-
Therapy

Skin bleaching is one application of galvanic electro-therapy. The electro-therapy device will force certain substances through the skin without breaking the surface of the skin. This process is called **phoresis.** There are two forms of phoresis. They are cataphoresis and anaphoresis.

Cataphoresis is a treatment that **pulls** the solution into the skin tissue. In cataphoresis the client is in contact with the negative probe of the device. The cosmetologist uses the positive electrode. The positive electrode is usually wrapped with a cloth. The cloth is soaked in the solution. When you touch the skin with the solution-soaked cloth, the solution is drawn into the skin.

Anaphoresis gives an effect that is opposite of cataphoresis. In **anaphoresis** the solution is **pushed, or forced, into the skin,** instead of being "pulled." This is the most effective way to bleach your client's skin. Although a solution-soaked cloth is also used in this method, this time the cloth is **wrapped around the negative electrode.** The positive electrode pushes the alkaline bleaching solution into the skin.

Electrolytic-Suction-Cup
Treatment

Another skin treatment using the galvanic electro-therapy device is called the electrolytic-suction-cup treatment. This treatment is said to **soften the skin, open the pores, and increase glandular activity,** all at the same time. While the specially constructed suction cup is in contact with the client's skin, the pores will open and skin tissue will soften. At the same time, a very gentle gravity-forced stream of water vapor removes sebum and dirt. This leaves the skin cleaner, fresher, and feeling wonderful.

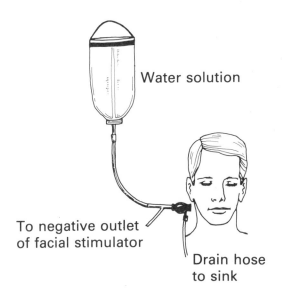

Water solution

To negative outlet
of facial stimulator

Drain hose
to sink

In this treatment, the special cup is connected to the negative electrode. The client is connected to the positive electrode. This causes a negative galvanic current to pass through the skin. After you have cleansed the skin, the electrodes are usually reversed. The positive galvanic current will close the pores, firm the tissue, and restore the skin to its natural state of acidity.

The galvanic current can be changed on most machines by simply "flipping a switch," so the D.C. current is changed back to A.C. **Faradic current** is used to exercise the muscles. Alternating current (A.C.) will activate muscle tissue. You may already be wondering how and why your client may benefit from this treatment.

Faradic Electro-Therapy

Background Information   In an age of wellness and physical fitness, most of us are aware that exercising our muscles is necessary to keep our bodies functioning at their best. This is also true for facial muscles. One way often used to exercise facial muscles is stretching them in front of a mirror. Models often do facial exercises to keep their facial muscles in good tone. Unfortunately, few people continue to do these exercises. So, many people choose to go to the salon for their facial exercises. Massage and electrical stimulation are two ways to aid in preserving facial muscle tone.

Massage is an excellent way of soothing and relaxing facial muscles. It is not as effective at making the muscles work as electrical stimulation, but it is one which may help preserve the skin from "wrinkling" longer than if you did nothing.

It is believed that faradic electro-therapy is the most effective way to make facial muscles work to their potential. Electro-therapy causes the muscles to contract, then relax. There are two forms of A.C. electro-therapy you can use: (1) faradic current, and (2) sinusoidal current.

Faradic current alternates like A.C. household current. It is different because of the special way it is produced. It is called an **induced current**. It is a way of producing A.C. current from D.C. current. Faradic devices aren't as popular as sinusoidal devices.

Using Faradic Electro-Therapy

Safety Tip

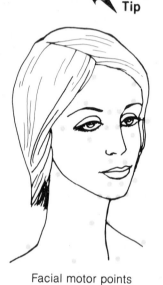

Facial motor points

When using faradic current, the cosmetologist can choose between the direct method or the indirect method. In the **direct method**, both electrodes are placed on the client's skin. The felt-covered electrodes are soaked in a conductive solution. **The electrodes should never touch each other.** The current should be set at "0" at first, then gradually increased until the client's comfort/tolerance level has been reached. For the best results, the electrodes are applied to the motor points of the face to stimulate the muscles. The current traveling between the electrodes through the motor nerves causes the muscles to flex for a part of a second. How long the current flows through the muscle before it is automatically turned off can be determined by the setting on your machine.

The **indirect method** of faradic electro-therapy places the cosmetologist between the electro-therapy device and the client. So, the current flows through the client and travels to the cosmetologist's fingers. In this method, you usually wear a wrist band. This band is one of the electrodes. The other electrode is a solution-soaked pad, which is attached to the client's neck (usually between the shoulders, or held by the client). After this is done, you place your fingers on the face and adjust the current to a comfortable level. Then you massage the motor points according to the procedure taught in your school.

Safety Considerations

Safety Tip

Whether the direct or indirect method is chosen, it is important to check your meter to make sure the current adjustment is set at "0." If not, the client will get a small "shock" when touched. You should remember to remain in contact with the face once the current has been turned "on." Reach over with one hand and turn the current to "0" before removing the other hand.

Sinusoidal Electro-Therapy

This therapy is similar to faradic electro-therapy. In both modes of operation, the A.C. current causes the muscles to contract and relax. Some cosmetologists prefer the faradic current because it is thought to be the **most soothing** and least irritating type of therapy. The 120-volt A.C. current used in all salons is sinusoidal. The word **sinusoidal** describes how the current changes from positive polarity to negative polarity. The frequency (how often) that it changes is regulated by the power company. You have already read earlier that it changes 60 times per second (60 hertz). Generally, sinusoidal devices also change the frequency of current. Some devices allow you to change the frequency as well as the amount of current.

Usually, a pure sinusoidal wave is not used. Instead, it is modified (changed) slightly. This is done in an effort to make the therapy more effective. The result is that it produces a longer muscle contraction and is considered to have a better massaging action on the muscles.

The cosmetologist uses sinusoidal therapy in the same way that faradic therapy is used. The same electrodes are used, and it may be used directly or indirectly. It produces very smooth and repeated contractions of the facial muscles. Because it is able to affect both voluntary and involuntary muscles, it may be used for scalp treatments as well as facial treatments. It is considered to be especially good for stimulating **deeper muscles** because it **penetrates more than faradic current.** Thus, it is used on middle-aged clients who have facial wrinkles.

A word of caution is necessary. **The treatment period should be no longer than 30 minutes.** If the muscles become fatigued, the benefits of the treatment will be lost. Also, don't give facial treatments of this type to unhealthy skin. **For example, refuse a service on skin with open cuts or red, open sores!**

The use of high-frequency by cosmetologists isn't intended to stimulate muscles. High-frequency treatments use A.C. current that changes **thousands of times per second.** Because the frequency change is so fast, no muscular reaction is produced. Instead, these high-frequency currents **produce heat** as they move through the skin. When used correctly, heat can have a definite therapeutic effect on the skin.

There are different high-frequency currents. The one used the most is called **tesla current.** High-frequency tesla currents are at a very high voltage, but the current is very small (low). The device can look very different, depending on who makes it. It may have one or two electrodes. Small,

Using a Sinusoidal Electro-Therapy Device

 Safety Tip

High-Frequency Therapy

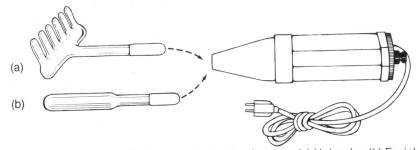

High-frequency unit with glass electrode attachments. (*a*) Hair rake. (*b*) Facial disk electrode

hand-held units are the most popular because of their low cost. These units are one-electrode devices. Sometimes these devices are called **violet rays** because of the violet-colored light that comes from the electrode. Many of these devices have a selection of plug-in electrodes. Often they are clear glass. The size and shape of the electrode will allow them to be used on different parts of the body. For example, a rake-shaped, glass electrode is used for the scalp.

Indirect Treatments

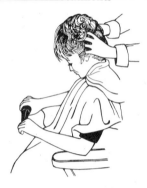

These treatments are given to clients who have dry skin or scalp. **It is believed that the indirect treatments will prevent the skin from becoming drier.** Like the indirect method we just talked about, in this treatment the electrode is held by the client, or it is attached to the client. In high-frequency indirect treatments, the current flows through the client's skin to the massaging fingertips of the cosmetologist. Heat is produced where the fingertips come in contact with the client. The cosmetologist will have a tingling sensation in his/her fingertips. As a safety precaution, **make sure the machine is set at "0" to start,** and **then** adjusted to the comfort/tolerance level for the particular client you are working on, and your own comfort/tolerance level.

The Direct Method

Safety Tip

Just like galvanic and faradic therapy, high-frequency therapy follows similar safety rules. Always keep the current turned down to the lowest possible setting to begin with, then gradually increase the current **after the current** is applied to the skin. When the current has been adjusted to a comfortable level, the glass electrode is moved slowly across the skin. Before using the glass electrode, some cosmetologists prefer to use an emollient skin cream because it transfers the heat so it is more evenly distributed across the skin. Using the cream also helps the glass electrode to slide across the skin more easily during the treatment. Special care should be taken when using cream on the scalp or skin. **Be sure that the cream doesn't contain alcohol,** which can be **flammable.** If a cream with a flammable base were used, a spark from the high-frequency unit would ignite the alcohol and start a fire!

It is believed that the high-frequency treatment stimulates the nerves in the skin and promotes circulation of blood through the vessels. It is also considered to increase circulation in the lymph systems and overall glandular activity, as well as increase the general metabolism of the body.

When a high-frequency treatment is being given, there will be an odd smell in the air. This odd smell is **ozone.** The ozone is created as the tesla current "breaks down" the air around the electrode. As the ozone drifts up to your nose from the electrode, you smell "something different" in the air. It is believed that ozone has a therapeutic effect. The high-frequency treatment is considered to have a germicidal effect on the skin, so disorders such as a blackhead or simple acne tend to clear up when treated regularly. Tesla high-frequency therapy can also be used to remove warts, moles, or other tissue growths, but this is **not to be done by the cosmetologist!**

Often cosmetologists are asked to recommend a treatment for the removal of unwanted hair. Because this happens, it is important for the cosmetologist to be familiar with the options available to the client. Although the cosmetologist isn't licensed to remove unwanted hair with electrical methods in most states, it is a good idea to be informed about how some of these other methods work.

By definition, **electrolysis** is the removal of unwanted hair using an electrical method. The person who performs this service is an **electrologist**. Electrologists also combine electrolysis with another method called **thermolysis** (diathermy). When the electrologist combines electrolysis with thermolysis, the resulting technique is called **the blend**, or **dual method**. Electrolysis, and thermolysis, used individually, has its own advantages and disadvantages. The blend, or dual method, tends to take the best of the advantages and put them together; however, the result also combines the disadvantages.

Define electrolysis and thermolysis (diathermy) terms.

Electrolysis and Thermolysis

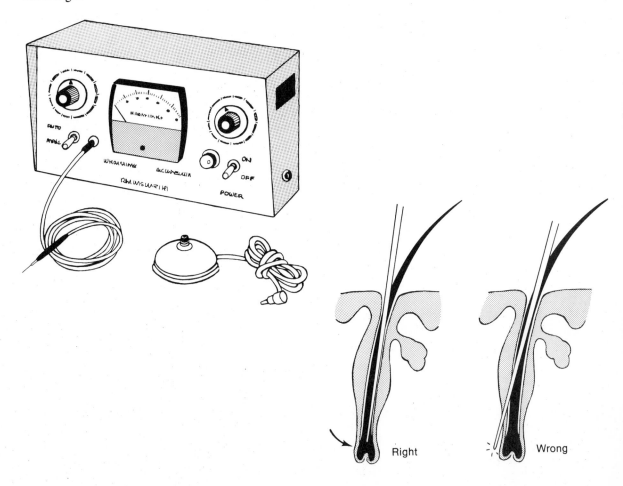

Right   Wrong

Electrolysis uses a low-frequency **galvanic** current. It is thought that body salts and water in the skin are broken down by the current, causing a chemical reaction between the water, salt, and the skin. The result is that **lye (sodium hydroxide)** is formed at the bottom of the hair follicle. The lye destroys the hair bulb over a period of time, and the hair stops growing. So, the current activated in the follicle causes the formation of chlorine, hydrogen, hydroxyl ions and sodium chemicals. These chemicals combine to form sodium hydroxide (lye) and hydrochloric acid. It is the sodium hydroxide which finally causes the **papilla** (nerve and blood supply) to die. And no more hair can grow from that follicle.

It is believed that **the negative electrode causes an alkaline reaction** within the skin, forming sodium hydroxide. When the electrologist's needle is withdrawn from the hair follicle, the sodium hydroxide is left in the bottom of the follicle to dissolve the tissue in there and prevent the regrowth of hair. Although this system is thought to work quite well, it can be somewhat painful because the treatment on an individual follicle may take from 50 seconds to one and one-half minutes, depending on the resistance of the skin and the moisture content of the tissue. So, it is very time consuming. The process can be made to go faster by simply increasing the galvanic current, but the pain may be too uncomfortable for the client.

Thermolysis (Diathermy)

Thermolysis uses high-frequency current to produce heat in the tissue. Thermolysis uses heat, rather than a chemical reaction like the galvanic method. As a matter of fact, the high-frequency current used in this method is in the megahertz range. A megahertz is a million alternations per second.

The setting for the thermolysis needle before it is inserted into the follicle will depend on how much tissue will be destroyed. Often the device will have both a manual control for the time the current remains "on," as well as an automatic timer control. The automatic setting is good because it prevents the current from being accidentally left on for too long a time. Seldom does this method require a time period longer than 30 seconds in the manual mode, or 1/2 second in the automatic mode. The disadvantage of this method is that if the angle at which the needle is inserted is slightly out of line with the walls of the follicle, the area of destroyed tissue won't be in the area necessary to stop hair from regrowing. Another disadvantage is trying to determine how long to leave the current on. So, if either the angle of insertion of the needle is wrong, or the duration of time the current is left on is too short, the unwanted hair will grow again. If you're not extremely careful, scarring of the skin may occur.

The **blend** or **dual method** combines galvanic current with low-level high-frequency current. The result is a method considered to be as effective as electrolysis and as fast and painless as thermolysis.

It is thought that the use of high-frequency improves electrolysis in four ways: (1) The tissue around the follicle is made porous by the heating action of the electrode applied to the tissue so that the lye produced by the galvanic current is absorbed by the tissue better. (2) High-frequency causes the lye to liquify, so it moves around and fills up the follicle cavity. (3) It heats up the sodium hydroxide trapped under the skin, which speeds up the dissolving action of the hair-growing tissue. (4) High-frequency current reduces the painful effects of long periods of electrolysis, because the high-frequency current has a numbing, anesthetic effect on the skin.

KNOWING SUBOBJECTIVE 5

An important application of high-frequency electro-therapy is scalp treatments. High-frequency scalp treatments may be given after silking but before the curling service, as well as in other situations. Consult your instructor about other applications of this type of scalp treatment.

The high-frequency scalp treatment is considered to be beneficial in several ways:

1. It **normalizes** the activity of the sebaceous glands and the apocrine and eccrine sweat glands.
2. It increases the circulation of the blood by **stimulating** the scalp.
3. It destroys germs by causing the air bubbles to release ozone and nitrous oxide.
4. It **relaxes** the muscles of the scalp to relieve itchiness, tightness, or falling hair.

Describe the benefits of a high-frequency scalp treatment.

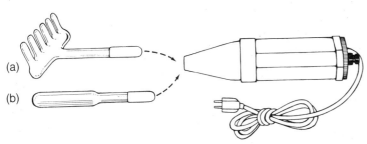

(a)

(b)

High-frequency unit with glass electrode attachments. (*a*) Hair rake. (*b*) Facial disc electrode

The high-frequency appliance is used in one of two ways: (1) directly or (2) indirectly.

In the **direct method,** the glass scalp rake or the glass facial disc is applied directly to the scalp.

The **indirect method** can be used for both skin and scalp applications. The client holds the metal electrode, and the current travels through the client's body and through the hands of the cosmetologist, who acts as a ground for the current. This method is seldom used. If this method is used, the client should not touch any metal object, such as the frame of a metal chair.

DOING SUBOBJECTIVE 6

Give a high-frequency
scalp treatment.

Supplies

☐ high-frequency unit
☐ 1 glass-rake electrode
  attachment (direct treatment)
  or

☐ 1 glass-rod electrode
  attachment (indirect
  treatment)
☐ timer

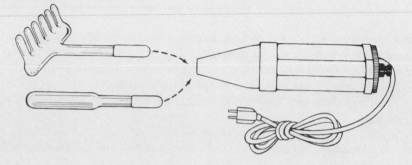

Direct Method

<table>
<tr><td>

PROCEUDRE

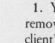 **Safety
Tip**

1. You and your client should
remove all jewelry. Place the
client's valuables in a safe place,
not on the styling station.

2. Attach glass-covered
electrode to the power unit;
then plug it into the electrical
outlet.

**Safety
Tip**

3. Set the timer for 3
minutes.

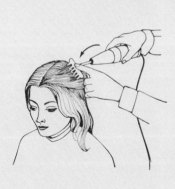

4. Turn the knob at the end
of the power unit very slowly
to start with the smallest
possible amount of current
through the glass rake.

5. **Place your index finger
on the top of the glass rake;**
then lower the rake to the
crown area of the client's head,
then remove finger.

</td><td>

RATIONALE

1. As a safety precaution,
remove all jewelry because it is
a good conductor of electrical
current. It could cause a shock.

2. To prevent electrical
shocks, make all adjustments of
the electrode attachment before
you plug the unit in.

3. Overexposure to high-
frequency current can burn the
skin.

4. This is safe procedure.

5. Placing your index finger
on the rake decreases the
sparking effect and grounds the
electrical current.

</td></tr>
</table>

6. Move the glass rake back and forth on the scalp. Work from the forehead to the nape and side to side until the entire scalp area has been stimulated. Move the rake lightly all over the scalp for a small amount of time. Do not break contact.

6. If you are going to give several treatments, the first one should take 2 or 3 minutes; gradually increase the treatments **to a maximum of 5 minutes**. This treatment improves circulation for a more healthy, normal scalp.

 Safety Tip

Indirect Method

1. Give the glass- or metal-rod electrode to the client. Advise the client to hold it in both hands.
2. Turn on the unit slowly.
3. Give scalp manipulations without breaking contact with client.

1. This is standard procedure.

2. This is standard procedure.
3. Give scalp manipulations while the client holds the electrode. The electrical current passes through the client's body and through your hands and body; since you are standing on the floor, the current is grounded.

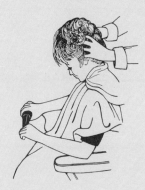

GLOSSARY

A.C.   See Alternating current.

Alternating current   An intermittant flow of electricity that moves in one direction and then in the opposite direction.

Ampere   A measure of electrical current.

Anaphoresis   An electro-therapy process by which a solution is pushed into the skin (for bleaching).

Anode   The positive electrode of an electro-therapy device.

Blend   A technique combining electrolysis with thermolysis. Also called the Dual method.

Cataphoresis   An electro-therapy process by which a solution is pulled into the skin (for bleaching).

Cathode   The negative electrode of an electro-therapy device.

Circuit breaker   A safety device which stops the flow of current.

Complete circuit   The route that an electrical circuit travels from its source of generation via conductors and back to the source.

Conductor   A material which will allow electrons to move through it.

Converter   A mechanical electrical device used to change direct current so it can be used to power alternating current appliances. (This term is now obsolete.)

Current   Moving electrons.

Cycle   See **Hertz.**

D.C.   See **Direct current.**

Diathermy   See **Thermolysis.**

Direct current   Current which moves in only one direction, such as that produced by a battery.

Direct method   A faradic electro-therapy technique in which both electrodes are placed on the client's skin.

Double-insulated appliance   A type of appliance which is not grounded, but is safe to use because of the type of insulation used around its wiring.

Dry cell   A type of battery.

Dual method   See **Blend.**

Electrologist   A person who uses different kinds of electrical current that travels through a very fine needle to permanently remove unwanted facial and body hair.

Electrolysis   Removal of unwanted hair through an electrical method.

Electrolyte   A nonmetallic electrical conductor.

Electrolytic suction-cup treatment   A skin treatment using the galvanic electro-therapy device.

Electron   A particle which rotates around the nucleus of the atom.

Electro-therapy   The use of electricity to stimulate the body.

Faradic current   Alternating current used to exercise the muscles through electro-therapy.

Faradic therapy   A type of electro-therapy used on the skin and muscles.

Fuse   A safety device which stops electrical current.

Galvanic electro-therapy   A therapy which uses D.C. current, produces heat, and causes muscles to contract and relax.

Galvanic therapy   See **Galvanic electro-therapy.**

Generator   A device which produces A.C. voltage.

Grounding   A safety procedure for wiring which minimizes the possibility of getting a shock from electrical appliances.

Hertz   A unit measuring the alternation of current.

High-frequency treatments   Therapy using A.C. current to produce heat.

Indirect method   A faradic electro-therapy technique in which the cosmetologist is placed between the device and the client.

Insulator   Material which will not allow current to pass through.

Nucleus   The center of an atom.

Ohm   The measurement of resistance in a conductor.

Phoresis   A process of forcing substances through the skin without breaking the surface of the skin.

Photoelectric cells   Cells made of materials which will produce a voltage when exposed to any light.

Piezoelectric crystals   Crystals which will develop a voltage if pressure is applied in the form of twisting or bending.

Power   Voltage multiplied by current in a circuit.

Rectifier   A device which changes alternating current into direct current (usually now, an electronic device).

Resistance   Opposition (measured in Ohms) to electrical flow.

Rheostat (REE-oh-stat)   A device that regulates the flow of electricity.

Short circuit   The condition created when a conductor interferes with a circuit.

Sinusoidal   See **Sinusoidal therapy.**

Sinusoidal therapy   A treatment using A.C. current to contract and relax muscles.

Skin bleaching   A technique using galvanic electro-therapy to bleach the skin.

Sodium hydroxide   A chemical compound also known as lye.

Tesla current   A high-frequency current sometimes used in therapy.

Thermocouple   A junction between two dissimilar metals which generates a voltage when heated.

Thermolysis (diathermy)   A technique which uses high-frequency current to produce heat in the tissue.

Transformer   A device which can raise or lower A.C. voltages; normally used to lower voltage down to 120 or 240 volt.

Vaso-constrictor   Something which reduces the flow of blood in blood vessels.

Vaso-dilator   Something which increases the flow of blood in blood vessels.

Violet Ray   A small hand-held electrode device used in high-frequency therapy.

Volt   A unit of electrical potential.

Voltage   Electrical potential.

Wall plate   A portable appliance used in electro-therapy which can produce galvanic, faradic, or sinusoidal currents (not to be confused with the wall plate around an outlet).

Watt   A unit of electrical power.

Wattage   A designation sometimes used to refer to electrical power of appliances.

Wet cell   A type of battery.

QUESTIONS

1. What term is used to explain how much electrical potential is available for use?
2. Are 120 volts and 240 volts of electricity used in North America?
3. A.C. is the abbreviation for what electrical term?
4. Would copper be a good conductor of electricity?
5. Name the center of an atom.
6. Name the rotating particle of an atom.
7. Name the term which indicates opposition to the flow of electrical current.

8. What device lowers the power line voltage for household use?

9. If you try to draw too much current through a wire, what "blows" or is "tripped?"

10. Is galvanic current an A.C. or D.C. current?

11. Does galvanic current produce a chemical reaction as well as heat?

12. What is the positive electrode called?

13. What is the negative electrode called?

14. Name the process that causes chemicals to be forced through unbroken skin.

15. Is it believed that the positive electrode produces an acidic reaction on the skin?

16. Is it believed that the negative electrode produces an alkaline reaction on the skin?

17. Do we think that the positive electrode hardens and firms up the skin?

18. Is it usually best to begin a treatment with the meter set on 5 milliamperes?

19. Does cataphoresis pull the solution into the skin?

20. Does anaphoresis push, or force, the solution into the skin?

21. Does faradic therapy exercise the facial muscles?

22. Define the direct method and indirect method of electrotherapy.

23. Is high-frequency therapy a form of galvanic current?

24. Is it thought that indirect treatments prevent the skin from becoming drier?

25. Is removal of unwanted hair using an electrical method called the blender?

26. Using galvanic current, does the electrologist cause lye to form in the follicle of the hair?

27. Does thermolysis involve the use of high-frequency current to produce heat in the skin tissue?

28. Is it thought that the use of high-frequency current improves the effectiveness of electrolysis?

29. True or false. High-frequency scalp treatments are considered to be beneficial by normalizing the activity of the sebaceous glands and the apocrine and eccrine sweat glands.

30. True or false. It is not necessary to remove all jewelry before giving your client a high-frequency scalp treatment.

ANSWERS

1. Volt 2. Yes 3. Alternating Current 4. Yes 5. Nucleus 6. Electron 7. Resistance 8. Transformer 9. Fuse; circuit breaker 10. D.C. current 11. Yes 12. Anode 13. Cathode 14. Phoresis 15. Yes 16. Yes 17. Yes 18. No, "0" 19. No, 20. Yes 21. Yes 22. (Check your answer with the text) 23. No, tesla current 24. Yes 25. No, electrolysis 26. Yes 27. Yes 28. Yes 29. True 30. False

Describing Nail Anatomy, Disorders, and Diseases

26

This knowledge chapter contains important facts about nail shapes, growth, structure, disorders, and diseases of the nails of the human hand and foot. You will need to know this information in order to give manicures and pedicures successfully. Being able to recognize certain nail disorders is necessary so that you can answer a client's questions about them. Some knowledge of nail diseases is needed in order for you to protect yourself from performing services on clients that have a highly contagious disease. If you give a service to a client who has a contagious disease, you may spread the disease to yourself and to the other clients visiting the salon. Therefore, this chapter will describe what you need to know about the nails, and the next chapter will describe how different nail services are given.

Purpose

Use the information in this chapter to recognize, describe, and label nail shapes, disorders, diseases, and the main bones of the arm and hand.

Major Objective

Score 75 percent or better on a multiple-choice exam on the information in the chapter.

Level of Acceptability

1. Describe 4 basic nail shapes and the anatomy of the fingernail, its surrounding structures, and nail growth.
2. Describe nail irregularities.
3. Identify nail diseases.
4. Recognize and label the main bones of the arm, hand, foot and leg.
5. Describe disorders and diseases of the feet.

Knowing Subobjectives

KNOWING SUBOBJECTIVE 1

Describe 4 basic nail shapes and the anatomy of the fingernail, its surrounding structures, and nail growth.

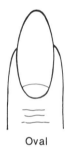

Oval

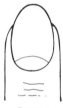

Round

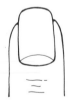

Square

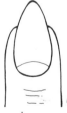

Pointed

Although nail shapes may vary, there are four generally recognized nail forms: square, round, oval, and pointed.

The **oval shape** is usually the most complimentary, but current fashions, finger shape, and the needs of the client have to be considered. (Rather long nails can interfere with a client's work or recreation. For example, a client who plays basketball may experience frequent nail breakage unless the nails are somewhat short and rounded, instead of long and oval.)

The fingernail is an **appendage (ah-PEN-dij) of the skin**. It includes a nail plate and the tissue that surrounds it.

The **nail plate** (nail body) is the visible (almost clear) hard keratin portion on the top of the finger (like hair, the nail is made of keratin). The area of tissue directly under the nail plate is called the **nail bed**. A healthy nail looks **pink** because the blood that flows to the nail bed can be seen through the nail plate.

The **free edge** of the nail is the part that extends beyond the end of the fingertip and can be seen from both sides of the hand.

The tissue that surrounds the nail is: cuticle, eponychium, nail wall, nail groove, nail mantle, and hyponychium.

The **cuticle** is a thin semicircular piece of skin that overlaps the nail.

The **eponychium (ep-oh-NIK-i-uhm)** is the inside point where the nail enters the skin.

The **nail wall** is a semicircular fold of skin that overlaps the nail plate on either side and extends to the first knuckle.

The **nail groove** is the channel (slit) on each side of the nail plate. This is where the nail moves when it grows.

The **nail root** is beneath the skin at the base of the nail in a deep fold of skin called the **nail mantle**.

The skin located directly **beneath** the nail's free edge is the **hyponychium (high-poh-NIK-ee-uhm)**.

The skin that surrounds the entire nail is called the **perionychium**.

The **matrix (MAY-triks)** is the inner part of the nail. It affects the nail's shape, size, regeneration, and growth. It contains the lymph, blood vessels, and nerves that help the nail grow. Keratin grows and hardens in the matrix. This process produces the **nail body**. A bacterial infection involving pus in the matrix is called **onychia**. The light arc at the base of the nail is called the **lunula**. It has a half-moon shape. The light color results from an air pocket between the nail plate and the nail bed at the base of the nail.

If the matrix is injured, the growth and shape of the nail can be distorted. Unlike hair, nails grow continuously at the rate of .1 millimeter per day (1/8 inch per month). (They grow faster in summer than in winter.) If a nail is lost or removed, it will take about 3 months to restore the fingernail and 9 months for toenails. The middle fingernail grows fastest, the thumbnail slowest.

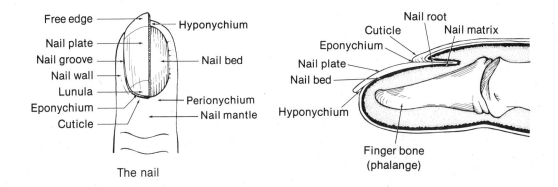

The nail

Finger bone
(phalange)

Nail growth can be slowed during serious illnesses and old age. It can be increased through nail biting from nervous tension. The general physical and emotional condition of the individual is somewhat indicated by the fingernails.

KNOWING SUBOBJECTIVE 2

Although there are 4 basic nail shapes, you probably will encounter nails of many different appearances. If you know the basic shapes, you will be able to suggest services that will improve the appearance of the client's hand, but even more important, you will be able to recognize disorders. **You must refuse service to clients who have contagious diseases**. Advise them to consult a doctor. A **disease** is a disorder that interferes with the normal state and/or function of the body. **Onyx (ON'x)** is from the Greek word for fingernail, **onycho**. This subobjective describes various irregularities and diseases of the nail. A simple, easy-to-follow format is used:

Onychosis (on-ee-KOH-siss) is a term used to describe any nail disease.

The **prognosis (prahg-NOH-siss)** for a disease (or irregularity or some other condition) is the outlook, or forecast, for recovery from it.

Treatment, of course, is the procedure needed to avoid or stop the disease.

Onychophagy (on-ee-KOF-aj-ee) is the technical term for nail biting. The condition involves slightly deformed nail shapes, with no inflammation (redness) or other abnormal signs.

Cause   It is a nervous habit of many individuals.

Prognosis   The condition will subside if the person stops biting the nails. If the habit is continued, the individual risks getting a disease from bacteria found on the nails or infection of the cuticle from mouth bacteria.

Describe nail irregularities.

Safety Tip

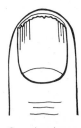
Onychophagy

Treatment Having regular manicures helps stop biting because nail polish is unpleasant to taste. Other distasteful chemicals may be applied to discourage it, but willpower is the only effective solution to the problem.

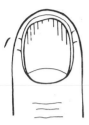

Onychatrophia

Onychatrophia (on-i-kat-ROH-fi-ah), atrophy of the nails, is characterized by the wasting away of the nail plate. The nail loses sheen; the plate becomes smaller and may separate from the nail bed.

Cause Injury to the nail matrix or internal disease can result in onychatrophia. Also called **onychia**.

Prognosis Nail regeneration depends on the extent of the injury to the matrix or the illness of the client.

Treatment Use only a fine emery board. Do not use a metal pusher or a file during the manicure service. Advise the client to avoid highly alkaline soap or detergents.

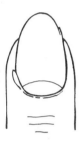

Hangnails

Hangnails involve small skin tears or nail splits. The skin can bleed and be painfully raw. Also called **agnails**.

Cause The skin tears in the cuticle area result from dryness or from injury, sometimes caused by improper manicuring techniques.

Prognosis If only a very small area is affected, the skin rebuilds quickly. Larger areas require more treatment and time for correction.

Treatment Soaking in an antiseptic solution and application of antiseptics are in order for small areas. A large area of skin should be treated only by a doctor since surgery may be required. If caution is not exercised, bacterial infection may result.

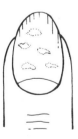

Leukonychia

Leukonychia (loo-koh-NIK-i-ah) is characterized by white spots on the nail plates on fingers or toes.

Cause Heredity or minor injury may cause leukonychia. One theory suggests that the white spots are tiny air bubbles caused by incompletely keratinized cells.

Prognosis Spots may disappear when nail grows out.

Treatment None.

Onychorrhexis (on-ee-koh-REX-iss) is a split, brittle nail condition. It includes longitudinal splits parallel to each other on one or more fingernails. No inflammation is present around or under the nail.

Cause   The condition may result from heredity and, in some cases, from use of permanent-type polishes or strong solvents for removing nail polishes. Injury to the nail may also cause splitting.

Prognosis   A 3-month treatment will usually improve the condition of the nails.

Treatment   Advise the client to see a doctor to make sure that disease is not present. Drinking an envelope of gelatin mixed with fruit juice each day may help improve the nails. Hot oil manicures may also help.

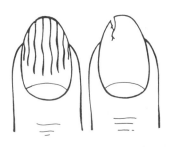

Onychorrhexis (brittle nail)

Onychauxis (on-ee-KAWK-siss), hypertrophy, is a thickening of the nail plate. It is an overgrowth in the thickness or the depth of the nail.

Cause   It may result from injury and internal disorders, or from minor nail injury.

Prognosis   The client should be advised to see a doctor for prognosis.

Treatment   Advise the client to see a doctor. If infection is not present, a manicurist may buff nails with pumice powder.

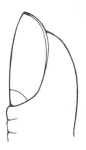

Onychauxis

Pterygium (ter-IJ-ee-uhm) is a condition in which the cuticle sticks to the surface of the nail base.

Cause   Unusually dry skin around the fingernail may result in this condition.

Prognosis   The condition may recur.

Treatment   Hot oil manicures will soften the cuticle and make unneeded growth easy to remove. Carefully remove it with a sanitized cuticle nipper.

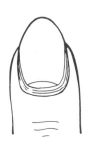

Pterygium

Corrugations (kor-uh-GAY-shuhnz), also called beau's lines or transverse furrows, are characterized by wavy horizontal lines across the nail.

Cause   The condition may result from heart disease, pregnancy, emotional shock, or some acute infections. It may also be caused from minor injury to nails.

Prognosis   The nail usually grows out normally in three months, but this may vary with the individual's condition.

Treatment   Advise the client to see a doctor for the underlying cause of the nail condition. Buffing may make some improvement, but it cannot completely smooth most corrugated nails.

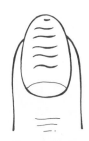

Corrugations

Blue nails appear bluish instead of healthy pink. The client with blue nails can receive a manicure.

Cause   The condition results from heart trouble or other circulatory (blood flow) problems.

Prognosis and Treatment   The client should ask a doctor about the internal cause of blue nails.

Bruised nails have dark spots caused by dried blood underneath the nail plate.

Cause   The condition occurs from an injury to the nail.

Prognosis   Whether the new growth will be normal depends on the extent and nature of the injury.

Treatment   A client with a badly bruised nail may need to see a doctor. In manicuring, the nail must be handled carefully to avoid further injury or pain.

KNOWING SUBOBJECTIVE 3

Identify nail diseases.

In general you can recognize nail diseases by **inflammation** of the skin surrounding the nail, extreme discomfort from soreness, and other signs of infection.

A client may not realize that the disease exists until you point it out. Tell the client to ask a doctor about the condition. **Do not try to treat diseased nails**. By referring a client to a doctor, you will protect yourself and your clients from the possible spread of contagious or infectious disorders.

When manicuring, you should be extremely careful not to damage the nail or surrounding tissue. Damaging the nail can cause a local infection. If bleeding should occur from accidental improper use of a manicuring implement, an antiseptic should be used immediately. If an antiseptic is not used on an injured matrix, bacteria may enter the matrix and cause onychia. Some of the diseases that cosmetologists are likely to encounter follow.

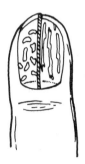

Onychomycosis

Onychomycosis (on-ee-koh-migh-KOH-siss), tinea (ringworm) of the nails on fingers or toes, is a disturbance of the nail growth due to a vegetable fungus (parasite). It is not very common, but it is very contagious. The condition is characterized by thickening and deformity and finally loss of the nail. Also known as **Tinea Unguis** (UNG-gwis).

Cause   Heredity can be a factor, but this disease is usually the result of nail injury coupled with an invasion of a fungus.

Prognosis   The nail usually requires three months to grow back if it is treated by a doctor. Although the condition is resistant to treatment, competent dermatologists treat it with success.

Treatment   Tell the client to get a doctor's advice immediately.

Safety Tip

Tinea of the hands is **not** a nail disease, but you must be aware of it. It is sometimes called the **one-hand-two-foot disease**. It is a rare infection that affects only one hand but both feet. Its acute form is characterized by blisters on palms and fingers at the edge of inflamed areas. In its chronic state, it can be identified by dry, scaly lesions, usually in one large patch instead of several areas.

Cause   It is a fungus infection.

Prognosis   It is resistant to treatment.

Treatment   Tell the client to get a doctor's advice for treatment.

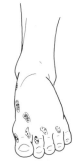
Tinea

Onychocryptosis (on-ik-oh-krip-TOH-siss) is the technical term for an **ingrown nail**. It is characterized by lateral growth of the nail plate into the edge of the nail groove, usually occurring in the big toe, but also in the fingernails.

Cause   Improperly fitted (tight) shoes and incorrect nail trimming can cause the condition.

Prognosis   It may recur after treatment.

Treatment   It may be remedied by trimming the nail in a semi-lunar manner so that the corner of the nail may raise it above the skin surface. In cases of extreme discomfort, a doctor should be consulted for surgical relief and/or advice about bacterial infection.

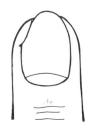
Onychocryptosis

Onychogryposis (on-ee-koh-gri-POH-siss), also called **claw nails**, involves marked thickening of the nail. The nail plate becomes elongated and twisted (curved).

Cause   It results from trauma (shock); other causes are unknown.

Prognosis and Treatment   Tell the client to get a doctor's advice.

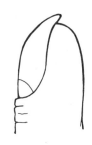
Onychogryposis

Onycholysis (on-ee-KOHL-eh-siss) involves a spontaneous separation of the nail plate from the nail bed, without actual shedding.

Cause   Local or general infections and treatments with certain types of antibiotic drugs may cause the condition.

Prognosis and Treatment   Tell the client to get a doctor's advice.

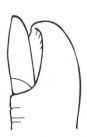
Onycholysis

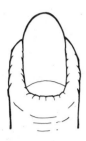

Paronychia

Paronychia (par-on-NIK-ee-ah), felon, is a bacterial infection of the tissue around the nail. It is characterized by pain, redness, and swelling of skin around the nail plate, without nail loss. This is very contagious, so it is not treated in the school or salon.

Cause   People who have their hands in water for long periods of time get this condition. Housewives and cosmetologists are particularly likely to have it.

Prognosis   It usually responds well when treated by a doctor.

Treatment   Tell the client to ask a doctor for advice.

Eggshell Nails—Hapalonychia (hap-palo-NIK-ee-ah) involves very thin fragile nails that are white in color. These nails split and break easily. A defect in the nail matrix causes this.

Cause   Rare, but can result from aging and/or use of acetone or hydroxide solutions in manicuring.

Prognosis   Nail hardeners or polish (enamel) adds strength to these nails to prevent splitting.

KNOWING SUBOBJECTIVE 4

Recognize and label the main bones of the arm, hand, foot and leg.

You should be able to identify the main bones of the arm and hand in order to understand the manicuring task.

You should know the 3 bones in the arm and 3 types of bones in the hand.

The 3 bones in the arm are humerus, ulna, and radius. The **humerus** is the **large bone** in the upper part of the arm. The **ulna (UHL-nah)** and **radius** are the 2 bones that form the forearm. The ulna, which is attached to the wrist, is on the same side as the **little finger**. The **radius (RAYD-ee-uhs)** is the bone that attaches to the wrist on the **thumb side**.

The wrist is the flexible joint between the forearm and the hand. The wrist is made of 8 bones called carpals (KAHR-puhlz). Metacarpals **(met-ah-KAHR-puhlz)** are the long bones that form the palm of the hand. **Phalanges (FAY-lanj-ez)** are the bones that form the fingers **(digits)** of the hand. There are 14 of them, 3 for each finger and 2 for the thumb.

KNOWING SUBOBJECTIVE 5

Describe disorders and diseases of the feet.

Care of the feet and toenails is very important because they are subjected to many shocks and germs every day. Sports and other exercise, such as tennis, jogging, racquetball, roller/ice skating, aerobic dancing, and walking, leave the feet open to a lot of different disorders and diseases. Several of the more common disorders and diseases that appear on the feet are callouses, ingrown nails, athlete's foot, and plantar warts.

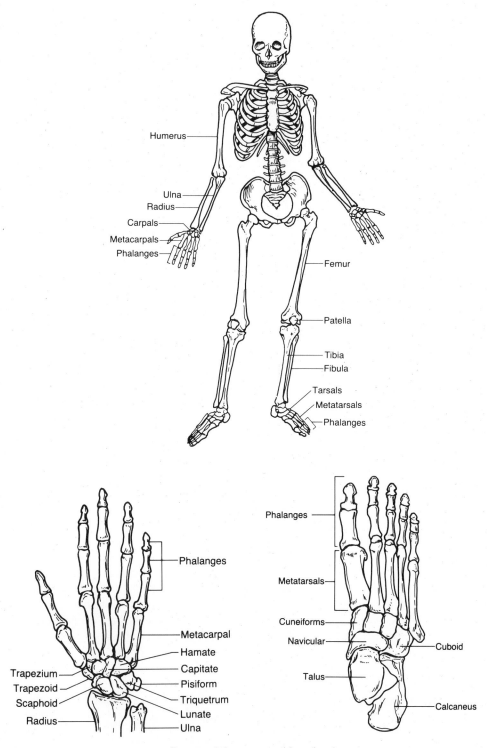

Humerus

Ulna
Radius
Carpals
Metacarpals
Phalanges

Femur

Patella

Tibia
Fibula

Tarsals
Metatarsals
Phalanges

Phalanges

Metacarpal
Hamate
Capitate
Trapezium
Pisiform
Trapezoid
Scaphoid
Triquetrum
Lunate
Radius
Ulna

Phalanges

Metatarsals

Cuneiforms
Navicular
Cuboid
Talus
Calcaneus

Bones of the arm and hand

A **callous** is an abnormal thickening of the skin commonly found on the heels and around some part of the edge of the foot. (It is also commonly found on the elbow(s), knee, or somewhere on the hands.) A callous is caused by repeated shocks to a particular area of the skin. These "shocks" can be caused by a shoe that doesn't fit properly, rubbing against the skin of the foot in the wrong way. In order to protect itself, the skin "thickens." Extra thick socks, or even two pairs of socks, will often prevent callouses from forming.

An **ingrown nail** occurs when the side of the toenail overgrows into the nail fold of skin along the edge of the toe. This is usually caused by cutting the nail too deeply into the corner of one or both sides of the nail. If the nail is left more square at the corners, an ingrown nail sometimes can be avoided.

Diseases of the foot are very common because feet create a natural environment for the growth of bacteria, funguses, and viruses. Particularly during exercise, the feet become hot and perspire. Inside shoes, they are shielded from the germicidal effects of the sun's ultraviolet rays. Special care of the feet must be taken during and after bathing. After they have been washed, feet must be thoroughly dried, particularly between the toes.

Athlete's foot is a common fungus-type disease that can be particularly bothersome. It is caused by a type of fungus known as **ringworm**. Since it is very contagious, it is important that **a client who has this disease not be given a pedicure**. The symptoms of this disease are itching and the appearance of one or more clear, watery blisters. White scaling and thickening of the skin, as well as cracks (fissures) between the toes, may also be seen. Athlete's foot should always be treated by a doctor.

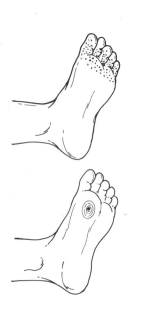

Plantar warts, which are caused by a virus, are found on the sole of the foot. These warts are contagious. For example, when a person with a plantar wart walks through a shower area, the virus causing the wart is left behind on the floor. If another person walks on the spot on the floor where the virus is present, that person probably will develop a plantar wart, too. Plantar warts look like circles within a circle—like a small circular target. These flat warts have a small spot right in the center. Plantar warts are painful, and removing them isn't always easy because they can go deep into the skin. A doctor must always treat plantar warts. Different kinds of treatment are used, depending on where the warts are located. Pedicures should **not be given to a client with plantar warts**. Refer the client to a dermatologist.

Disorders and diseases of the feet are so common that this is a major field of study, which is called **podiatry**. A doctor who specializes in disorders and diseases of the feet is called a **podiatrist** (PEH-digh-trehst).

GLOSSARY

Agnail See **Hangnails**.

Athlete's foot A highly contagious fungus-type disease.

Atrophy Wasting away or withering of a part of the body, as atrophy of the nails.

Blue nails   A condition where nails apear bluish instead of healthy pink; caused by circulatory problems.

Bruised nails   Nails with dark spots underneath the nail plate; caused by injury to the nail.

Callous   An abnormal thickening of the skin.

Carpals (KAHR-puhlz)   The eight bones in the wrist.

Corrugations (kor-uh-GAY-shuhnz)   Wavy lines or furrows across the nail; caused by heart disease, pregnancy, emotional shock, acute infection, or minor nail injury.

Cuticle   The thin semicircular piece of skin that overlaps the nail.

Disease (diz-EEZ)   A disorder that interferes with the normal state and/or function of the body.

Eggshell nails (hapalonychia)   Thin, white, fragile nails resulting from defect in the nail matrix.

Eponychium (ep-oh-NIK-ee-uhm)   The inside point where the nail enters the skin.

Free edge   The part of the nail that extends beyond the edge of the fingertip.

Hangnails   Skin tears or splits in the cuticle area due to skin dryness, injury, or improper manicuring.

Humerus (HYOO-meh-ruhs)   The large bone in the upper part of the arm.

Hyponychium (high-poh-NIK-ee-uhm)   The skin located directly beneath the nail's free edge.

Ingrown nail   A toenail which has grown into the fold of skin along the edge of the toe.

Leukonychia (loo-koh-NIK-i-ah)   White spots on the nail plates caused by heredity or minor injury.

Lunula   The light arc (half-moon) at the base of the nail.

Mantle   The deep fold of skin at the base of the nail that contains the nail root.

Matrix (MAY-triks)   The inner part of the nail that contains the lymph, blood vessels, and nerves.

Metacarpals (met-ah-KAHR-puhlz)   The long bones that form the palm of the hand.

Nail bed   The area of tissue directly under the nail plate.

Nail body   See **Nail plate**.

Nail plate   The visible (almost clear) hard keratin portion on the top of the finger.

Nail root   The place where the nail begins beneath the skin at the base of the nail in the mantle.

Nail wall   The semicircular fold of skin that overlaps the nail plate on either side and extends to the first knuckle.

Onychatrophia (on-i-kat-ROH-fi-ah)   The wasting away of the nail plate, due to injury of the nail matrix. Also called onychia.

Onychauxis (on-ee-KAWK-siss)   A thickening of the nail plate caused by injury, internal disorders, or minor nail injury.

Onycho (on-IK-oh)   (Prefix.) Pertaining to the nail.

Onychocryptosis (on-ik-oh-krip-TOH-siss)   An ingrown nail caused by improper trimming or tight shoes.

Onychogryposis (on-ee-koh-gri-POH-siss)   Elongated, twisted, thickened nails caused by trauma. Also called claw nails.

Onycholysis (on-ee-KOHL-eh-siss)   A spontaneous separation of the nail plate from the nail bed, without actual shedding, caused by local or general infections or certain types of antibiotic drugs.

Onychomycosis (on-ee-koh-migh-KOH-siss)   Ringworm of the nails caused by a vegetable fungus.

Onychophagy (on-ee-KOF-aj-ee)   A slight deformation of the nails caused by nail biting.

Onychorrhexis (on-ee-koh-REX-iss)   A split, brittle condition caused by heredity, permanent polishes, or strong polish-removing solvents.

Onyx   From the Greek word for fingernail, onycho.

Onychosis (on-ee-KOH-siss)   Any nail disease.

Paronychia (par-on-NIK-ee-ah)   A bacterial infection of the tissue around the nail.

Pedicuring (ped-eh-KYUR-ing)   Care of feet and toenails.

Phalanges (FAY-lanj-ez)   The bones that form the fingers.

Plantar warts   Virus-caused warts on the sole of the foot.

Podiatrist   A doctor who specializes in the disorders and diseases of the feet.

Podiatry   Study of the disorders and diseases of the feet.

Prognosis (prahg-NOH-siss)   The outlook, or forecast, for recovery from a disease.

Pterygium (ter-IJ-ee-uhm)   A condition in which the cuticle sticks to the surface of the nail base; caused by unusually dry skin.

Radius (RAYD-ee-uhs)   The bone of the arm that attaches to the wrist on the thumb side.

Tinea Unguis (UNG-guis)   Ringworm of the nails. See Onychomycosis.

Ulna (UHL-nah)   The bone of the arm attached to the wrist on the little-finger side.

QUESTIONS

1. What is the part of the nail which extends beyond the fingertip called?
2. Give the name for the skin directly beneath the free edge of the nail.
3. What is the channel on either side of the nail called?
4. What part of the fingertip affects nail growth and regeneration?
5. Can nail growth slow as a person grows older?
6. Are contagious diseases treated in the salon?
7. What term is used to describe any nail disease?
8. Does onychophagy mean ingrown nail?
9. What is the term for a condition in which the nail plate wastes away?

10. Is the forearm bone that leads to the thumb called the radius?
11. What is a condition characterized by a thickening of the nail plate?
12. Should tinea of the hand and nail be treated in the salon?
13. Is paronychia a bacterial infection of the tissue around the nail?
14. What are the bones called that make up the wrist?
15. What name is given to an abnormal thickening of the skin in the areas of the elbows, and heels of the feet?
16. What name is given to a contagious foot disease caused by a virus?

ANSWERS

1. Free edge 2. Hyponychium 3. Nail groove 4. Matrix 5. Yes 6. No 7. Onychosis 8. No 9. Onychatrophia 10. Yes 11. Onychauxis 12. No 13. Yes 14. Carpals 15. Callous 16. Plantar warts

Manicuring/Pedicuring the Nails 27

Most people like to have a total "look." Some things are very obvious; they set the style. Others, like the details in a picture, fill in the overall impression and make it truly complete. These kinds of details could be eliminated, but the total effect, the total "look," wouldn't be the same. Manicuring and pedicuring are two of these details. **Manicuring is the art of caring for the hands and fingernails.** Manicuring completes the appearance of a well-groomed client and complements high-fashion hairstyling and clothing. While most full-service schools and salons offer manicuring, some also provide pedicuring. **Pedicuring is the art of caring for the feet and toenails.**

Many state licensing agencies or boards have a special separate license for persons who have been trained to be manicurists. So, a person who is not taking the entire cosmetology program can obtain a license for manicuring. Most states automatically allow a licensed or registered cosmetologist to perform manicuring services.

Manicuring in particular has become a large part of the beauty world. Many new products and services have been developed to enhance, beautify, or strengthen the fingernails. Of course, these new services will bring many more dollars and profit to the person performing them, as well as to the schools/salons.

Using professional manicuring implements, supplies, and procedures, shape and apply polish to the nails. Your instructor may also require you to identify and be able to give special nail services.

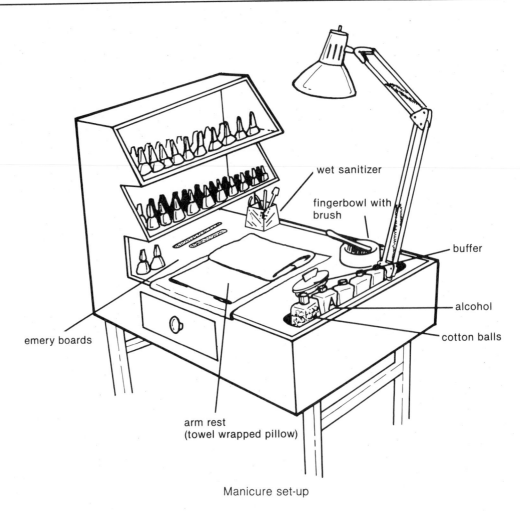

wet sanitizer

fingerbowl with brush

buffer

alcohol

cotton balls

emery boards

arm rest
(towel wrapped pillow)

Manicure set-up

Level of Acceptability

Use the proper safety precautions and sanitation methods to manicure the fingernails. Give a plain manicure in 25 to 40 minutes and an oil manicure in 45 to 50 minutes. Score 75 percent or better on a multiple-choice exam on the information in this chapter.

Knowing Subobjective

1. Identify different nail services and when they are given.

Doing Subobjectives

2. Give a plain or oil manicure (including hand and arm massage).
3. Give a nail wrap.
4. Apply different types of artificial nails.
5. Give a pedicure.

The basic manicure service is given to men and women when their fingernails are in a normal condition. "Normal" in this case means that the nails grow normally and don't have any unusual problems, such as brittleness and cracking. The skin surrounding the nail is also healthy. This service usually includes nail polish removal, cleansing, filing, nipping excess skin around the cuticle, applying cuticle/nail builder, applying polish, and applying a sealer coat to protect the polish.

Identify different nail services and when they are given.

The service usually does differ, depending on whether the client is a man or a woman. For example, a man would probably have either a clear polish, clear paste polish, or a powder polish to simply add sheen to the nails. A nail buffer is used with the nail paste or powder **pumice** polish. Buffing is done from just below the nail cuticle to the free edge of the nail. By contrast, a woman would probably request polish with color.

The oil manicure service is similar to the basic manicure, except that a special skin moisturizing cream or lotion is used to supply or keep moisture in the skin surrounding the nail. The oil manicure prevents hangnails from occurring, or it will help heal them if they are present.

Nail wrapping is a service to strengthen the fingernail. Different fibers, such as very thin sheets of linen or silk, etc., are glued and then shaped to the nail. The fiber is sealed over the free edge of the nail. **Nail wrapping protects the nails,** and it is helpful for the client who has trouble growing longer nails because of splitting. Clients feel that longer nails will give their fingers a longer, thinner, more graceful appearance—and they are right! When a fingernail is cut or filed too far down into either side of the nail groove, the free edge of the nail is weakened; breakage or cracks may result. The nail wrap must be done again after 2 to 3 weeks, depending on the growth rate of the nail and how much "wear and tear" the nails are given.

Artificial nails is a general term used to describe any one of three or more services. These services would include, but not be limited to: acrylic sculptured nails, nail tips, nail caps, and artificial nail shells made from porcelain, plastic, or nylon.

For example, **acrylic sculptured nails** really aren't nails at all. They are made from a powder mixed with a special chemical hardener to make a paste. Then, a special form is secured around the nail. The acrylic paste is applied to the nail and then shaped and molded with a brush into a nail shape before it dries. After the acrylic powdery paste has completely dried, the special form is removed, and the nail is filed into the desired shape.

(A few words of caution) should be noted when using artificial nail supplies, as well as regular manicuring supplies. **Most nail polish removers (acetone),** hardeners, glues (adhesives), etc., **are very flammable.** To avoid the threat of fire, **do not smoke, and do not allow clients to smoke** during any of these manicuring services!

Safety Tip

DOING SUBOBJECTIVE 2

Give a plain or oil manicure (including hand and arm massage).

Supplies

- □ manicure table
- □ cosmetologist's chair
- □ client chair
- □ finger bowl
- □ closed cotton container
- □ manicure tray
- □ small glass implement container
- □ hot oil heater
- □ 2 new emery boards
- □ metal pusher
- □ manicure scissors
- □ buffer
- □ orangewood stick
- □ cuticle nipper and scissors
- □ nail brush
- □ spatula
- □ a new paper cup for hot-oil heater
- □ 2 laundered towels

- □ cotton
- □ cuticle softener
- □ cuticle remover (solvent)
- □ base coat
- □ sealer (top coat)
- □ hand lotion or creme
- □ absorbent tissue
- □ enamel thinner
- □ enamel remover
- □ disposable plastic bag
- □ 70 percent alcohol
- □ soap
- □ nail builder
- □ nail enamel
- □ aerosol enamel dry
- □ powder or paste nail polish
- □ manicure oil
- □ pumice powder

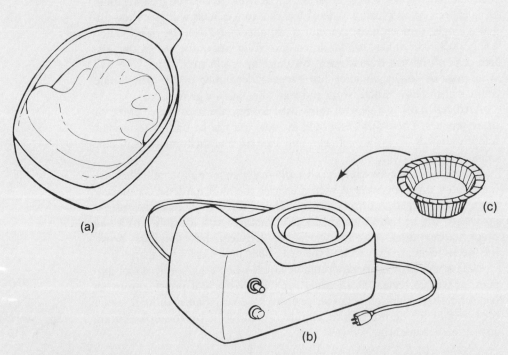

(a) Finger bowl, (b) electric heater, (c) paper or plastic cup for lotion (oil)

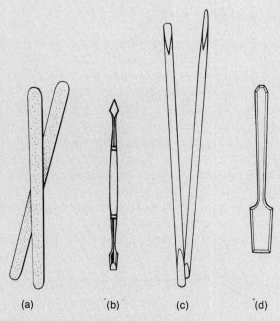

(a)   (b)   (c)   (d)

(*a*) Emery boards, (*b*) metal pusher (*c*) orangewood sticks, (*d*) spatula

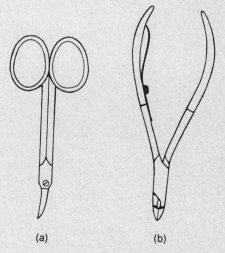

(a)   (b)

(*a*) Cuticle scissor, (*b*) cuticle nipper

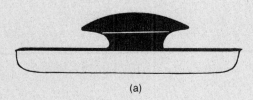

(a)

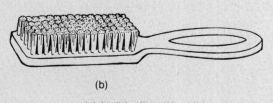

(b)

(*a*) Nail buffer, (*b*) nail brush

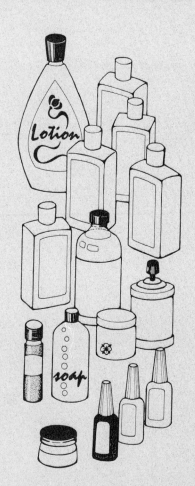

A. Polish removal and shaping of the nail

PROCEDURE	RATIONALE
1. Examine the client's nails for irregularities or disease.	1. Never work on a client with an infectious or contagious nail disease. Ask your instructor or manager if you are unsure about the condition of the client's nails.
2. Help the client decide on a nail shape and an enamel color.	2. Some clients may select a clear or neutral enamel rather than a color.
3. Saturate a small piece of cotton with nail polish remover. Hold the cotton between the middle and index fingers of your right hand.	3. If you hold the cotton this way, you will protect your own nails from the polish remover.
4. Hold the client's wrist in one of your hands. Hold the client's finger between your thumb and index finger. Apply the remover to one of the client's nails for 5 seconds; then move cotton firmly down the nail toward the free edge. Repeat until all enamel has been removed from each nail.	4. Polish (enamel) will dissolve in 5 seconds. Moving the cotton toward the free edge is the easiest way to remove old polish. Polish must be removed from all nails prior to shaping.
5. Use a small piece of cotton rolled onto an orangewood stick and saturated with enamel remover to remove polish around the edge of the cuticle of each nail. **Keep remover away from heat or clients who are smoking.**	5. The cotton protects the client's skin, yet this allows for complete removal of old enamel. Nail polish remover is **very flammable.**

Safety Tip

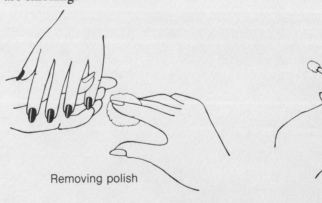
Removing polish

6. Make any necessary recommendations to the client regarding the best nail shape. Discuss suggestions and client's preferences.

7. Using a coarse emery board, begin shaping the nail on the little finger of the left hand. Always shape the nail from one side toward the center, then from the other side toward the center. Never use a back-and-forth sawing technique. Begin with the little finger and move toward the thumb.

8. Tilt the board slightly so that it touches the bottom side of the nail's free edge.

6. Consider client's occupation, leisure activities, age, and finger shape. The shape of the nail usually should conform to the shape of the finger.

7. If the nails are in good condition, the coarse side of the emery board will shape them quickly. Filing from each side to the center of the nail helps the nail to grow evenly. Filing back and forth can cause the nail edge to split or crack as it grows from the finger.

8. If you hold the emery board this way, any mistakes you make will be beneath the free edge. These errors can be corrected and will not be visible when enamel is applied.

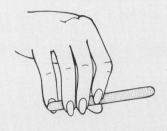

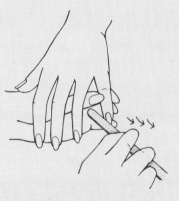

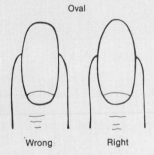

Oval

Wrong   Right

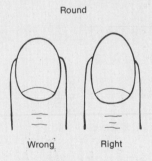

Round

Wrong   Right

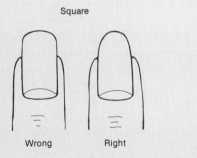

Square

Wrong   Right

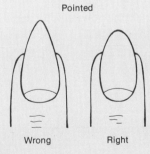

Pointed

Wrong   Right

Correct and incorrect nail shapes

PROCEDURE	RATIONALE
9. Always file from the corner to the center of the nail. Use quick, smooth, short strokes.	9. Filing in one direction at a time avoids splitting nails.
10. Use the fine side of the emery board to lightly file the edge of the nail downward.	10. The fine side neatly completes the shaping of each nail. The coarse side of the emery board will shred the free edge.

⚡ Safety Tip

11. Place the client's left hand in a bowl containing warm soapy water when you have finished the nails. If you are giving an oil manicure check the temperature of the oil in the heater cup. Place the client's fingers in the oil cup.	11. The soapy water or hot oil softens the cuticle so that it can be shaped more easily. It is possible for the heater to overheat, so **check the temperature of the oil.**
12. Shape the nails of the right hand.	12. This is standard procedure.
13. Remove the left hand from the finger bowl and towel-dry each finger. Place the right hand in the soapy water or heated oil.	13. Since both hands will not fit into the finger bowl or cup at once, soak the hands one at a time.

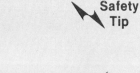

B. Apply cuticle remover and shape cuticle

PROCEDURE	RATIONALE
1. Use a cotton-tipped orangewood stick to apply cuticle remover to each free edge and cuticle of the left hand.	1. The cuticle remover softens the cuticle and dead skin beneath the free edge. Once softened, they can be removed easily.
2. Gently push cuticle back to the fold of the skin. Hold the nail (lunula) using metal pusher. Apply styptic powder if the nail bleeds.	2. The cuticle is fragile, so sharp metal instruments must be used carefully. **Styptic (STIP-tik) powder** (with alum) or antiseptic astringent will stop minor bleeding. Never use styptic pencils because they are **not sanitary**: they may carry bacteria from one client to another.
3. Reapply cuticle remover as needed.	3. Cuticle remover may dry out.

⚡ Safety Tip

4. Use a metal pusher to loosen the dead cuticle around each nail of the left hand. Return the pusher to the alcoholized cotton in glass container.

5. Use a cotton-tipped orangewood stick to clean under the nails of the left hand.

6. Use a towel to remove excess cuticle remover from the left hand.

7. With a clean orangewood stick, apply a small amount of nail builder (cuticle creme) to the back of your left hand.

8. With your index finger apply creme to each nail. Using the thumb and index finger of both hands, massage the creme into the nails.

9. Massage the client's thumbnail with your left hand. Use your right hand to massage the client's little finger. Use circular movements to massage the nail builder into the nails.

10. Massage all the nails of the left hand.

11. Use an orangewood stick to gently shape the softened cuticle.

12. Carefully use the manicure nipper to remove the ragged cuticle of each nail. Put the nipper in alcoholized cotton at the bottom of the implement container.

13. Remove the right hand from the finger bowl and towel-dry it.

4. The metal pusher makes it easier to shape the cuticle. The 70 percent alcohol keeps metal implements sanitized, preventing the spread of pathogenic bacteria.

5. Cotton protects skin from the sharp orangewood stick. The cotton also absorbs the cuticle remover and soil from nails.

6. This will keep the client's hands from becoming too slippery.

7. The orangewood stick must be clean and free from bacteria.

8. This works the creme into the nail plate and surrounding tissue.

9. The nail builder, or cuticle creme, strengthens the nail and surrounding tissue. Circular movements help the nail builder penetrate the nail. Nail builder discourages development of hangnails.

10. All nails must have nail builder, or cuticle creme, worked into the surface of each nail plate.

11. This prevents nail injury.

12. This is standard procedure.

13. This is standard procedure.

Safety Tip

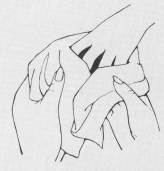

Thoroughly dry fingers and nails

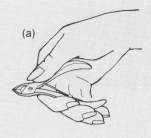
(a)

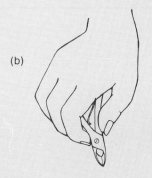
(b)

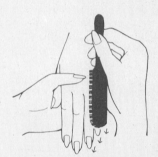

Brush in one direction toward free edge of nails

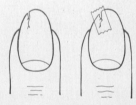

Nail patch if artificial epoxy type nails are not available

14. Place the client's left hand in the finger bowl or heated oil and repeat steps 1 through 12 on the right hand.

15. After you have manicured the client's right hand, apply hand lotion to client's left hand and work the lotion from the fingertips to above the elbow. Begin the massage at the elbow. Use both hands in a circular motion toward the wrist.

16. Massage down each fingertip and push cuticle around each finger.

17. Repeat procedures 15 and 16 on the right hand.

18. Use nail brush to scrub the nails of left hand; towel-dry. If an oil manicure is given, a finger bowl and warm soapy water will be needed now. Repeat this procedure on the right hand.

19. Check the appearance of the cuticle and the shapes of the nails. Reshape if necessary. Apply cellophane tape to torn or split nails.

20. Apply a small amount of nail polish remover to a piece of cotton. Use nail bleach or peroxide to remove any stains. Wipe the nails of both hands.

14. The same procedure must be followed on both hands.

15. This service is added to a manicure.

16. It is easier to push back the cuticle at this point in the manicure.

17. This is standard procedure.

18. The nail brush removes bits of dead skin and the cremes or oils that have been applied.

19. Nail cuticles and free edges should be shaped the same. Tape is applied and trimmed to repair split or broken nails. A cold-wave end paper also works well for patching split nails.

20. The base coat and enamel will not stick unless all traces of oil and cremes are removed.

C. Application of base-coat polish

PROCEDURE

1. Apply a clear base coat to the nails of the left hand. Apply the base coat first on the little fingernail and work toward the thumbnail.

RATIONALE

1. The base coat serves as a primer, or foundation, for the nail enamel.

2. Hold the base-coat brush between your thumb and index finger. Place your little finger on the manicure table. Hold the client's other fingers with your left hand.

3. Apply base coat in 3 strokes—just below the cuticle down the center to the free edge and then along each side of the nail from just below the cuticle to the free edge.

4. Repeat procedures 1 through 3 until you have put a base coat on all nails.

5. Roll enamel bottle between palms and fingers of both hands.

6. Begin applying liquid enamel polish on the little fingernail of the left hand. If clear polish is used, apply it to buff the nails.

7. Follow procedures 2 and 3 to apply polish to the nails of the left hand.

8. Repeat procedures 2 and 3 to apply polish to the nails of the left hand.

9. Apply additional coats of polish as needed.

10. Use a cotton-tipped orangewood stick and nail polish remover to remove polish from the cuticle or the surrounding skin of each finger.
11. Carefully spray nails as directed with aerosol enamel.

2. Placing your little finger on the manicure table will steady your hand so that you will not apply the base coat to the cuticle of the nail.

3. Applying the base coat in this way minimizes the possibility of streaking and promotes even drying.

4. This is standard procedure.

5. This movement mixes the enamel.

6. Most enamels are lacquers, which give a shiny, varnish-like coating. They are made of a variety of compounds. Many new ones are being developed to give translucent, frosted, and pearl effects. Buffing the nails helps circulation.

7. This is standard procedure.

8. This is standard procedure.

9. Deep colors may require 2 or 3 separate applications to produce the proper color or shade.
10. Do not allow client to leave with enamel on the nail's cuticle or surrounding skin.

11. Aerosol drying products shorten drying time ordinarily required for nail enamel.

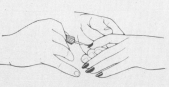

Hand positions for applying polish

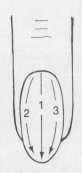

Polish strokes

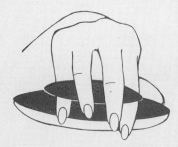

Position of buffer

12. After nails are dry, apply a top, or sealer, coat. Use procedure employed for enamel application.

12. Top coat, or sealer, will prevent enamel from chipping or cracking between manicures.

13. Sanitize work area, implements, all bottles, and your hands.

13. This is standard procedure.

Hand and Arm Massage

Manicuring usually includes hand and arm massage. The purpose of hand and arm massage is to increase the circulation of the blood in those areas and stretch the muscles of the hand and arm. This service also moisturizes the skin, helping it retain its elasticity and flexibility.

The hand and arm massage is performed **after the basic manicure** has been completed and after the top coat of polish or sealer has dried completely. Because the objective is to increase circulation to the arm and hand, the procedure begins at the elbow and finishes at the hand. Insofaras the drawings are easy to follow and the steps should be simple to use, a rationale for each step has been omitted. Each of the **manipulations of the hand and arm may be repeated three times.** So, for example, if the procedure calls for massaging the elbow, you may massage it three times before going to the next step. The exact procedure you use will be determined by your instructor.

1. Sanitize your hands.
2. Pour a small portion of lotion into your hands and rub it around to warm it to a comfortable temperature.
3. Apply lotion along one arm from elbow to hand of client. Add more lotion, if necessary.
4. Hold the client's wrist with one hand and cup the client's elbow with your other hand. Use a circular motion to masssage the client's elbow.
5. With both of your hands, use a circular thumb motion in alternating directions to work around the arm from the elbow to the client's wrist.
6. On the forearm and elbow, use a **chucking movement**, which may be compared to the friction used in wringing out a large **wet** bath towel. Give attention to massaging the elbow because the skin there is often very dry, and a callous may be forming.
7. After massaging the elbow and forearm, begin a circular chucking movement on the wrist. Then, with the thumbs of both hands, use circular movements to work your way down the back of the hand to the knuckles.
8. Repeat the circular thumb movement from the wrist to the knuckles on the palm of the hand.
9. Continue with the circular thumb movements of both your hands along each side of the client's hand until all the fingers have been massaged.

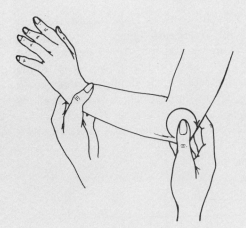

Use a circular motion to massage elbow

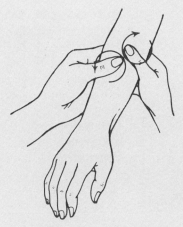

Use alternating directions with circular thumb motion from elbow to wrist

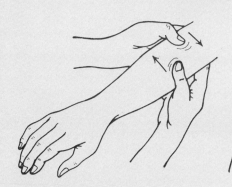

"Chucking movement"

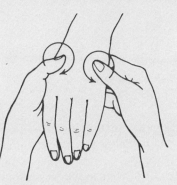

Circular movements down back of hand to knuckles

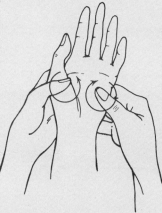

Massage from wrist to knuckles on palm

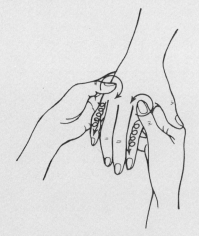

Massage each finger

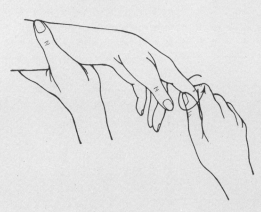

Finger rotation

10. After resting the client's elbow on the manicure table, support the wrist with one of your hands and gently rotate each finger.

11. Now, take each of the client's fingers (one at a time) between your thumb and index finger. Begin close to the palm and work toward the fingertips. Use a gentle squeezing action, slide along the finger about 1/4 inch, and squeeze again. Repeat until all fingers on this hand are done.

12. Gently flex the hand back and forth to relax and limber up the muscles of the hand.

13. Repeat steps 1–12 on the other hand.

DOING SUBOBJECTIVE 3

Give a nail wrap.

The supplies used in the nail wrapping process will depend on the particular "kit" or products used by your school. At least a partial list of supplies that is common among the different manufacturers would include:

Supplies

- fast-drying glue (usually 5-second type)
- linen or silk wrapping fiber
- round file/buffer
- emery board
- small scissors
- orangewood stick

Safety Tip

The exact steps you will use for a nail wrap will be given to you by your instructor. Unless strict sanitation practices are followed, the nail can develop a **fungus**.

If a client were in the process of having a regular manicure, the nail wrap would be done before the application of a base coat and/or the nail polish. A rationale has not been given for each of these short nail wrapping steps.

1. Apply adhesive (glue) across tip of **dry** fingernail.

2. Apply linen or silk fiber to nail. The fiber should be applied only to the first 1/4-inch of the nail's tip.

3. Now, apply glue to top of fiber covering nail and briefly hold each side of fiber across nail (the glue will "set-up" in 5–10 seconds and is called "5—second glue").

4. Trim excess fiber, but leave enough to tuck under the free edge of the nail. Remember, if you are using a silk fiber, do **not** tuck it under the free edge. Apply more glue under the free edge of the nail. Use the flat end (some prefer the pointed end) of an orangewood stick to smooth the linen under the free edge.

5. Use downward strokes of your emery board to shape excess fiber to match the shape of the nail's sides and free edge.

6. Using the round file/buffer, shape and smooth the nail seam on the top of the nail and the nail tip.

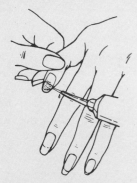

Apply adhesive across tip
of **dry** fingernail

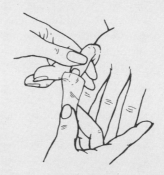

Fiber (linen or silk) applied
only to first ¼-inch of nail

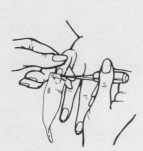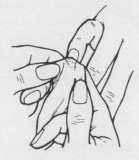

Apply glue to top of fiber and hold till "set-up"

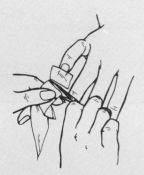

Trim as per manufacturer's
instructions

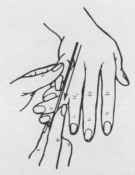

Shape with emery board

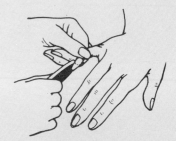

Shape and smooth with
round file/buffer

Apply additional glue as
necessary, filing after each
application

7. Apply additional glue to insure proper bonding between the nail and the fiber.
8. Repeat application of glue/file procedure until the seam becomes almost invisible. The seam should "feather" from below the seam through the nail tip.
9. Repeat steps 1–8 for each nail.
10. Your client has the option of having polish or simply leaving the nails natural.

DOING SUBOBJECTIVE 4

Apply different types of artificial nails.

There are many artificial nail products available for professional use. This subobjective will explain two types. The first kind is called **acrylic sculptured nails**, and the second kind is called **nail tips** (also called caps). **The purpose of both products is mainly to extend the length of the fingernails,** thus giving the fingers a more slender, graceful appearance. This service would normally follow the basic manicure, except that no polish or base coat would be applied before application of either type of artificial nails.

 Safety Tip

Remember that many of these products are flammable! You should not allow smoking in the immediate area in which you are working! Store supplies away from heat.

Since most of these nails come in a "kit" from the manufacturer, it is difficult to identify a supply list for these services. One kit may have a powder or hardener that another kit doesn't contain. At least a partial list of supplies needed would be as follows:

Supplies

- ☐ manicure scissors
- ☐ nail forms or tips
- ☐ adhesive (glue)
- ☐ brush
- ☐ round nail file/buffer
- ☐ emery board
- ☐ orangewood stick
- ☐ solvent

Note that your instructor will have the best list of supplies and the particular procedure you should follow.

Acrylic Sculptured Nail Procedure

1. Use the emery board to roughen the surface of the nail plate.
2. Apply nail forms and secure along sides of fingertip. Be careful not to slant the tip of the forms in a downward direction. If you do, the finished nail will have an unnatural downward slope that will be unattractive.
3. **Carefully read and follow the manufacturer's mixing directions.** Begin application with a clean brush from the free edge to the end of the nail form.

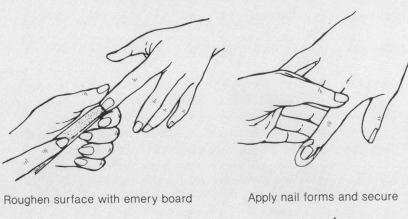

Roughen surface with emery board   Apply nail forms and secure

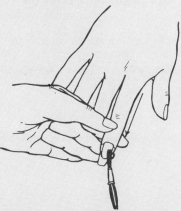

Starting in center of nail plate, work across entire nail. Blend into nail form and dry

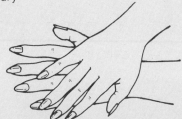

File, seal and apply enamel or buff for "natural" nails

4. Now apply to center of nail plate and smoothly work across entire natural nail, blending into nail form. Allow nails to dry for 5 minutes, or as directed.
5. Carefully remove forms.
6. File each nail to desired length and shape. Seal and apply nail enamel or buff and allow nails to appear natural.

Note: Do not use regular polish remover (acetone) to remove a sculptured nail. Follow manufacturer's directions. Pulling may injure the nail permanently! Brush and mixing container must be cleaned immediately after use, or they become unuseable. Tightly cover all bottles.

Safety Tip

Nail Tip Procedure

1. Give basic manicure procedure up to base coat/polish step.
2. Match nail tip to client's nails. File to adjust small differences.
3. Apply glue to nail groove of nail tip to be used.
4. Place tip across free edge of nail and adjust placement with an orangewood stick. Hold client's finger in a downward position so that the glue doesn't run onto cuticle. Polish remover on the end of a cotton-tipped orangewood stick can be used to clean up small amounts of glue.
5. Use your manicure scissors to trim straight across tips that are too long.
6. Use emery board to shape nail for the contour of client's finger.
7. Pay particular attention to the nail seam when buffing to achieve a "natural" look from the nail plate to the sculptured extension.
8. Apply glue to seam and tip for added durability, strength, and smoothness. Repeat as needed.
9. Proceed until all nails have been done.

Note: Patches are available to fix a tip that has split or cracked.

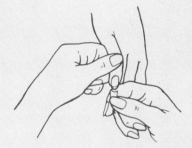

Match tip to client's nails and file to fit

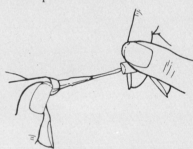

Apply glue to nail groove of nail tip

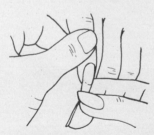

Place across free edge and adjust with orangewood stick

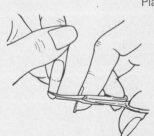 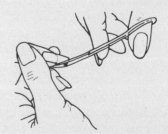 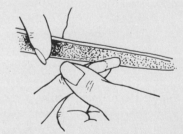

Trim with manicure scissors and shape with emery board

Since the pedicuring steps are so similar to those of manicuring, the rationale has been omitted.

Give a pedicure.

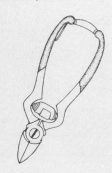

Supplies

- three terry towels
- emery board (nail file)
- antiseptic/disinfectant
- toenail clipper
- cuticle remover
- nail polish
- cotton
- nail polish remover
- nail massage cream
- moisturizing lotion
- two foot bath containers
- orangewood stick
- plastic refuse bag
- nail builder cream
- alcohol

Pedicuring Procedure

1. Soak one of the client's feet in disinfectant solution for 4 to 5 minutes. (The solution should cover the ankle.) Then dry with terry towel.
2. Use nail polish remover to remove polish from toenails.
3. Shape toenails with the emery board and/or toenail clipper, depending on how long the nails are. Remember not to file or clip the nails too far into the corners, or the client may develop an ingrown nail. Shape the nails straight across, then gradually round the corners.
4. Begin soaking the other foot at this time.
5. Apply cuticle remover and use orangewood stick to carefully remove unneeded cuticle. Be careful not to injure the matrix of the nail. Do not use metal pushers.

Preliminary Steps

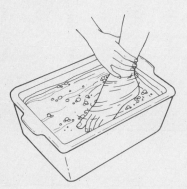

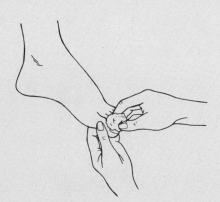

Remove old nail polish

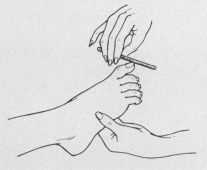

Shape with emery board or toe nail clipper

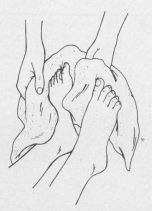

Soak feet in disinfectant for 4-5 minutes and dry with towel

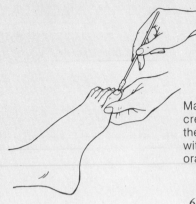

Massage with nail cream around cuticle, then clean free edge with cotton tipped orangewood stick

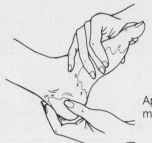

Apply moisturizer and massage

6. Apply and massage nail cream around cuticle. Then, clean free edge of nails, using cotton tipped orangewood stick and polish remover or solvent.
7. Apply moisturizing cream to the foot and massage. Give extra manipulations to the heel and sides of the foot.
8. Remove the other foot from the foot bath and dry thoroughly. Nip cuticle as needed.
9. Repeat steps 2, 3, 5, 6, and 7 on the foot you have just dried.
10. Using foot bath and nail brush, remove excess moisturizing lotion, massage cream, and cuticle cream from nails of each foot. Dry each foot.

Application of Nail Polish

1. Use cotton between toes to separate each toe for the application of polish to one foot; otherwise, nails may smear.
2. Double-check each nail to make sure all cream film(s) have been removed, or the polish won't stick to the nail. Remove any residues with alcohol on cotton.
3. Apply base coat to the toenails of one foot.
4. Repeat steps 1 through 3 on the other foot.
5. Apply nail enamel (polish) to one foot; then the other. Allow at least 20 minutes for the enamel to dry before permitting the client to put on footwear.
6. Sanitize your work area and discard soiled supplies, such as used cotton, refuse bags, etc. Sanitize foot bath containers, etc.

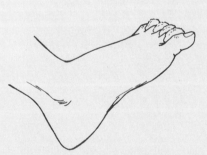

Separate toes with cotton

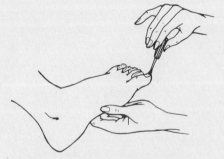

Apply base coat, then enamel

1. Rest heel of foot on footstool.
2. Evenly apply a small amount of massage cream from ankle to toes.
3. Using your thumbs in firm rotating movements, massage the skin from the instep of the ankle down to the first digit of the toes.
4. Return to the instep and repeat 3 times.
5. Continue until the entire top area of the foot has been massaged.
6. Support the client's heel with one hand and rotate each toe with the thumb and index finger of the other hand. Repeat 3 times.
7. Now rotate the foot from the ankle. Repeat 3 times.
8. Massage the entire sole of the foot, using a rotating manipulation with your thumbs.
9. Repeat steps 1 through 8 on the other foot.
10. Sanitize work area.

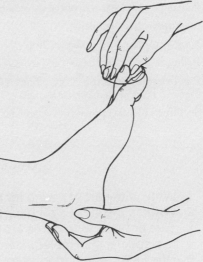

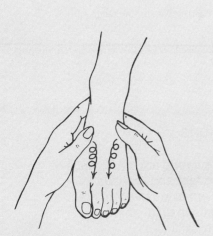

Massage from instep to first toe digit

Rotate each toe 3 times

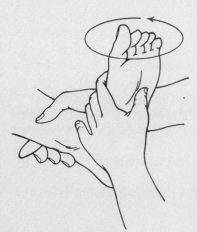

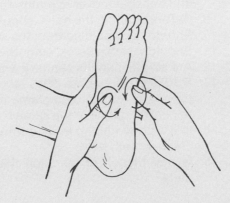

Rotate foot from ankle

Massage sole of foot

GLOSSARY

Acetone   The chief ingredient of nail polish remover.

Acrylic sculptured nails   Artificial fingernails which are formed from acrylic paste and shaped on the client.

Alum   Used in styptic to stop bleeding.

Artificial nails   Materials shaped to look like fingernails.

Artificial nail shells   A type of artificial nails made from porcelain, plastic, or nylon.

Chucking movement   A massage technique similar to wringing out a towel.

Manicuring   Care of the hands and fingernails.

Manicurist   A person trained in the care of hands and fingernails.

Nail caps   A type of artificial nails used to extend natural fingernails.

Nail tips   See **Nail caps.**

Nail wrapping   A service to protect the fingernails from breakage.

Pedicure   Care of the feet and toenails.

Powder pumice polish   Very fine powder used to polish (shine) fingernails and toenails, resulting in clear, shiny nails.

Styptic (STIP-tik) powder   A powder that will stop minor bleeding.

QUESTIONS

1. What is the art of caring for the hands and fingernails?
2. What is the art of caring for the feet and toenails?
3. True or false. Manicures are given exclusively to men.
4. Is a special skin moisturizer used in an oil manicure?
5. Does nail wrapping weaken the nail?
6. Are acrylic sculptured nails made in different sizes?
7. Are nail polish removers and adhesives likely to catch fire when exposed to a spark or flame?
8. Would you normally use a cotton-tipped orangewood stick and polish remover to remove polish from around the cuticle?
9. Before shaping the nails, should you remove all polish?
10. Should nails be filed from the side to the center?
11. Should you use quick, smooth strokes when filing the nails?
12. Are styptic pencils sanitary when used to stop bleeding?
13. If 70% ethyl alcohol (99% isopropyl alcohol) is used to sanitize metal manicure implements, will this be an effective way to control germs in the salon?
14. Is it a good idea to leave a thin film of polish around the cuticle to protect it?
15. Is nail bleach or peroxide used to remove stains from the nails?

16. Will nail polish adhere properly to a nail that is NOT thoroughly dry?
17. Is "chucking" a massage movement?
18. Are nail tips also sometimes called nail caps?
19. If you aren't careful during the application, can an acrylic sculptured nail end up sloped in an unnatural downward direction?
20. True or false. Manicure scissors are never used to shorten nail tips that are too long. They should only be filed.
21. Are small toe towels used between the toes during the application of nail polish when giving a pedicure?
22. Is a base coat used on the toenails as well as the fingernails?

ANSWERS

1. Manicuring 2. Pedicuring 3. False 4. Yes 5. No; strengthens it 6. No 7. Yes 8. Yes 9. Yes 10. Yes 11. Yes 12. No 13. Yes 14. No; remove all polish from cuticle 15. Yes 16. No 17. Yes 18. Yes 19. Yes 20. False 21. No; cotton 22. Yes

Styling Wigs and Hairpieces 28

Men and women have worn wigs and hairpieces for thousands of years. Until only 10 or 15 years ago, hairpieces were something of a status symbol. They were very expensive, and only very wealthy people could afford to buy them. Recently, modern manufacturing methods have lowered the cost of hairpieces so that most people can buy them.

Today, people wear wigs for many different reasons. Some wear wigs to cover baldness. Others feel that a hairpiece gives them a new look, which improves their appearance. Many people who have fast-paced lives find that wearing a wig is the only practical way to have a good appearance and meet the demands of a hectic schedule.

Making hairpieces has become such a large industry that many states have separate licenses for the care and styling of hairpieces. Cosmetologists usually receive instruction and have practiced on caring for hairpieces as **part** of their training, so that additional licensing and training is not really necessary.

Since most beauty salons try to offer a full range of services to their clients, knowledge and skills in servicing hairpieces are an important part of any basic training program. Caring for and styling hairpieces has created a new source of income for schools and salons.

Using professional wiggery supplies and implements, fit, shape, clean, set, and style a wig and hairpiece.

Major Objective

Level of Acceptabilty
Use the proper steps and safety precautions to clean a wig in 20 minutes, set it in 25 minutes, and comb it into a finished hairstyle in 20 minutes. Also, clean a hairpiece in 15 minutes, set it in 10 to 20 minutes, and comb it into the client's hair in 15 to 30 minutes. Score 75 percent or better on a multiple-choice exam on the information in this chapter.

Knowing Subobjectives
1. Describe the various types of wigs and hairpieces, explaining how they are made, colored, and styled.
2. Explain how wigs are measured and altered.

KNOWING SUBOBJECTIVE 1

Describe the various types of wigs and hairpieces, explaining how they are made, colored, and styled.

Types of Wigs and Hairpieces The terms **hairpieces** and **hairgoods** are used to describe any of the following: wigs, toupees, postiches, wiglets, cascades, chignons, switches, falls (or minifalls), etc.

Wigs usually are hairpieces that cover 80 to 100 percent of the head. A **toupee** is also a wig, but it is considered a special kind of hairpiece. It ordinarily covers **less** than 80 percent of a client's head.

Postiches (pos-TEESH-ez) are small hairpieces made from angora and yak hair. They are round at the base. They are used in an ornamental way, usually in competition hairstyling. Pastel colors can be applied to them for "fantasy" styling effects.

Wiglets vary in size and length. They are put on different areas of the head to complement or enhance the hairstyle. It is common to use more than one wiglet in the hair for "cocktail" or "evening" styles.

Cascades have oval-shaped bases. They can vary in length from 4 to 8 inches, and they are worn in the upper and lower crown sections. They are larger than a wiglet, but smaller than a fall.

Chignons (SHEEN-yahnz) and **switches**, which are long tresses of hair secured at one end, are used to build height or volume in hairstyles. They are arranged in knots, braided, or woven through the hair.

Falls are long hairpieces which vary in size. A fall has a base that is larger than a cascade but smaller than a wig. Usually secured in the crown section of the head, a fall may be arranged casually or set and combed into a very elaborate "haute coiffure." Minifalls are simply small falls.

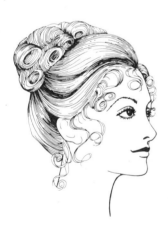

Hairpieces are made from human and synthetic hair. **Human hair** is classified as European, Oriental (Asiatic), and less often, West Indian. The consensus seems to be that **European hair** is the easiest to arrange. It also is the most expensive. Oriental or Asiatic hair is usually coarser. It has a tendency to curl too much unless rather large rollers are used. These types of hair, in addition to that from West India, are less expensive, but they are somewhat more difficult to style than European hair. Most hairpieces are made in Japan, Korea, or Europe.

Hairpieces made of **synthetic** (man-made) **fibers** are much less expensive than pieces using human hair. In the past, synthetic fibers that were used to make hairpieces were too shiny and unnatural appearing; however, modern technology has improved their appearance so much that many professional synthetic hairpieces are sold in schools and salons. Professional hairpieces may be purchased directly from the manufacturer in some instances or from some professional beauty and barber suppliers.

You can use a simple test to find out if a wig is made of human or synthetic hair.

Cut a single piece of hair from the hairpiece. Burn it with a lighted match. If it is synthetic it will melt, and a bead will form on the end of it. Very little odor will be noticed. If the hair is human, you will notice a strong sulfur-like odor (from sulfur in the hair).

Human and synthetic hairpieces are made in one of two ways—hand-tied or machine-wefted. **Hand-tied hairpieces** are usually quite expensive because, as the name implies, each hair is sewn one at a time to the mesh (netting) cap that forms the base. Machine-made hairpieces are less expensive because a machine sews the hair around a strip of material called a **weft**. The wefts are then sewn together in ¼-inch lengths to a mesh cap.

In the 1960s, at the beginning of the modern wig boom, many people preferred hand-tied wigs because machine-tied wigs often were bulky, heavy, and difficult to style. Modern technology, however, has developed "ventilated," light, natural-appearing machine-made wigs, so now the market is evenly divided between the two types. The same is true of human and synthetic hairpieces. Synthetic hairpieces dominate from time to time because they are made with a permanent curl in them. They only have to be cleaned, dried, and then combed. They do not have to be set.

Hand-tied hairpieces **must** be cleaned with a special **dry cleaning** fluid made just for hair. The dry cleaner is necessary so the wefting doesn't loosen up and cause hair loss from the cap of the wig. You should be very careful with dry cleaning fluids because many of them are **flammable**. For this reason do not work around anyone with a lighted cigarette or other things that could start a fire. Try to use this fluid only in open and well ventilated areas of the salon. Synthetic wigs are cleaned with a nonflammable cleaner that is like, but not the same as, shampoo.

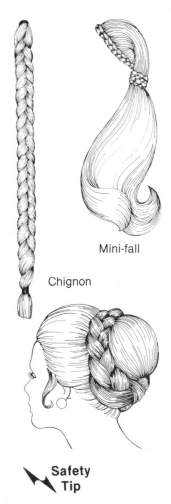

Chignon

Mini-fall

Safety Tip

Hairpieces are colored (dyed) to match the 70 color choices on the **JL color ring.**

All hairpieces have "processed" colors, rather than natural ones. Human hair (regardless of color) is boiled many hours in chemicals that clean and take out its color. When the hair is pure white, the hair is dyed with a fabric color **(not a tint)** that matches one of the colors on the JL color ring. Synthetic hair also is dyed with a fabric color to match one of the colors on the ring. **Hairpieces need conditioning** because the sun causes those processed colors to become lighter, in the same way that natural hair can become "sun-bleached."

Coloring of Hairpieces

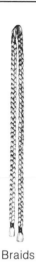

Braids

Human hairpieces can be colored with professional temporary, semipermanent, or permanent products. However, since the hair has been "processed" as previously described, **coloring is risky** and the results are unpredictable, at best. If a hairpiece requires a drastic color change, you should tell the client that the results cannot be guaranteed. Since mass production has substantially lowered the cost of hairpieces, you might advise the client to purchase a new hairpiece. Considering supply costs and the cost of your time, coloring a hairpiece may be a very expensive service for the client.

Synthetic hairpieces may be dyed with over-the-counter fabric or vegetable colors. Professional tints and bleaches **should not** be used on synthetic hairpieces.

When any type of hairpiece is colored, you must be sure to protect the mesh cap or wefting from any contact with tint, bleach, or toning material. Oxidizing tints, bleaches, and toners will deteriorate (damage) the wefting fabric.

KNOWING SUBOBJECTIVE 2

Explain how wigs are measured and altered.

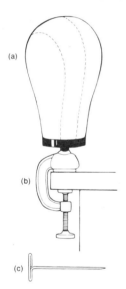

(a) Canvas block (head) for styling wig; (b) wig clamp for supporting canvas block; (c) T-pin for securing wig to canvas block. Note: a plastic bag is usually put over the cloth canvas block to protect it from water and setting lotions, etc.

Several basic pieces of equipment are needed to measure and alter hairpieces. The wig is placed on a **canvas block** (a) that is held in place on the styling station by a **wig clamp** (b). A **T-pin** (c) is used to keep the wig on the canvas block. The block is usually covered with a plastic bag to protect the canvas cloth from water and setting lotions.

You can use several simple steps to measure a hairpiece.

Measure the distance from the **front** center hairline to the center **nape** hairline (measurement 1). Measure from each side hairline to the beginning of the crown section (measurement 2), then from each side hairline to the beginning of the nape section (measurement 3). Transfer the measurements to the canvas block. Use a pencil to write on the plastic cover.

Measure the distance around the head (measurement 4) and the width of the nape hairline as shown (measurement 5). Transfer both measurements to the canvas block.

Follow figures a, b, c, d, e on the opposite page to alter a hairpiece that is too large for client's head.

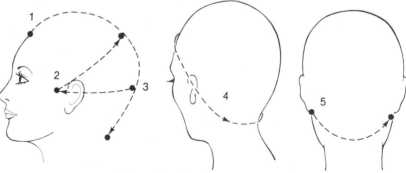

Measuring the client's head size

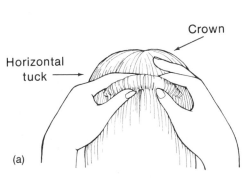

Crown

Horizontal tuck →

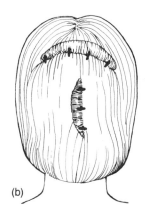

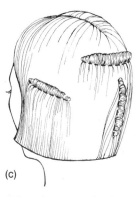

(a)

Gather extra wefting in the crown section first and carefully mark it horizontally with T-pins

(b)

Gather extra wefting and mark a vertical tuck

(c)

If the wig comes down over the tops of the client's ears, put horizontal tucks on each side of the wig

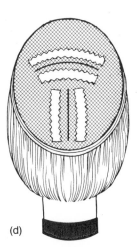

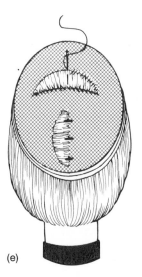

(d)

Remove the wig and place hair-set tape on the **inside** of the wig along the fold of each tuck. Pull the T-pins from the outside of the wig. Turn the wig inside out again, and pull the tuck to the inside of the wig. The **base** of the tuck should come between the hair-set tape marks

(e)

Use a needle and special thread to stitch the base of the tuck. Then sew the top of the tuck flat against the wefting of the wig

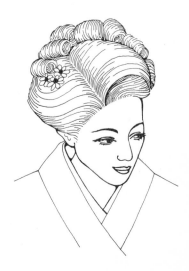

Finished style

GLOSSARY

Cascade   A hairpiece from 4 to 8 inches long with an oval-shaped base worn in the upper or lower crown section.

Chignon (SHEEN-yahn)   A long tress of hair secured at one end; used to build volume or height to a hairstyle.

Fall   A long hairpiece with a base larger than a cascade and smaller than a wig.

Hand-tied hairpiece   A hairpiece that has each hair sewn individually to the mesh cap.

JL color ring   The 70 standardized colors used to dye human and synthetic hairpieces.

Postiche (pos-TEESH)   A small hairpiece that is made from angora and yak hair; used as an ornament.

Switches   Long tresses of hair secured at one end.

Synthetic fibers   Fibers that are made of materials other than natural animal or human hair; used to make wigs.

Toupee   A hairpiece that covers less than 80 percent of a client's head.

Weft   The strip of material to which hair is sewn in a machine-made hairpiece.

Wig   A hairpiece that covers from 80 to 100 percent of the head.

Wiggery   The services of fitting, shaping, cleaning, setting, and styling wigs and hairpieces.

Wiglet   A hairpiece that may vary in size and length and may be put on different areas of the head to complement or enhance a hairstyle.

Yak hair   An animal hair used to make postiches.

QUESTIONS

1. What are human hair wigs cleaned with?
2. What is a weft?
3. What is the difference between a wig and a toupee?
4. If a hairpiece is hand-tied, does it mean the hair is actually sewn entirely by hand to the mesh base?

ANSWERS

1. A special wig dry cleaning fluid 2. Material to which hair is sewn in a wig or hairpiece 3. A toupee only covers part of the scalp, and a wig usually covers the entire scalp 4. Yes

Planning a Salon 29

In the early part of this book you read that cosmetology is an art, a science, and a business. At this point you may be wondering, "I've seen how an artistic imagination and creative flair will help me as a cosmetologist; I've seen how knowing some science is helpful; and I've seen how important it is to have technical skill; but what about business? Except for selling a few products to a client who comes into the salon anyway, I haven't learned anything about starting my own business."

You need to know quite a few things about planning your own business. Some of them can only be learned through experience, and you will be able to pick them up when you work in a salon. However, there are some basic principles that you can learn now.

Purpose

Describe the basic principles needed to plan a salon as a successful business.

Major Objective

Score 75 percent or better on a multiple-choice exam on the information in this chapter.

Level of Acceptability

1. Identify the basic forms of ownership.
2. Explain how to select a good salon site and building.
3. Explain how to figure the amount of rent you can afford to pay.
4. List things to consider in negotiating a salon lease.
5. List things to consider when purchasing an existing salon.
6. Identify salon insurance needs.
7. Describe the importance of the salon reception area.
8. Describe the importance of retailing in the salon.

Knowing Subobjectives

KNOWING SUBOBJECTIVE 1

Identify the basic forms of ownership.

Salon ownership by one person is called **sole proprietorship**. Salon ownership by **two or more persons** without the issuance of stock is called a **partnership. A corporation** salon is usually a large establishment or chain of salons that may be owned by one or many persons called **stockholders**. A **corporation** is a legal entity that can protect people against certain liabilities. It also has tax advantages for larger operations. Your lawyer can tell you more about this when the time comes. When you start your own salon, it will probably be small, so you needn't be concerned now.

In a business formed as a **sole proprietorship**, the proprietor (or owner) is solely **responsible for all liabilities** (debts) of the business but also is entitled to **all profits** from the business.

In a **partnership**, the owners are liable for an **equal share of the debts** of the business and entitled to an **equal share of the profits**.

One difficulty with a partnership is that each partner may be held liable for debts incurred by the other partner(s). For example, A and B have formed a partnership. B charges $1000 worth of goods at a local department store in the name of the salon and leaves for another state to begin a business there. Partner A must pay for the goods charged to the business by partner B.

Another problem is that few partners take in exactly the same number of dollars for any given period of time, yet each partner is entitled to an equal share of the profits. For example, partner A's total take-in money from beauty services is $300 per week, and partner B's take-in is $200. If the profit from staff covers all fixed and variable costs, would A receive $300 and B $200? No. The totals would be added together and divided by 2 ($300 +

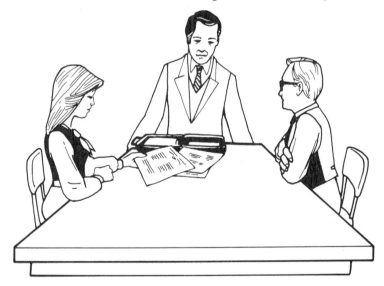

Consult an attorney before signing any agreements

$200 = \$500 \div 2 = \$250$), so each partner would receive $250, less state and federal taxes, etc. Should this be a continuous thing, and it usually is, A has to give $50 of his or her money to B every week.

Partnerships can operate smoothly (although few do) if a lawyer draws up a **partnership agreement**. This document should spell out what partners A and B are agreeing to do or not to do. It will usually state:

1. Number of (and which) days and hours per week each partner will work.
2. Amount of money each will invest in the business.
3. Division of profits based on each partner's take-in dollars.
4. Requirement that **both partners must sign** business checks.
5. Provision for dissolving the partnership in the event that one partner dies. The wife or husband of the deceased partner is paid an amount of money equal to the share of the business.

A partnership should never be formed without a partnership agreement approved by a lawyer.

KNOWING SUBOBJECTIVE 2

There are 2 important decisions you will have to make when you plan a salon: Where should the salon be located, and what kind of building is best?

When selecting a location, you should consider several things:

1. **Population density** means the number of people living in an area. A rule of thumb is that the more people there are in a particular area, the more desirable it is for a salon location. A high-income neighborhood that also has large apartment buildings is a good location, particularly if those buildings are within walking distance of the site you are thinking about. If there are only a few apartment buildings in the immediate area, a different location might be better.

Explain how to select a good salon site and building.

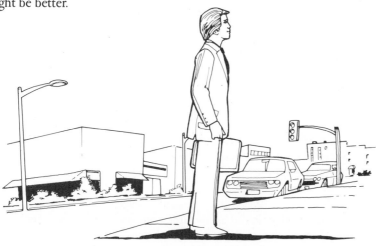

Selecting a possible salon location

When choosing a location, you must consider more than the available buildings and your preferences. Most cities and towns have zoning restrictions (ordinances) that involve the use of property in various locations. The location for a salon that will employ more than one person in addition to the owner must be zoned for commercial use.

2. **Accessibility** is an important factor. The location should be easy to find. Clients should not have to cross unusually busy streets or take complicated routes to reach the salon. The building should be visible from the street and should be near public transportation.

3. **Traffic patterns** relate to established routes used to travel from one part of a community to another. People use these routes when going to work, recreational facilities, grocery stores, church, etc. The location being considered should not be "off the beaten track."

4. **Socioeconomic factors** are important in two respects. What is the average income level of possible clients who live in the area? If the income level for these potential clients is very low, you should select a different location.

5. **Physical advantages** or features of the location selected should include adequate plumbing for shampoo bowls and a 100-gallon fast-recovery hot water heater. There should also be good lighting and an adequate number of electrical outlets for hair dryers, air wavers, curling irons, and thermal heaters.

The most successful salons are always located on the ground level of the building. **Second-floor** or **basement** locations have not been nearly as successful as the street-level ones because clients dislike walking up or down stairs.

The salon sign and phone number should be visible from the street so that appointments can be made by phone. In most cities, ordinances restrict the size, height, shape, and location of outside business signs. In some cases, you may have to appear before the local zoning board to describe the sign you want to put up and get permission to display it. If the type of sign you want to put up is prohibited, you can ask for, and sometimes receive, an **exception (called a variance)** to the ordinance.

The outside, as well as the inside, of the building should be attractive and in good condition.

Ample parking for clients is a must for almost any salon. A recent survey showed that few persons will walk more than about 900 feet to conduct any kind of business.

The building owner should agree to maintain a year-round temperature of 72 degrees in the beauty salon. Air conditioning is important because of the heat generated by the hair dryers.

6. **Existing businesses** in an area provide clients for each other. A drugstore, for example, is an excellent business neighbor for a salon because many shoppers will visit the salon after completing their business in the drugstore. Medical and dental offices also work out well next to beauty salons.

Since you will probably remain in the same location for quite a few years, you should carefully consider all 6 of the factors mentioned before you select a location.

Another economic factor is the monthly rent. This will vary greatly with the social and economic level of the neighborhood. **Rent** is probably the most important factor in determining whether a salon will make money. The amount of money paid for rent should **not exceed 4 to 6 percent** of all the money taken in during the year. If you are thinking about renting a building for $400 and want this to be no more than 6 percent of the money you take in during the year, you can calculate how much business (dollars) must be done to justify that monthly rent:

Explain how to figure the amount of rent you can afford to pay.

$$
\begin{array}{rl}
\$\ 400.00 & \text{monthly rent} \\
\underline{\times 12} & \text{months per year} \\
\$4800.00 & \text{yearly rent}
\end{array}
$$

This amount, $4800, is the amount of rent you would have to pay during the year. It should be equal to 6 percent (.06) of all the money brought into the salon. You can use this method to calculate the amount of money the salon must bring in.

$$
\begin{array}{rl}
x = & \text{total money earned in one year} \\
.06x = & \$4800.00 \\
\overline{.06} & \overline{.06}
\end{array}
$$

$$
x = \quad 06.\overline{)\,\$480,000.}^{\ \ \$\ 80,000.}
$$

$$
x = \quad \$80,000
$$

The salon will have to take in $80,000 in one year. The average-size salon has four operators and takes in about $40,000 to $50,000. Thus, it is unrealistic to expect to take in this much money; so you would have to get the landlord to lower the rent quite a bit or find a different location. **Rent is a "fixed cost"**; it stays the same whether you have one client or two thousand in a month.

Percentage rents are not desirable for the beauty industry. Some building owners attempt to encourage this kind of agreement from salon owners, but it will not be in your best interest. In a percentage agreement, the building owner and cosmetologist agree in writing that 10 percent of all the dollars collected will be paid to the building owner. The effect of this agreement is that 10 cents of every dollar collected is paid to the building owner; the result is that a "fixed cost" becomes "variable." The more dollars that are collected for services, the more money is paid for rent, so you have to share the rewards of building up your business with someone who had nothing to do with it. Percentage rents should be avoided!

The need to carefully choose a rent bracket cannot be overemphasized. Once you have signed a lease, the amount you pay for rent will not decrease, but like most things, it will probably increase over the years.

KNOWING SUBOBJECTIVE 4

List things to consider in negotiating a salon lease.

The legal agreement between the owner of a building and a renter is called a **lease**. The person granting the use of the building or space is called a **lessor**. The person using the space to operate a business is called the **lessee**. The lessor is also called the **landlord**, although this term will not appear on a lease agreement. The **lessee** may casually be referred to as a **tenant**, but this term will not appear on a lease agreement either.

The desirable term (length of time) for a beauty salon lease is 7 years with an option (chance) to renew the lease for 7 more years at the same monthly rent. A long lease is needed to:

1. Prevent increases in rent.
2. Prevent eviction (a legal order to move out).
3. Continue to operate and to establish a clientele.
4. Give the owner something of value to sell in the event he or she decides to stop owning the salon. The time remaining on a lease that has a low monthly rent makes a business very salable.

Most landlords will ask you to sign a "form" lease, which you should **not** sign until you have added amendments to it. **Amendments** are items in writing that the landlord agrees to provide at no charge. The amendments are part of the lease. Honest landlords (lessors) who say they will do certain things to make the property more usable for a beauty salon will put the items in writing **if** they actually intend to do them. **Do not sign a lease agreement until your lawyer has approved it!**

You should add the following minimum amendments to a lease.

The lessor will:

1. **Supply and maintain appliances** to provide a year-round temperature of 72 degrees in the salon.
2. **Provide** an adequate supply of **hot and cold** water for the efficient operation of the salon.
3. **Supply and maintain parking places** (whatever number is needed) for the exclusive use of beauty salon clients and post parking signs if needed.
4. **Maintain sidewalks** and common areas that connect or are next to the salon.

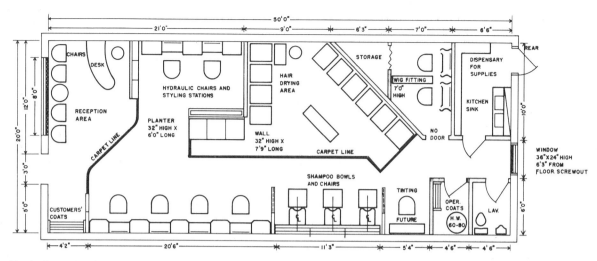

Basic floor plan for a 6-station beauty salon. Notice how walls are used to define main working areas: reception, hair styling, hair drying, shampooing, and tinting. Equipment and counter space are placed against the walls so clients and employees can move from one area to the next in a direct line. Supplies are located out of the main traffic pattern, at the back of the salon. Carpet line shows that only the reception area and drying area are carpeted

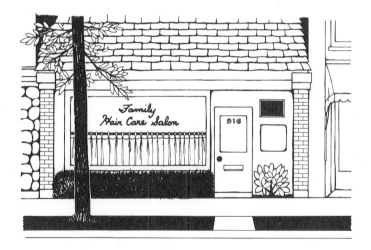

5. **Supply and maintain necessary plumbing** (including a dispensary sink), electrical power, and outlets for a _____-operator beauty salon.
   (fill in number)

6. **Repaint or wallpaper the interior** of the salon every 3 years.

7. **Supply and maintain shelving** for storage.

These amendments are **absolutely necessary**; changes in wording may cost you a lot of money. Some landlords require a deposit of 3 months' rent in advance to cover any damage to the building. At the end of the lease, this money is refunded if no damage has been done. Ordinary wear from use is **not** considered damage.

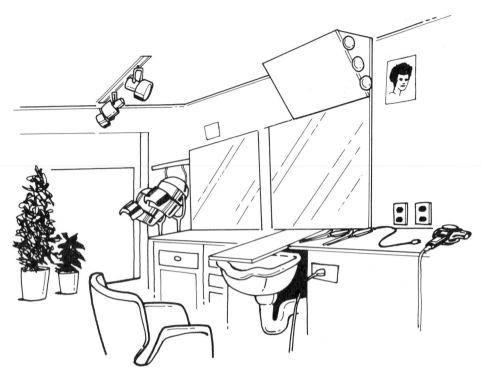

Modern shampoo/styling station

Most leases contain a **tax escalator clause**, which simply means that if the lessor's property tax increases, the rent will increase, but only in proportion to the tax levied for the space used.

KNOWING SUBOBJECTIVE 5

List things to consider when purchasing an existing salon.

Purchasing an existing salon can be risky business. The most important things are:

1. How much time remains on the lease?
2. What are the assets (what is owned) and liabilities (what is owed), including monthly rent?
3. How old is the equipment?
4. How much would it cost to replace it and open a new salon?
5. How much good will has the salon developed?
6. How many operators will continue to work after the salon is sold?
7. Does the owner plan to move out of the area or across the street?
8. What outstanding bills would the new owner be responsible for paying?
9. Decide if the location is excellent.
10. What does your lawyer think of the deal?

This Agreement, *Made the* _____ *day of* _____ *19* ____

between _____

_____

as Landlord, party of the first part, and _____

_____ *as Tenant   , part   of the second part,*

WITNESSETH, *That the said Landlord lets unto the said Tenant   , and the said Tenant*

hire   from the said landlord, that certain apartment or suite of rooms designated as _____

on the _____ *floor in the building known as* _____

_____

with the appurtenances thereof, including water and steam heat,

TOGETHER *with the following fixtures and furniture, viz.:*

_____

_____

_____

for the term of _____ *months* _____

to commence at 12 M. on the _____ *day of* _____ *19* ____

and to end at 12 M. on the _____ *day of* _____ *19* ____

at the _____ *rental of* _____ *Dollars,*

payable at the office of the said Landlord as follows, viz.: _____ *Dollars*

on the _____ *day of* _____ *19* _____, *and* _____

Dollars on _____ *day of each and every* _____ *thereafter*

during the full term of this Lease.

_____

AND IT IS FURTHER AGREED, *By and between the parties, as follows: That should the said*
part   of the second part, _____ *heirs, executors, administrators or assigns, fail to make the*
above mentioned payments as herein specified, at the time and in the manner herein specified, or fail to
fulfill any of the covenants herein contained, then and in that case it shall be lawful for, and said part

of the second part do   hereby consent that the said party of the first part, his _____
or assigns, may re-enter and take full and absolute possession of the above rented premises, and all of
the same, and hold and enjoy the same fully and absolutely, without such re-entering working a for-
feiture of the rents to be paid and the covenants to be performed by the said part   of the second part

as herein specified or by _____ *heirs, executors, administrators or assigns, for and during the full*
term of this Lease.

The said Premises are also Leased upon the Further Covenants and Conditions:

1st. That this lease contains all that has been agreed to by said Landlord or his agents, and there are no verbal agreements or promises other than those appearing on this lease.
2nd. The said Tenant   shall pay for the gas and electricity and said Landlord for the water used on said leased premises.
3rd. That the Tenant   shall take good care of the apartment and its fixtures, and suffer no waste or injury; shall not drive picture or other nails, or screws, into the walls, ceilings or woodwork of said premises, nor allow the same to be done, and shall at _____ own cost and expense make and do all repairs required to walls, ceilings, paper, plumbing works, pipes and fixtures belonging thereto, whenever damage or injury to the same shall have resulted from their misuse or neglect; and shall at _____ own cost and expense, amend, restore and make good all damage or breakage of any glass, window shades or screens, chandeliers, or any other of the property whatever, appertaining to said premises.
4th. That the Tenant   shall not expose any sign, advertisement, awning, illumination or projection on or out of the windows or on the exterior of the said building, in any place, except such as shall be approved and permitted in writing by the Landlord or his authorized agent   , and the said Tenant   shall use only such shades in the windows of said apartment as are put up or approved by Landlord.
5th. The Tenant   shall use and occupy said premises as not to annoy or interfere with the rights of other tenants in said building.
6th. That the Tenant   shall not assign this agreement, or sublet the premises, or any part thereof, or make any alterations or additions in or to the apartments or premises without the Landlord's or agent's consent in writing; or permit or suffer upon the same, any act or thing deemed extra hazardous on account of fire; and shall comply with all the rules and regulations of the Board of Health and City Ordinances applicable to said premises; and that _____ will not use nor permit to be used the said premises, nor any part thereof, for any other purpose than that of a private dwelling apartment for _____ and family, and conformably to the Rules and Regulations printed on the back of this Lease.
7th. That the said Landlord will furnish, at his own expense, steam heat to warm the leased premises to a comfortable temperature, unavoidable delays excepted, during the months from October to April, inclusive.
8th. The Landlord shall not be liable for any loss of property or effects by theft, or otherwise, from the building or the demised premises, or any accident or damage to the person or property of the Tenant   in or about the building or the demised premises.
9th. There shall be no surrender of said premises before the expiration of this Lease by the part   of the second part, except by agreement with the party of the first part, provided that if said building should be destroyed by fire, this Lease shall thereupon terminate, but without rebate of rent paid, or due and unpaid.
10th. The Tenant   will conform to and observe the Rules and Regulations printed on the back of this Lease.
11th. _____

_____

_____

SAVINGS CLAUSE

The provisions of this lease shall remain in force pursuant to the terms thereof, except insofar as those provisions are inconsistent with the Housing and Rent Act of 1947, as amended, the Rent Regulations under said Act, as amended, and the Registration Statement on file in the Area Rent Office.

IN WITNESS WHEREOF, The parties to these presents have hereunto set their hands and seals the day and year first above written.

Signed, Sealed and Delivered in Presence of

_____   _____ [SEAL]

_____   _____ [SEAL]

_____   _____ [SEAL]

                                            _____ [SEAL]

Sample lease agreement

1. If there are 7 to 10 years left on the lease, the deal may be workable. If only 1 or 2 years remain, the landlord may raise the rent when the lease runs out. Be careful. The landlord could require an entirely different lease or could refuse to rent to you at all.

2. Your accountant should review the salon's books to determine how much profit the business is making.

3. Carefully check the condition of the equipment. If it is depreciated, it should have been done over a 5-year period, since that is the useful life expectancy (how long it will work properly without major repairs) of salon

equipment. If it is new or fairly new, find out if it is paid for or how much is owed on it.

4. If it is a 6-operator salon, it would cost $2,000 to $2,500 to put in new equipment, so the prospective buyer should not pay more than $12,000 to $15,000 for it.

5. Most businesses attach a dollar value to the good will (their good reputation) they have developed over the years, but the beauty service business is highly personal. The good will developed by the old salon may not carry over to yours. A client who has come to Mary Ann (or George) for 10 years may not continue to go to the salon if you own it. Good will is not as important in this situation as it would be in the case of one soft drink company purchasing another. Your accountant has formulas for working out the value of good will.

6. If the salon has a certain number of busy staff members, there is no reason to believe they will stay and work after the salon is sold. Indeed, perhaps the reason it is being sold is that several staff members intend to start their own salons a short distance away.

7. Consider the deal only if the present owner signs an agreement not to operate within a radius of 3 to 5 miles of the salon.

8. Be sure that all bills are paid. Your lawyer can and should find out this information.

9. Decide if the location is excellent. A good profit shown on the books of the present establishment is the best evidence of a good location. (Other factors of management are of course involved.)

10. A qualified lawyer can give you good advice about how to handle the transaction legally. If an agent is involved in the sale, his or her commission, which ranges from 6 to 10 percent, is paid by the seller.

Selecting a name for a salon is an important step in planning. **Do not use your name** for the name of the salon. Using your name has the following **disadvantages**:

1. Clients calling for an appointment always want the owner to style their hair. The result is unprofitable because you work while your staff watches.
2. New employees do not get as many appointments because, again, the owner is "requested"; it is difficult to convince the client that the new employee is competent, too.
3. If the salon carries your name, signs, stationery, checkbooks, etc., must be changed if it is sold.

It is much better to call the salon "My Fair Lady Beauty Salon," or "Beauty Spot Hair Designers," or something similar that tells everyone what kind of service the business offers.

Business liability insurance is necessary to protect the salon from a lawsuit made by a person injured in front of or in the salon. This may involve a client tripping on a sidewalk or falling on a slippery floor. Most leases specifically state that the **lessee** must carry liability insurance.

The owner may also wish to carry fire, wind, and glass-breakage insurance; these, too, are often required by the lease agreement.

The salon owner is expected to carry **malpractice insurance** for accidents that may result in injury to the client—for instance, cold-wave solution dripping into the client's eye or a scissor point in a client's ear. People sue others for good reason and for **no** reason. Salon owners can spend a lot of money proving their innocence. They must have the financial protection of good insurance that **covers all salon employees**. This type of coverage is usually available through the National Hairdressers and Cosmetologists Association.

Identify salon
insurance needs.

The reception area of the salon is very important to the operation of any good salon. This area is basically the "nerve center" of the salon. Consider the following points about the reception area:

Describe the
importance of the
salon reception area.

1. The **client's first impression** of you and your business is based on this area.
2. The **appointment book is located in the reception area.**
3. The **telephone** is at the reception desk for receiving appointments.
4. The **cash register** is conveniently located here also.
5. Client color/permanent wave cards are usually filed near the reception desk.
6. Shelves and displays for **retail items** are often located in the reception area.

The person that "directs traffic" in terms of greeting clients, scheduling appointments, collecting money, handling complaints, etc., at the reception area is the **receptionist**. As you might imagine, the receptionist must be a person who is enthusiastic, polite, diplomatic, and smart enough to keep things at the desk running smoothly. Of course, this person should be neatly groomed at all times, as well as willing and able to assist the client. Assistance may include (but is not limited to) explaining a new product, answering the phone, handling a client's complaint, and bringing a lunch snack in for other busy staff members.

KNOWING SUBOBJECTIVE 8

Describe the
importance of
retailing in the salon.

Retailing in the salon usually includes products such as shampoos, conditioners, hair sprays, nail care items, unique hairstyling appliances (curling irons, hair dryers), combs/brushes, and cosmetics. Other items for retail could include special hair ornaments, scarves, jewelry, and many other things that the clients will buy on a regular basis. The information that follows will help you decide how to go about selecting and selling retail items in the salon. Some salon owners are so successful at retailing, that they pay the salon rent with these profits.

Selecting a Retail Item   It is much easier to sell an item which is **used in the salon**. For example, retailing an excellent shampoo that is used every day in the salon is usually successful. **Packaging/labeling** of the shampoo is also important. The package should be neatly and attractively done. Of course, **by law**, the **ingredients** in a shampoo sold to the client **must be listed on the label**.

   After finding an excellent shampoo, some salon owners **private label** the shampoo with their own name. In such cases the label should be attractively designed and should include the salon name, address, and phone number. Private labeling protects the sale of the shampoo, since the client can be assured of getting exactly the same product only at the salon whose name appears on the label.

Pricing a Retail Item   Price is a very important concern for clients. Special care should be taken when determining the price of the shampoo in the example. It is necessary to **price your retail item(s) competitively** with similar ones available to the client. However, it is also the goal of the salon to make a profit so the selling price should include a mark up.

What is a Fair Profit?   A fair profit has to take into consideration the cost of the product to the salon, as well as a commission paid to the employee for recommending and selling the product to the client. Since the product has been paid for, the money spent for it is "tied up" on the shelf until the item is sold. Furthermore, the receptionist or other employees must take the time to individually **give each retail item a price sticker, display the product, and keep all the merchandise clean and neatly organized**. Therefore, a fair profit should probably be AT LEAST 50%-100%. For example, if a bottle of shampoo costs the salon $1.00 and the profit will be 50%, the shampoo will sell to the client for $1.50. If the profit on the shampoo will be 100%, the selling price will be $2.00. This may seem like too much profit, but considering the cost connected with selling the shampoo, it is fair.

How Much Should the Salon Retail?   The amount of retailing done in a salon will be determined by the size and location of the salon. A small one- or two-stylist salon may want to retail only three or four items, while the large, chain-type (10-20 stylists) salons may choose to retail 15 or more items.

Retailing Professional Products   Rather than selling private label products, some salons successfully sell brand name professional products. The rationale is that clients will be more willing to spend money for brands advertised in a magazine or seen on television. The only negative thing about this practice is that some manufacturers establish an identity of being sold exclusively in the professional salon and later begin selling the product to drugstores and discount stores. Salons can't sell the product for a price that is competitive! The drugstore or discount store can afford to sell the product at a lower price than the salon because these stores do high-volume buying at a lower cost to them.

Retailing is important, but it must be approached in an orderly, businesslike way. It's best to begin retailing gradually until you can figure out what will sell and what won't.

GLOSSARY

Amendments   Items in writing added to the lease that the landlord agrees to provide at no charge.

Corporation   A business owned by a number of stockholders.

Lease   A legal agreement between the owner of a building and a renter fixing the amount of rent, how long it will remain at that amount, and the rights and responsibilities of the owner and the renter.

Lessee   The renter; the tenant.

Lessor   The building owner; the landlord.

Malpractice insurance   An insurance that protects the cosmetologist against being sued for accidental injury of a client during the performance of a service.

Partnership   Ownership of a business by two or more people without the issuance of stock.

Partnership agreement   A document outlining the rights and responsibilities of each partner in a business.

Private label   Salon's name and address on a product that it is retailing.

Proprietorship   The amount the business is worth.

Sole proprietorship   Ownership of a business by one person.

Stockholders   People that have a partial ownership in a corporation through their purchase of one or more stock certificates.

QUESTIONS

1. What is the name given to a business that has two or more owners, but no stock is issued?
2. Should two people start a partnership and open a salon without a partnership agreement?
3. Is it a good idea to consult a lawyer before signing important legal papers?
4. If you like a particular area for the location of your salon, should population density remain an important factor?

5. True or false. If the building is particularly nice for a salon, accessibility really isn't very important.
6. What is the special name for local zoning restrictions?
7. What does the socioeconomic factor mean?
8. Are percentage rents desirable for salon owners?
9. Does rent tend to decrease over the years?
10. What is the term for the person who rents a space in a building?
11. What is the term for the person that authorizes the use of their building for a particular purpose, such as a salon?
12. Name the legal document of agreement written between the landlord and the renter.
13. Will a lease generally prevent increases in rent for the term of the agreement?
14. In the absence of a written agreement, must the landlord provide adequate air conditioning for a salon?
15. True or false. Plumbing and electrical work are the cheapest things you can have done in a salon?
16. Should you use your name when opening a new salon?
17. If the client slips on a puddle of water in the salon, which type of insurance covers this situation?
18. If bleach blisters the client's scalp, which type of insurance covers this situation?
19. What is the name given to the person at the front desk who answers the phone and schedules appointments?

ANSWERS

1. A partnership 2. No 3. Yes 4. Yes 5. False 6. Ordinances 7. The income level of families in a certain area 8. No 9. No; remain the same or increase 10. Lessee 11. Lessor 12. Lease 13. Yes 14. No 15. False 16. No 17. Liability insurance 18. Malpractice insurance 19. Receptionist

Operating a Salon 30

Now that you have some idea of what goes into planning a salon, it's time to learn about actually operating a salon. The objectives that follow are very thorough, but they certainly don't cover all possible salon operating situations. Your instructor may have additional information that is very important too. However, the information in this chapter will be very helpful. Learning and using this information may well determine whether your salon is a success or a failure.

Describe the basic principles involved in the operation of a new salon. **Major Objective**

Score 75 percent or better on a multiple-choice exam on the information in this chapter. **Level of Acceptability**

Knowing Subobjectives

1. Explain factors involved in purchasing salon equipment and supplies.
2. Identify considerations involved in designing salon operating policies and using techniques for interviewing prospective employees.
3. Describe salon operating costs.
4. Explain basic economic principles of supply and demand.
5. Explain the client supply charge system.
6. Explain basic accounting and taxation principles.
7. List advantages for accepting credit cards.
8. Explain the booth rental system.

KNOWING SUBOBJECTIVE 1

Explain factors involved in purchasing salon equipment and supplies.

The cost of operating a salon is normally figured in "per-operator" dollars. Usually, the cost per operator of opening a new salon is $2,000 to $2,500. This dollar range should easily include the usual operating equipment and supplies, such as the reception desk, dryer lounges, hydraulic styling chairs, shampoo bowls, shampoo chairs, and so on. You can always spend more money per operator if you want custom-made equipment. Ordering standard equipment from catalogues will keep costs below or at $2,500 per operator. Always get bids for equipment from several beauty supply dealers. You can do this by submitting a written request for bids including:

1. Color, fabric, and style of equipment.
2. How many pieces of each kind of equipment are needed.
3. Opening supplies needed.
4. Date bids will be opened.
5. Date equipment is needed to open the salon.

Dealers may give a discount if the equipment is paid for in cash. Some dealers give a discount if you make your first purchase through them. Study the bids carefully to select the best deal!

You may wish to purchase the equipment on an installment agreement through the dealer. After you make a down payment, you must make

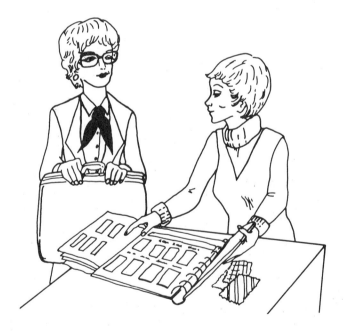

Selecting decorating samples for the salon

monthly payments, usually for a period of 1 to 5 years. There is usually a **service charge** for **late payments**. Depending on the signed sales agreement, if more than 3 payments have not been made, the dealer may be able to call for all of the money due immediately (usually referred to as a **balloon clause**)! If the balloon payment is not made in full, all of the equipment may be repossessed by the dealer. **Never sign any legal agreement unless your lawyer has approved it!**

Equipment may also be financed through a bank, probably at a lower interest rate (the cost of using money) than a dealer will charge. Small loan companies usually charge the highest rate of interest and should be avoided.

Operating supplies are also called "consumable supplies" because they are **used completely** in the performance of a service. **They cannot be reused**. Consumable supplies will ordinarily represent about **8 percent** of the total dollar sales for any given year. If a salon spends $8,000 per year for supplies, its total sales are about $100,000. This is determined from the fact that 8 percent equals $8,000 in supplies:

Step 1: $8\% = .08$

Step 2: $.08x = \$8,000.00$

Step 3: $\dfrac{.08x}{} = \dfrac{}{.08}$

Step 4: $x = \dfrac{\$8,000}{.08}$

Step 5: $x = .08\overset{100,000.}{\overline{)\$8,000.00}}$

Answer: $100,000

If another salon did $72,000 in sales and spent $12,000 on consumable supplies, something would be very wrong with your supply costs because $72,000 \times .08 = \$5,760$, or 16 to 17 percent, which is **too high!** This percentage is figured by:

Step 1: $\dfrac{\$12,000}{\$72,000} = \dfrac{1}{6}$ or $6\overline{)1}$

Step 2: $6\overset{.166}{\overline{)1.000}}$

Answer: .166

The answer can be rounded off to .17 or 17 percent.

Most salon owners have salespersons calling on their business. These salespersons may seem to be a bit of a nuisance, but they are **not**. The **supply salesperson** is the **important link** between the manufacturer and the salon owner. Advertisements of new products are available, but they are not substitutes for discussing the real advantages and benefits of a new product with a salesperson who can answer questions. The salesperson may also give advice on choosing a salon location.

Any reputable sales representative for a supply dealer will **guarantee** a product. Products that do not perform according to claims by the salesperson may be **credited** to the salon account if the empty container or unused portion of the new product is returned. The dealer will issue a credit to the salon and return the product to the manufacturer.

A salon owner should **not divide** (split) his or her **supply business** between more than 2 or 3 supply dealers because:

1. **Bookkeeping becomes difficult.**
2. **Too much time** is spent chatting with sales representatives.
3. If the volume of business is **large enough** and bills are paid **promptly,** a **discount** may be given.
4. There is less **product duplication** because you can become familiar with the stock of only two or three suppliers.

1. **Bookkeeping becomes difficult** when many suppliers are used since detailed records must be kept on all products and the firms that supplied them.

Some salons buy supplies on credit; but remember, a **charge account is a privilege** that should not be abused because doing so is both unethical and unwise. Credit ratings can be checked between almost any two cities in the world. If you cannot pay the full amount of a bill, explain the situation to the dealer's credit manager and make a partial payment.

Some salons prefer to pay for supplies C.O.D. (cash on delivery). This is all right, but there is a charge for handling a transction in this way. So, it is important to order weekly rather than every other day.

When the supplies are delivered to the salon, there is an invoice that states:

(a) salon name
(b) address
(c) invoice number and date
(d) quantity ordered
(e) description of supply
(f) price
(g) tax
(h) delivery charge

Always check **invoices against supplies accompanying** them and pay only according to these **checked invoices.**

Beauty Supply Co.
XXXX Hairstyle Lane
Anytown, USA 00001

Ship to: Family Hair Care Salon
XXXX Green St.
Everytown, USA 00000

Bill to: (if different)

Invoice #00000___

Purchase Order No. XX___

Terms Net___

Quantity	Item No.	Description	Unit Price	Extension
12	QA1	Q hair color	$1.67 per each	$20.04
12	AA1	A hair color	1.67 per each	20.04
6	123	Shampoo	1.25 per each	7.50
6	876	Conditioner	1.42 per each	8.52
		Total		$56.10
		Transportation (if applicable)		5.00
		Sales Tax (if applicable)		2.75

Total items	Packed by	Wt. Shipped	Please pay this amount
36	XYZ	15 lbs.	$63.85

Sample invoice from beauty supply house

Salon owners **do not** pay for supplies from a **statement**, which usually comes at the end of each month, unless the invoice numbers listed on the statement and corresponding dollars coincide exactly with the invoices collected through the month.

It is a good practice to always make checks **payable only to the company, not** the salesperson. The number of the invoice that the check is covering should **always** be written above the date in the upper right-hand corner of the check. Also, write the check number and date on the invoice(s). This system serves as an accurate cross-reference. Always write the date, company, invoice numbers, and the amount of the check on the check stub. Invoices, check stubs, and cancelled checks should remain on file.

2. Salespersons can be valuable resources for assisting the salon owner in solving problems, contacting schools for graduates, learning about new products, and finding a new location if another salon is to be opened. Most experienced salespersons are quite knowledgeable about the industry and are good sources of information. If many suppliers are used, however, talking to these persons about legitimate concerns can become too time consuming.

Always treat salespersons **courteously. Respect their time** as well as your own. If you cannot leave the work area, invite the salesperson to come over to that area and describe products, or **write** prices of items on the back of the order book. If you cannot talk, explain this and ask the salesperson to return later.

3. Discounts, which are common among large-volume accounts, can be useful. However, an owner can spend too much time bargaining for lower prices. Some salon owners spend 20 hours a week trying to tie up a lot of money to bring the unit price of an item down. Even if they are successful, the effects on the percentage of dollars spent for supplies are **not** great. The owner could probably make much more money by spending that time dressing hair.

Regardless of price, **any** supply that cannot be used within **90 working days** should not be ordered. To do otherwise is using too much cash. The cost of borrowing money to pay dealers for a large discount order may **be greater than** the saving made on that purchase.

4. **Product duplication** is the salon owner's worst enemy. Stick with the tried and proven products for **each** task. Avoid stocking many products that do **exactly** the same thing. Only small quantities of any new product should be purchased for trial use.

It's helpful to **develop an index card system** on products that are **ordered often** so that the quantity and unit price are available for reference. Matching the cards against each other will show price differences and product duplication. Nothing is "free." If the "deal" is 6 cold waves for $60 and 6 cold waves free, the result is 12 cold waves at a cost of $5 each. Use a small, inexpensive calculator for figuring such unit prices.

KNOWING SUBOBJECTIVE 2

Identify considerations involved in designing salon operating policies and using techniques for interviewing prospective employees.

All salon owners, large or small, should have a list of **operating policies**. This kind of a list lets all employees know exactly **what they are responsible for** and **what they are expected to do**. Policies also include things that the salon owner will do for them. In making up the list, the owner must ask what he or she can offer a prospective employee. In turn, an owner must consider what an employee has to offer.

For example, an individual will be employed because he or she:

1. Sanitizes his or her work area at the end of each day to prepare for the next day's work so that clients will not be kept waiting.
2. Arrives 15 minutes before the first appointment to be ready for the client.
3. Is cheerful and courteous to **all** the clients in the salon.
4. Willingly helps other employees and the owner in an emergency so that everyone remains "on schedule" for appointments.

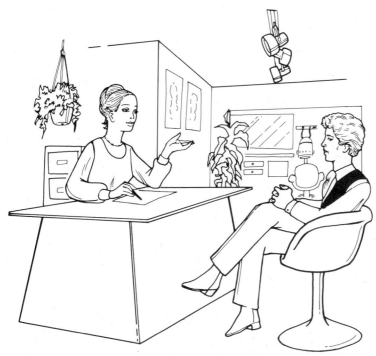

Inverviewing a prospective employee

5. Writes legibly and accurately in the appointment book so scheduling does not become confused.
6. Stays late for a client on special occasions.
7. Does not order supplies without consulting the owner.

An employee looks for a working arrangement that includes the following:

1. The salon is neat, clean, and kept in good repair, and new equipment is purchased as needed.
2. The salon owner pays malpractice insurance and hospitalization.
3. Paid vacations equal to ½ – ¾ of the individual's average weekly take-in dollars (and according to how long he or she has been employed) are provided.
4. The owner pays for professional seminars and has self-improvement styling classes once a month.
5. Only the best supplies are purchased for use in the salon.
6. Staff meetings are held to discuss and take care of operating problems.

All professional businesses put their **operating policies in writing**—the salon is no exception. Employees and employers can avoid many misunderstandings if policy lists are given to new employees.

You will need to learn good interviewing techniques when you talk to prospective employees. Two techniques are particularly important: close observation and note-taking.

Some of the **basic things you should look for are:**

1. Is the applicant on time?
2. Is the hair attractively styled?
3. Are clothes neat and clean and are shoes shined or polished?
4. Is the applicant poised and alert?

Some questions you should ask an applicant are:

1. What school did you graduate from?
2. Where were you last employed?
3. What other salons have you worked for?
4. Why did you leave your last position?
5. Would you object if I called your previous employer? If so, why?
6. Do you have a particular specialty?
7. What is your address and phone number?
8. How far do you live from the salon?
9. What commission do you expect?
10. What else do you expect?
11. Are the working days and hours acceptable?
12. Do you realize the importance of **working Saturdays?**
13. Will you consent to cut, set, or comb a model's hair to demonstrate your skills?
14. Do you have any questions regarding operating policies?

You may wish to type these questions as a questionnaire for the applicant to complete. Written notes are best; they should be carefully filed for future reference.

KNOWING SUBOBJECTIVE 3

Describe salon operating costs.

You can probably guess that one of the most important problems of planning and running a business is helping keep expenses under control. There are two general categories of expenses that you should keep in mind when you plan your salon:

1. Fixed costs
2. Variable costs

Fixed costs remain the same. Whether you have one client or a thousand, you will have to pay the same for these expenses. And they remain the same all year long. **Some good examples** of fixed costs are rent, insurance, dues, license fees, and basic legal fees. These expenses must be paid every month to keep the salon open for business. These expenses can change; for example, insurance rates, rent, or licensing fees can increase. But these increases will come at one time and will cover a specific period of time. So, if your insurance is increased from $50 a month to $75 a month, you will know that your insurance will cost $75 a month for the next 6 months or a year. These expenses won't change from day to day or week to week.

Variable costs change according to the number of clients you have. As the number of clients you serve increases, so will your variable costs. Supply costs are probably the best example of variable costs. They change directly with the number of clients served. For example, if you serve 12 clients, you will use twice as much shampoo as you would use for 6 clients.

Other examples of variable costs are commissions, laundry, utilities (water, light, power), interest, and repairs and maintenance.

You should be aware that the beauty-salon business is peculiar in salaries to employees (other cosmetologists). Think about this difference for a moment. If you buy a shirt in a department store, the clerk does **not** receive 50 percent of the purchase price paid for the shirt! The cosmetologist, on the other hand, is paid 50 percent of the price of the service.

You must base decisions to add new services on what they cost. Although most salons must provide a fairly wide range of services to please their clients, you need to recognize which services are most profitable. You can develop your skill in those areas and become known as an expert.

Here is one example about the difference in costs. The time it takes to give a shampoo/hairstyle is about the same as the time needed to give a haircut. You charge $7 for the shampoo/hairstyle and $8 for the haircut. Obviously the shop (and the stylist) can make more money giving haircuts than shampoo/hairstyles because the price is higher, and it **costs** the shop **less** to give haircuts. If you are good at cutting hair, you can provide 15 shampoo/hairstyles or 15 haircuts per day. Table 1 illustrates the possible gross income that you can earn from various combinations of these 2 services rendered by 1 stylist in an 8-hour day (see page 472).

You will need to think about other types of services. An **example** follows:

1. 15 shampoo/hairstyles at $7.00 = $105.00
2. 6 shampoo/hairstyles at $7.00 plus 3 cold waves at $32.50 = $139.50

In this case, you took in $34.50 more, but you have served 6 fewer clients.

The usual salon operating expenses are shown in table 2 on page 472. You can use the percentages of variable and fixed costs as a guide in planning your own salon.

TABLE 1. Possible Combinations of Gross Income Earned by a Stylist in One Day.

COMBINATIONS OF SERVICES		INCOME		
SHAMPOO/HAIRSTYLES	HAIRCUTS	SHAMPOO/HAIRSTYLES ($7.00)	HAIRCUTS (@ $8.00)	TOTAL SERVICE DOLLARS
15	0	$105.00	$ 0.00	$105.00
14	1	98.00	8.00	106.00
13	2	91.00	16.00	107.00
12	3	84.00	24.00	108.00
11	4	77.00	32.00	109.00
10	5	70.00	40.00	110.00
9	6	63.00	48.00	111.00
8	7	56.00	56.00	112.00
7	8	49.00	64.00	113.00
6	9	42.00	72.00	114.00
5	10	35.00	80.00	115.00
4	11	28.00	88.00	116.00
3	12	21.00	96.00	117.00
2	13	14.00	104.00	118.00
1	14	7.00	112.00	119.00
0	15	0.00	120.00	120.00

TABLE 2.

	Percentage
VARIABLE COSTS	
Salaries and commissions (staff and owner)	56
Service supplies	7
Retail supplies	1
Towel service	1.50
Utilities (water, heat, power, light)	3.50
Repairs and maintenance	1
Interest and carrying charges	.25
Legal services (including accounting)	1.25
Taxes	4
FIXED COSTS	
Rent*	6
Advertising	2
Depreciation	1.50
Insurance (malpractice, liability)	1.50
Telephone	1.50
Association dues, magazines	.50
Education and travel	.50
TOTAL COSTS	89.00
PROFIT	11.00
	100.00

*Note that rent is the highest fixed cost percentage

Even if you only listen to the news once in a while, you have heard an announcer say, "Economists are predicting a recession," or "Economists are predicting an upturn in the economy," or a variety of related things.

Economics involves studying the economy and why it works the way it does. It is a very complicated science, and economists themselves probably disagree about many more things than they agree about. (Harry Truman is supposed to have once said that if you laid all the economists in the country end to end they would point in different directions!)

However, there are some basic principles that economists agree on, and they are what you will learn about in this subobjective. To begin with, a simple working definition of economics you can remember is: **Economics is the description and analysis of the production, distribution, and consumption of goods and services.** What this means in a simpler way is that economics concerns **the study of who buys what, where, when, and why, and what happens when they do or don't.**

These questions involve a lot more than you might think, but there are 3 basic terms you can learn that will help you understand a little more about economics. They are **market, demand,** and **supply.** The market (or marketplace) is where people buy and sell. For your concerns, the market is all cosmetologists and people who use or might use their services. You can use the term "market" to describe a large or small area, for instance, the entire country, your state, city, or neighborhood. Your greatest interest will probably be in the market in your city or neighborhood.

The beauty market can be described as a "pure market" for several reasons:

1. It offers the **same** (or very similar) services in most places of business.
2. It is made up of many **small** economic units called salons. (An economic unit is where a product is made or provided.)
3. A single salon cannot affect the prices charged by other salons.
4. Its prices are not regulated by the federal government.
5. It offers **free entry**. Anyone can attempt to meet the minimum legal requirements set by the state board and operate a salon.

Before you decide to open a salon, you must decide what the **demand** is. The amount of demand is the number of people who want to buy a service or product. In other words, how many people want your services? What you will be concerned about, of course, is that there are enough people.

How much demand there is or will be **for these services** will depend on:

1. The **price** of the service.
2. The **price of similar substitutes**. Are similar home services or lower prices offered by other salons in a location?

Explain basic economic principles of supply and demand.

3. The **income of an average family** in the location you are considering.
4. The **personal choices** (tastes) of the clients in the general area.
5. The techniques of **advertising**, including those used by salons in the area.
6. The price **increases** you can expect for beauty-salon services in the area.

Some people use a graph like the one in chart 1 to decide on the demand for services. The figure of $6 is used for this example as the average price of a shampoo/hairstyle in the United States. (Possible prices in different cities are shown in table 1.) Chart 1 shows the number of clients willing to receive services at different prices.

If you join the different points that show how many people will buy a service at a particular price, you will have a **demand curve** (chart 2). You have probably figured out that **more** clients will ask for services if the price is lowered and that **fewer** clients will request them, if the **price is higher**.

The completed graph of the demand curve is shown in chart 3.

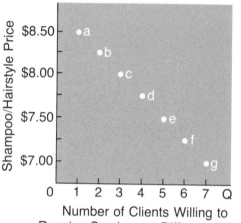

CHART 1.

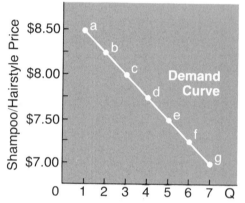

CHART 2.

TABLE 3. Possible Prices for Shampoo/Hairstyles in Various U.S. Cities

City and State	Possible Price of a Shampoo/Hairstyle
Minneapolis, Minnesota	$7.00
Chicago, Illinois	7.25
Pittsburgh, Pennsylvania	7.50
Akron, Ohio	7.75
Hollywood, California	8.00
New York, New York	8.25
Detroit, Michigan	8.50

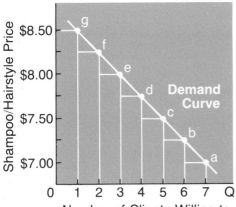

Number of Clients Willing to
Receive Services at Different Prices
(expressed in hundreds or Q)

CHART 3.

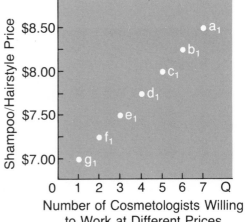

Number of Cosmetologists Willing
to Work at Different Prices
(expressed in hundreds or Q)

CHART 4.

TABLE 4.   Prices for Shampoo/Hairstyles

Price of a Shampoo/Hairstyle	Cosmetologists Willing to Work
$8.50	700
8.25	600
8.00	500
7.75	400
7.50	300
7.25	200
7.00	100

If other things that affect demand are **not** changed, the clients will determine the price you can charge for a service.

The third term, supply, also plays an important part in deciding on price. The **supply** is the number of people who provide a product or service. It is no secret that most people like to make money, the more the better. It is easy to see that if the price of a cosmetologist's services is high, more people will want to work as cosmetologists than if prices are low (see table 4 and chart 4). If you put the information in table 4 on a graph, it would look like chart 4. By connecting the points on that graph, you can make a line called the **supply curve** (chart 5 page 476).

If you put the demand curve onto the supply curve, they will crisscross. The point where they meet is called the **equilibrium** (chart 6 page 476). **Equilibrium** is the **highest price** that you can get from the **greatest number of clients** for a shampoo/hairstyle service.

If the supply of hairdressers remains the **same**, but the demand for more shampoo/hairstyles **increases**, the **price** will **go up**, for example, to $8.25 (chart 7 page 476).

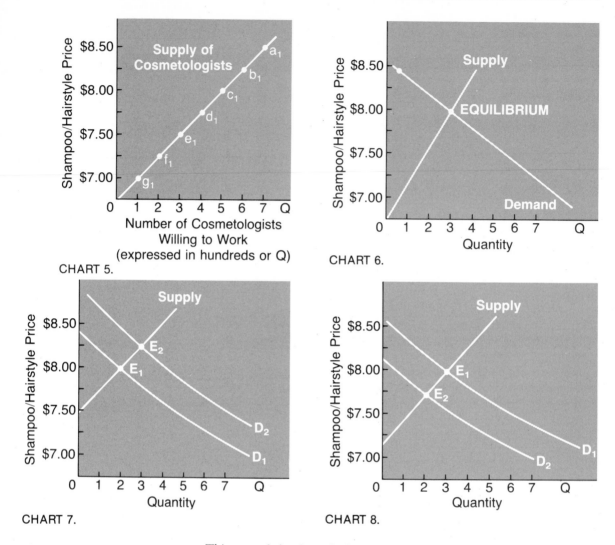

CHART 5.

CHART 6.

CHART 7.

CHART 8.

This example has been fairly simple and has included only basic concerns. These are important concerns, but you should remember that **price, substitutes, income, personal tastes, advertising,** and **anticipated price increases** all affect demand.

Prices can be affected by many things that you might not think would affect them. For instance, if you live in a small town, a large manufacturing plant could move into your area and create many new jobs. The plant would probably bring many more people to live in the town and the people who already live there might make more money. With this increase in income and in the number of people, there would be an increase in the demand for a cosmetologist's services.

One of two things would happen. Either more cosmetologists would move into your town and prices would stay the same, or you could raise prices and still probably have more business than you could handle. One of

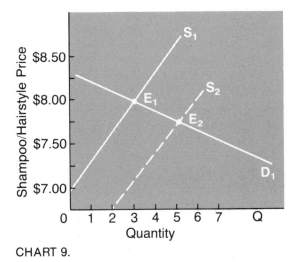

CHART 9.

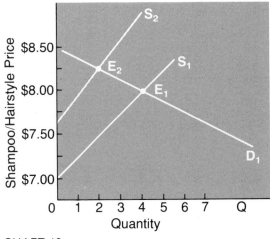

CHART 10.

two things would have to happen: increased supply (more cosmetologists) or decreased demand (higher prices). **The best way, in general, to control supply and demand is to increase the price until the demand is equal to the supply.**

The opposite is also true. If a large manufacturing plant in your town closed, many people would lose their jobs. They would have less money to spend, and demand would decrease (see chart 8 opposite page).

The examples you have just read show how prices can be influenced by changes in demand. Prices can change the same way if supply is changed.

For example, the number of cosmetologists available can cause prices to change. If the number of graduates from schools in the United States doubled, twice as many cosmetologists would be available for work. Price would **decrease**, for example to $7.75 (chart 9). There would be a **surplus** (too many) of cosmetologists.

On the other hand, if half of the schools in the U.S. closed and the number of graduates dropped by 50 percent, the price would **increase**, for example to $8.25 (chart 10), and there would be a **shortage** of cosmetologists.

You will need to understand these economic principles so you can (1) determine the **need** for a salon in a given area, (2) **set prices** that will attract clients, and (3) change (increase or decrease) prices as regularly as the factors that affect demand change.

KNOWING SUBOBJECTIVE 5

Client Supply Charges.   Historically, salon owners have paid a commission to the hairstylist based on the total amount paid by the client. For example, if the client had a permanent wave/hairstyle for $50.00, the stylist was paid 50% commission, which would amount to $25.00. The salon owner took the cost of the perm and other costs, such as rent, advertising, electricity,

Explain the client supply charge system.

etc., out of the other $25.00. This system worked well for many years. However, in the late 1970's and early 1980's, supply costs doubled, and the salon owners couldn't make a profit. A service charge program was started by many salons in order to stay in business.

This is how the supply charge is figured.   The salon figured the cost connected to the different services. Although the cost of a permanent wave varies with the product, an average price might be $5.00. If the salon had been charging $50.00 for a permanent wave/hairstyle under the old system, the price was increased to $57.00 to include a client supply charge. The client's service sales ticket would be coded with the supply cost for each service; in this example, the perm cost is coded $5.00. Therefore, the stylist would be **paid a commission after the supply charge has been subtracted** from the service sales ticket. So, if the client paid $57.00 for the service, the supply charge of $5.00 would be subtracted; then the stylist is paid a commission on $52.00.

Price charged client . . . $57.00
Cost of perm . . . .   − 5.00
                                 $52.00
                                      50% Commission
                                 $26.00   Amount paid to stylist

The service charge for supplies makes sense. Why should the stylist be paid for using a supply? The stylist is actually selling skills, talent, experience, and personality. After all, the salon owner is in business to make a profit!

KNOWING SUBOBJECTIVE 6

Explain basic accounting principles and taxation.

If you don't realize how important record-keeping is to a successful business, you will soon find out. You know some of the reasons for keeping **accurate records**. All of us pay income taxes, and so will your business. If you have employees, you will have to know when to pay them. You will also have to pay Social Security and other items for your employees. You will have to know when to pay your rent and many other bills.

You may have thought of this aspect of keeping good records, but there are other important reasons. Good records can **help** you **plan ahead** and help you operate your business more efficiently. For example, sometimes you can buy supplies for less at certain times of the year, and sometimes you can buy supplies for less if you buy larger amounts. Your records will show you the best time to buy supplies and the best amounts.

Also, your business may vary from time to time during the year. Records will show when you take in more money than at other times. If you know you are very busy during the spring or at Christmas but are rather slow during the summer, you may want to plan to hire temporary help for these periods.

TABLE 5. Family Hair Care Center, Balance Sheet, December 31, 19XX

Assets		
Cash	$30,000.00	
Equipment	15,000.00	
Supplies	5,000.00	
		$50,000.00
Liabilities		
Loan	15,000.00	15,000.00
Proprietorship	35,000.00	35,000.00
		$50,000.00

Why do you need to worry about records so much? After you have been in business for a year or two, you will know these things. That's true, but you have many things on your mind when you operate a business. If you don't have complete records, you will have to remember all of them—and you probably won't. Good records are your memory. **Record-keeping** is possibly the most unpopular part of running a business, but it is also one of the most important. You may want to have a professional bookkeeper or accountant or, even better, a certified public accountant (C.P.A.) to keep your records for you, but you still should be able to read and interpret your records. An accountant or C.P.A. will be able to help you.

So, you are not "helpless." There are a few simple formulas that you can use to interpret your records. They correspond to the two basic accounting statements. The first formula is called the **basic accounting equation**. It is: **Assets** = Liabilities + Proprietorship. These terms are very easy to understand. **Assets** are what the business **owns. Liabilities** are what the business owes. What is left over is **Proprietorship**, or what the business is worth. You can see how this equation works by looking at a **balance sheet** (table 5). The assets ($50,000.00) equal the total of liabilities ($15,000.00) and proprietorship ($35,000.00).

You can use this equation in several ways. For instance, you may know what you own (assets) and what you owe (liabilities), but do not know how much you are worth. You can find out by subtracting your liabilities from your assets like this:

Assets	$50,000.00
Liabilities	−15,000.00
Proprietorship	$35,000.00

There is another statement, and a formula that goes with it, that is also very important. It is called the income statement (see table 6). The **income statement** shows how much money you made. The basic income equation is this formula: **Gross Income − Expenses** = Net Income.

There are 3 terms that you need to know. **Gross income** is the money you receive from clients. As you may know only too well, what you earn

TABLE 6. Family Hair Care Center, Income Statement, December 31, 19XX

Gross Income		
Services—Shampoos, etc.	$14,000.00	
Miscellaneous		
Manicures, etc.	1,000.00	
Total Gross Income		$15,000.00
Expenses		
Salaries	$ 3,500.00	
Benefits	1,500.00	
Total Expenses		$ 5,000.00
Net Income		$10,000.00

and what you get are two very different things. You have rent to pay, clothes and food to buy, and other bills to pay. So that money is not really your own. The same thing is true for a business. Your business must use money it gets to pay for salaries, supplies, and other items that are needed to run the business. These are called **expenses**. They are the cost of doing business.*

If you subtract all expenses from gross income, you will get net income. **Net income** is the money you have left after you have paid the expenses of the business. You can do whatever you want with the net income. You can put it back into the business by using it to hire more employees, buy more supplies, or rent a bigger salon. Or you may save it as part of the business' proprietorship, in other words, how much it is worth. Or you may take it out of the business by paying it to yourself.

These two equations and statements should give you a basic idea of what accounting is about. But follow your own advice to your clients: get a professional. A client might be able to give a shampoo and set, but he or she is an amateur; there is, really, no telling what the results will be. The same thing is true for you when it comes to record-keeping and accounting. A professional will **know** what to do; a professional won't need to "hope it's right" or "guess" at the solution to a problem.

Students planning to become salon owners or managers should know a few important facts about tax laws. **Tax laws are made by the state or federal legislature.** These laws are called **Acts** because they are "enacted" (made by) the legislature. A violation (nonpayment) of tax law is a crime!

Certain taxes have to be paid by the employer (salon owner) out of his/her own pocket. Other taxes are paid by the employee in the form of a **payroll deduction** (subtracted from the employee's pay check). The employee's payroll deduction is sent to the government monthly, and reported to the government quarterly (four times per year). Employers generally **pay**

---

*Accountants make a technical distinction between an expense and a cost. Entire books have been written about the difference, but you don't need to worry about it here.

| Status __M__ Deductions claimed __0__ |
| Total earnings this pay period: $0.00 |

Status __M__ Deductions claimed __0__
Total earnings this pay period: $0.00
Taxes withheld:
  Federal $0.00
  FICA (Social Security) $0.00
  State (optional) $0.00
Total withholding: $0.00
Other deductions:
  Malpractice Insurance $0.00
Total other deductions: $0.00
Net earnings: $0.00
Year-to-date (optional)

Gross	Fed.	FICA	State	Ins.	Net
$0.00	$0.00	$0.00	$0.00	$0.00	$0.00

Family Hair Care Salon
XXXX Green St.
Everytown, U.S.A. 00000

Check Number
123456

Pay to the Order of *Jane Doe* $ *0.00*

Zero Dollars and Zero Cents

Joe E Moe
Joe E. Moe
Owner/Manager

Sample payroll check with stub attached. Withholding and "other" deductions vary from state-to-state, city-to-city, and salon-to-salon.

federal taxes to a local bank. The bank sends the tax money to the federal Government. State taxes are sent directly to the State's Department of Revenue (or Taxation).

The employer (salon owner) must pay the following taxes out of his/her own pocket in order to comply with these tax acts:

1. Federal Unemployment Tax Act (FUTA)
2. State Unemployment Tax Act (SUTA)
3. Federal Insurance Contribution Act (FICA)
4. Workman's Compensation Act.

FUTA (FEW'-TAH) requires all employers to pay .7% of the first $6,000 the employee earns to a maximum of $42.00 per month to the Federal Government. This money is used to pay the employee should he/she become unemployed.

SUTA (SOO'-TAH) **requires all employers to pay a percentage** based on the amount of the worker's earnings to the State Government. This percentage tends to be different from one state to the next. SUTA funds are used by the state to pay unemployment benefits.

FICA (FI'-Ka) is the **Social Security** tax that **requires all employers to match (an amount of money equal to) what the employee contributes** to the Social Security Fund. For example, if the employee's contribution is 6.13% of his/her earnings, the employer must put in an amount of money equal to that 6.13%. So, the **total money paid to FICA** would be an amount equal to 12.26% of what the employee earned. Percentages change from year-to-year, so check with the **Internal Revenue Service (IRS)**, or your accountant.

The Workman's Compensation Act requires that all employers must **pay** for an insurance policy that **protects employees that may be injured** while at work. The cost of this insurance policy will be different for various types of job categories. For example, insurance coverage for a hairdresser would most likely cost less than the coverage for a policeman. The reason being that a hairdresser is less likely to be injured on the job.

The employee must have the following taxes withheld from his/her pay check:

1. Federal Income Tax
2. State Income Tax
3. FICA Tax

The actual amount of money withheld from your paycheck will be determined by numerous factors, such as, amount of total earnings, marital status, and number of dependents etc., and whether the government percentage figures have changed from year-to-year.

Remember that as an employee you must **declare all tips of more than $20.00 per month, and pay the added tax.**

The salon owner should also realize that he/she is **responsible** for **unpaid taxes of a hairdresser who rents** space in the owner's beauty salon. For example, in the case "Wolfe v. U.S., No. 77–1434, United States Court of Appeals, Eighth Circuit, North Dakota" the Court held that the person renting space from a salon owner was **not** an independent contractor, but actually an employee of the owner; therefore, the owner would be held liable (have to pay) for the unpaid taxes owed by the hairdresser renting space in the beauty salon.

KNOWING SUBOBJECTIVE 7

List advantages for accepting credit cards.

The use of credit cards has become a multi-billion dollar per year industry. We live in a "plastic world." Many people feel more comfortable in charging services and products than in using cash.

Satellite communications make it possible for a person living in Minneapolis, Minnesota, to charge a piece of jewelry in Paris, France. A **credit check** is made by the store owner simply by using the **telephone.** The store call is relayed via satellite to the credit card company in Minneapolis. If the cardholder has good credit, the purchase is approved.

Salon personnel accepting credit card charges must check the expiration date and request other forms of identification. If salon personnel follow the correct steps for giving the card-company the charges, the business will be paid. It is assumed that the salon has given the card-holder a reasonable service or product in exchange for the amount charged.

Credit cards which are **convenient to use,** allow clients to avoid the "hassle" of cashing a personal check. Furthermore, paying for a service or a purchase with "plastic" eliminates the need to carry large sums of money in a purse or billfold, which could be lost or stolen.

The client using the card also has the advantage of delaying actual payment for the service until the salon part of the transaction is processed through the card company. So even though the client could probably pay cash for a product or service, he/she **will have had use of the money** until the monthly credit card billing is due.

Unlike a personal check that might be returned because of insufficient funds, payment for services charged on credit cards **is guaranteed**.

The only **disadvantage** in accepting credit cards is the **fee**. All credit card companies charge a user **fee**. The user fee is usually charged to the salon as a percentage of the amount of the service. The card company might charge an across-the-board fee of 8% on a $100.00 client charge, so the card company would pay the salon $92.00. Of course, the salons on a card program usually add the user fee into the cost of the service to the client.

Salons located in areas with a lot of "traffic," such as shopping centers, hotels, heavily populated areas, or tourist attraction/resort areas should probably use a credit card program. Figures clearly indicate that card use **increases overall salon sales**.

KNOWING SUBOBJECTIVE 8

Booth Rental   In the booth rental system stylists who have an established clientele **rent a booth** in a salon. Booth rental is not legal in all states. Check with your state board office. The stylist agrees to pay the salon owner a set amount of money every week or month. In exchange, the salon owner allows the stylist to use the salon's equipment, such as, shampoo bowls, styling stations, hydraulic chairs, telephone, restrooms, etc. The stylist must furnish his/her own operating supplies including shampoo, permanent waves, conditioners, etc. The stylist would be allowed to keep all money that the client is charged under the booth rental agreement. A person renting from a salon owner with this kind of agreement is called a **renter**.

A hypothetical example would be as follows: Mary rents a booth at the **Family Hair Care Center** for $200 per week. Mary collects only $150 from her clientele during the first week of her rental. She must pay the salon owner that $150, plus $50 from her savings account. But during the second week, Mary collects $800 from her clientele; however, Mary still has to pay the salon owner only the $200 agreed upon for the booth rental.

The advantages to the stylist would include: (1) no money paid out for equipment; (2) set working hours and preference of working days; (3) selection of uniform; (4) less bookkeeping for items such as phone, advertising, electricity, etc.; (5) control of prices for services, regardless of prices set for regular employees; and (6) no risk of going out of business and losing an investment, because no investment has been made.

The disadvantages to the salon owner are many, and for the reasons that follow, booth rental is **not** a good business management practice for an otherwise successful salon.

A brief list of **disadvantages** to the salon owner includes: (1) booth rental stylists don't have to follow salon operating policies; (2) regular salon employees may end up answering the phone for the renter and/or scheduling

Explain the booth rental system.

appointments; (3) salon equipment gets additional wear and will need replacement; (4) management is more difficult because the renter doesn't work a set schedule of hours/days per week; (5) other staff may become difficult to manage because "some" workers (the renters) don't have to obey operating policies; (6) newly-hired regular stylists (paid an hourly rate and/or commission) will have difficulty developing a clientele because the clients brought in by the renter have their hair done exclusively by the renter; (7) the salon owner must pay any tax due to the government that the renter has not paid; (8) if the renter moves to another salon in the neighborhood most, if not all, of the renter's clientele will also move to the other salon.

GLOSSARY

Assets   What is owned by a business.

Balloon clause   A statement in an installment purchase agreement that allows the dealer to demand full payment if more than three payments have not been made.

Basic accounting equation (Assets = Liabilities + Proprietorship)   A formula for interpreting the worth of a business.

C.O.D. (Cash on Delivery)   A shipping arrangement which requires full payment on delivery.

Demand   The number of people who want to buy a service or product.

Economics   The study of who buys what, where, when, and why, and what happens when they do or don't.

Equilibrium   The highest price that you can get from the greatest number of people for a service or product.

Expenses   The costs involved in doing business, such as salaries and supplies.

Fixed costs   Costs that remain the same and do not fluctuate with the number of clients served.

Gross income   Money received from services and products before expenses are deducted.

Liabilities   What is owed by a business.

Market (marketplace)   Where people buy and sell.

Net income   The money left after expenses have been paid.

Operating policies   A list showing what the employee and employer can expect of each other in respect to salon operations.

Operating supplies   Supplies that are completely used in the performance of a service.

Renter   A stylist who rents a booth from a salon.

Supply   The amount available of a service or product.

Supply charge   Cost of a supply which is subtracted from the price of the service before the hairstylist's commission is figured.

Tax escalator clause   A portion of the lease that allows the landlord to raise the rent in proportion to the tax increase on the building.

Variable costs   The costs that may change according to the number of clients served.

QUESTIONS

1. What type of supplies are completely used when giving the client a service?
2. What percentage of total sales should the operating supplies represent?
3. Name the communications link between the manufacturer, dealer, and the salon.
4. Is there usually a handling charge for C.O.D. supply orders?
5. True or false. The best way to accurately pay for supplies that are charged is to make your check out for the amount indicated on the statement.
6. Would you be smart to order enough supplies to last only 6 months?
7. Should you attempt to avoid product duplication?
8. Should a prospective employee arrive at 8:00 for an 8:00 appointment?
9. Should all employees in the salon order supplies?
10. True or false. An applicant for a new job should arrive a few minutes late so the salon owner will know the applicant's time is important, too.
11. Do variable costs remain the same?
12. Should a newly licensed person explain to the prospective employer that he/she likes to have Saturdays off?
13. Do fixed costs change, or do they remain the same?
14. What is the technical name for the description and analysis of the production, distribution, and consumption of goods and services?
15. What is the name for the point where supply and demand are equal?
16. If demand is too great for a particular thing, how can you reduce demand?
17. Does it make any sense for the salon owner to deduct the cost of the supply from the amount on which the operator's commission will be calculated?
18. Is the total amount of money taken into the salon called gross income?
19. True or false. Costs connected with doing business, such as supplies, are called expenses.
20. What are the abbreviations for the Federal Unemployment Tax Act, State Unemployment Tax Act, and the Federal Insurance Contribution Act?
21. For the Federal Insurance Contribution Act, what percentage of your share must the employer pay?
22. True or false. You must report all tips that exceed $20.00 per month.

23. Name two disadvantages to the salon owner of renting a styling station.

ANSWERS

1. Consumable supplies 2. 8 percent 3. Salesperson 4. Yes 5. False; on the invoice 6. No; 90 days 7. Yes 8. No; 15 minutes early 9. No 10. False; on or before the appointment 11. No 12. No 13. Remain the same 14. Economics 15. Equilibrium 16. Raise the price 17. Yes 18. Yes 19. True 20. FUTA, SUTA, and FICA 21. An equal percentage 22. True 23. a. Renter does not have to follow salon policies; b. salon equipment gets wear and tear, etc.

The Ethics of Cosmetology 31

How far could you get in life if you couldn't trust anyone? You could buy a burglar alarm to protect your house from robbers and count your change in the store to be sure that a cashier hasn't "cheated" you. There are laws against these kinds of actions, so you can call the police to catch a robber or report a dishonest salesperson.

You may have heard about the difference between the "letter of the law" and the "spirit of the law." This is what ethics really means. For instance, you have to trust that a doctor will give you the best medical treatment possible or that a pilot really knows how to fly a plane and handle it in an emergency. This is why ethics are important. All of us need to have faith in other poeple, that they will **act** ethically; in other words, that they will act **honestly** and in **good faith**. If you believe that most people act ethically, you will assume that a cashier gave you the wrong change by accident or that the person who got into your car was turning your lights off—and actually was doing you a favor. To put it another way, ethics help us have faith in people and give them the "benefit of the doubt" in a questionable situation.

Whenever you came across a new or important term in this textbook, you were given a formal definition of the term. As you may have figured out by now, a formal definition of ethics is almost a contradiciton in terms because ethics concerns the "spirit" of **your actions** at least as much as, if not more than, how your actions fit into a formal, legal pattern. But a formal definition spells things out and makes it clear what something is or does or what is expected of us. So, it is helpful and necessary.

Systems of ethics involve ways of judging human behavior and its effects. **Ethics** is involved with voluntary acts performed in a climate of knowledge and freedom of choice. What this means is that a person chooses to perform an act and that he or she should have the knowledge to judge whether or not he or she can perform it properly.

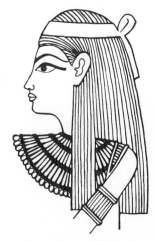

Egyptian—1350 B.C.

Professional Ethics

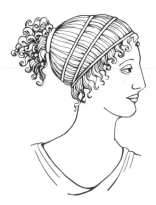

Greek—1000 B.C.–100 B.C.

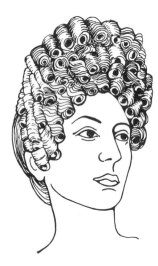

Roman—first century A.D.

Professions usually have boards or commissions that establish **codes of ethics. Professional ethics** are systems of rules that tell professionals how they should act when they offer their skills to the public. These boards or commissions can function on a state or national level, or both—for instance, the state and national bar associations and medical associations. These codes apply to all members of a profession. In cosmetology, state boards or commissions establish codes that all cosmetologists in the state must follow. You should be familiar with the code of ethics in your state.

Professional ethics are similar to ethics in general, but they are a little more clear-cut. If you think about it for a moment, the reason should be clear. If a salesperson lies to you about something that you buy or makes an honest mistake, you can get your money back; and at least in most cases, no harm is done. However, if you permanently damage a client's skin or hair, the damage cannot be repaired easily, if at all.

Another important point about professional ethics is what professions are all about. Professionals have knowledge and skill in very special fields that most people know little or nothing about. The general public is at the mercy of a professional. People need to have some kind of guarantee that they will be treated honestly and fairly. Thus, professional ethics protect the public. In this way ethics also help professionals by giving the public a reason to have faith in the profession.

There are three things that your client will expect from you as a professional cosmetologist.

Your **competence** involves the knowledge and information you learned as a student. However, cosmetology is a fast-moving profession. Things change rapidly. What was a "new" style 5 years ago might not even be used today. The "best" product in today's market might be considered "hopelessly old-fashioned" 10 years from now. Or 5 years from now scientists may discover that a chemical that they thought was safe has harmful side effects. Thus, you must keep up with advances in cosmetology. By presenting yourself to the general public and to your clients as a professional cosmetologist, you are saying that your knowledge and skills are up-to-date.

Responsibility comes down to a simple statement that you will recognize right away. It is the Golden Rule: Do unto others as you would have them do unto you. You want people to treat you responsibly, that is, to be reliable and to have integrity. Clients feel the same way. As a professional you are, and should be, expected to be honest and have a sincere concern about your work.

Having a desire to serve the public requires dedication and discipline. "The customer is always right" may be one way to look at dedication, but it might be even more important to think of your client as your friend. If your friend were "in a pinch" and needed help as a favor at the last minute, you would do everything possible to help. The same thing is true for a client who may need an appointment at a bad time or on short notice. Most clients will appreciate this kind of consideration and, like good friends, will be with you for a long time.

There is one important point to remember. Being a client's friend does not mean being chatty, gossipy, or too familiar. Clients expect to be treated in a courteous, professional manner. However, a client may tell you something personal—a problem, an interest, or a concern. Be a good friend. If your best friend told you something very personal, you wouldn't repeat it. The same thing is true for a client. Don't pry into your client's personal life, but if a client does mention something personal, keep it to yourself. By being a good friend to others, you are your own best friend.

Those things that will help you maintain professional standards and ethics toward your clients and the general public are listed below.

The Ethical Responsibilities to the Client and Public in General

Your responsibilities to clients are:

Give a full measure of service in the best interest of the client.

Learn new methods, receive new ideas, and improve techniques.

Render service on the basis of quality and price.

Make no charge for services that cannot be proved by valid evidence to be fair.

Refrain from false representation of services and misleading advertising.

Refrain from misrepresenting the type, quality, and manufacturer of products used in services.

Give the client, wherever possible, the benefit of the doubt in matters of differences.

Observe the rules of sanitation and hygiene set forth by law.

Refrain from discussing with one client the type of service rendered to another.

Hold as confidential personal matters entrusted by the client.

Render service in such a manner that a charge of gross negligence, incompetency, or misconduct would be unwarranted.

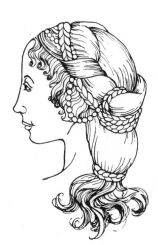

Renaissance—fifteenth century

Your responsibility to the general public is to do the following:

Place dedication to service before financial reward or other personal gain.

Stand ready to volunteer your special skills, knowledge, and training for the public welfare.

Endeavor to maintain a reputation in the community as an intelligent, honest, efficient, and courteous professional worthy of public trust.

See that those admitted to the practice of cosmetology are properly qualified by character, ability, and training, and that those who thereafter prove unworthy of these privileges are deprived of them.

Carry malpractice and public liability insurance.

Standards Among Professionals

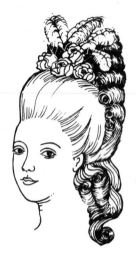

French—early eighteenth century

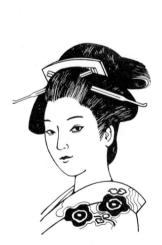

Japanese

You owe your colleagues and your employer the same ethical standards and practices that you owe your clients and the general public. These responsibilities are similar to those standards you offer to your clients, but they apply more specifically to the profession.

The most important thing to remember is that you are part of a "team." If you work in a salon with other cosmetologists, your work contributes to the salon's success or failure. So, getting along with the people you work with, working hard and conscientiously, being pleasant, and never downgrading your co-workers or employer helps make the salon a success. And that is something that benefits everyone.

The same thing is true if you work by yourself or are an employer. If you are an employer, making a pleasant atmosphere in your salon makes your employees feel important, and it encourages them to work well.

But even if you work all by yourself, you are in a "partnership" with other cosmetologists—even the one on the other side of town who is in "competition" with you for business. Have you ever heard a friend say "All lawyers are crooks" or "All car salesmen are crooks." If you ask him or her why he or she thought that way, the answer you get will probably be something like this: "This lawyer told me that the lawyer who was handling my father's estate was a crook, and I believed him. Then he . . . . " Or, "This salesman told me that he had had a chance to buy the car that the dealer down the street had interested me in, but that he had turned it down. He said it was a piece of junk. Then he showed me the same model car and offered to sell it to me for $100 less than the dealer down the street. But a week after I bought the car, I noticed that the . . . . "

It took one person one time to sour your friend on all lawyers, or salesmen–or cosmetologists. By running down the "competition" or charging ridiculously low—or high—prices, an entire profession lost a client. If you as a cosmetologist do this, every cosmetologist will lose.

The following list will give you guides for ethical conduct toward others in your profession.

Conducting yourself so that the spirit of fair dealing, cooperation, and courtesy shall govern relations between members of the profession.

Refraining from soliciting clients by offering services, through advertising or by other means, at a price below the range charged for like services by other professionals in the community.

Refraining from directly or indirectly offering employment to or hiring an employee of another salon. You may, however, negotiate with anyone who, of his or her own initiative or in response to public advertisement, applies for employment.

Refraining from advertising for help "with a following."

Refusing to endorse or permit the use of your name with publicity or advertising of cosmetic products made primarily for nonbeauty-salon consumption.

Refusing the use of your name in editorial or news items in which your professional knowledge is exploited to encourage self-application of a product or service.

Refraining from lending your talents to trade events of the industry that are not in the best interest of the profession.

Refraining from directly or indirectly, falsely or maliciously, discrediting the ability of a fellow cosmetologist or injuring his or her good name or reputation.

Keeping private any information given in confidence by a fellow cosmetologist in any matter of business and refraining from divulging or using it to the detriment of the informant.

Refraining from using an office in a professional organization for personal gain.

Refraining from performing any act tending to promote your own interests to the detriment of the profession or a professional organization.

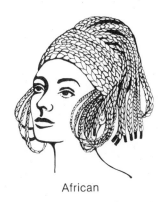

African

Responsibilities of the employer and employee to one another include the following:

Developing a mutual bond with employees that will result in reciprocal interest of employee and employer.

Assuming responsibility for the services rendered by the employee.

Instilling professional pride in the employee regarding the quality of performance.

Observing all wage and hour regulations—federal, state, and local.

Establishing salon charges that will permit a fair reward to the employee and employer.

Working with management and co-workers to maintain an attractive and sanitary establishment.

Taking pride in maintaining a good reputation for the establishment.

Providing financial incentives for the employees to increase their abilities, which results in gain for both the employee and employer.

Participating in training sessions provided by the employer.

Refraining from misrepresentation regarding conditions and permanency when advertising or offering employment.

Refraining from misrepresentation when accepting a position.

Giving reasonable notice when employment must be terminated.

Exerting reasonable effort to assist an employee who has not been dismissed "for cause" in securing employment elsewhere.

Encouraging attendance and participation in association activities.

Encouraging participation in civic, cultural, social, political, and religious organizations.

Responsibilities of the cosmetologist to the profession at large include the following:

Upholding the dignity and honor of the profession.

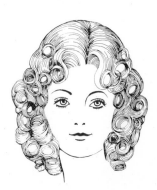

American

Affiliating with a unit of a recognized organization of the profession and contributing time, energy, and ability to it so that the profession may be advanced and ideals kept constant.

Safeguarding the profession so that only those qualified by education and good moral character may be admitted.

Lending one's best efforts in improving the educational standards of the profession.

Understanding and complying with laws, rules, and regulations of cosmetology, which contribute to the public health, welfare, and safety of the community; refraining from assisting others to evade these laws.

As we have discussed, the code of ethics goes beyond laws and regulations. Performing the art and science of cosmetology will be a stimulating and self-satisfying career only if you uphold both legal and ethical standards in an effort to serve the public interest.

State boards or commissions of cosmetology make up lists and codes of ethics that cosmetologists must follow. Check your state for the specific code that is used where you live. But more important, think of your friends. If you knew something special that could help your friend, would you use it selfishly to your own advantage by bending or twisting a rule? Of course not. The same thing is true when it comes to your clients and other professionals. Always deal ethically with others and you will be surprised at how many friends you will have in satisfied clients and co-workers. And you will have one friend you might not have even thought of—yourself.

GLOSSARY

Ethics System(s) of rules concerning voluntary acts performed in a climate of knowledge and freedom of choice. Professional ethics are systems of rules that tell members of a profession how they should act when they offer their skills to the public.

QUESTIONS

1. If you dislike someone you work with, should you say so to your clients?
2. Would it be reasonable for your employer to insist that you arrive for work 15 minutes before your first appointment?
3. Should you attend continuing education workshops—even though you have to pay for the ticket?
4. Should you tell your clients if you dislike your boss?
5. Are you practicing good ethics if you sell your clientele many services whether they need them or not?
6. What is it called when one acts honestly and in good faith?
7. Is ethical behavior a voluntary thing or mandatory?

8. What is the system of rules which tell professionals how they should act when they offer their skills to the public?
9. True or false. It is ethical to learn new methods, receive new ideas, and improve techniques.
10. Is it unethical not to carry malpractice insurance?
11. Is it ethical to gossip about your client?
12. Should you advertise cut-rate prices for services?
13. As a salon owner, should you set your prices so there is a fair reward to you and your employees?
14. Are you practicing ethics when you refrain from breaking laws formulated by your local city council?

ANSWERS

1. No 2. Yes 3. Yes 4. No 5. No 6. Ethics 7. Voluntary 8. Ethics 9. True 10. Yes 11. No 12. No 13. Yes 14. Yes

Relating Chemistry to Cosmetology 32

Chemistry is involved in all of the services a cosmetologist provides. A good cosmetologist should have a working knowledge of the basics of chemistry.

Have you ever had a course in chemistry or do you know someone who has? What was your impression? Difficult?

If you think chemistry is "hard," you are right—at least to a certain extent. Chemistry can be a very complicated field—some people spend many years learning to become chemists.

But before you think you are "in over your head," you should keep a few things in mind: (1) chemistry always has been an important part of cosmetology; (2) chemistry has become even more important in recent years because of new products that have been developed from complex chemical formulas; and (3) you or your friend may have had to study chemistry for no **particular** reason. It may have just been one of several courses you took along with English, history, and math. This situation is different. You will be able to apply what you know now. You have a **specific** reason for learning the basics of chemistry because you will use it while you are a student and later when you are a cosmetologist.

Does this mean that you must be a chemist? No! But it would be a good idea for you to learn the basic principles of chemistry that are explained in this chapter. Give this chapter a chance, and you will be surprised by how quickly you will learn the chemistry you need to know in your career. (Who knows? You may get really interested in chemistry once you see how it works in cosmetology.)

From time to time you may find that something is hard to understand. Stick to it! Chemistry can be difficult. But once you have gotten over this hump, you will have mastered a very important part of cosmetology.

Major Objective	Provided with the information in this chapter describe, define, and identify the basic principles of chemistry related to the practice of cosmetology.
Level of Acceptability	Score 75 percent or better on a multiple-choice exam on the information in this chapter.
Knowing Subobjectives	1. Define organic and inorganic chemistry, matter, substances, and the ways matter can be changed.
	2. Define elements, compounds, atoms, ions, and molecules.
	3. Define physical and chemical properties.
	4. Define the kinds of mixtures: solutions, colloids, and suspensions.
	5. Define acids, bases, salts, and pH.

KNOWING SUBOBJECTIVE 1

Define organic and inorganic chemistry, matter, substances, and the ways matter can be changed.

Chemistry   The first term you should know is chemistry. **Chemistry** is a science concerned with matter and the way it changes: This definition sounds simple, but the rest of this chapter will be devoted to showing just what this statement means.

Matter

It is a hot summer day. The room is "stuffy," so you walk over to the window and open it. A cool breeze blows in the window and the rooms feels much more comfortable. But now you are thirsty, so you go into the kitchen for a nice, cold glass of ice water. You turn on the faucet and watch the glass fill with water. Then you go to the refrigerator and put in a few ice cubes.

In these actions you have just come in contact with all 3 forms of **matter**. Matter is all around us—it is everywhere. In chemistry, **matter** is defined as anything that has **weight** and takes up **space**. The 3 forms of matter that you saw on that hot summer day are: **solid** (the ice cubes), **liquid** (the water), and **gas** (the air). A solid (ice cubes or powders) has definite shape and volume. A liquid (water or shampoos) has definite volume but indefinite shape. A gas (hydrogen peroxide evaporating) has indefinite shape and indefinite volume.

As a cosmetologist, you will work with all 3 forms of matter every day. You probably have already realized one category of matter you will work with: solid (a client's hair, fingernails, and skin). But the various products that you will use every day are other, maybe better, examples. They come in all forms—solids, liquids, and gases—and it is very important to know what kind of product you are using because they act differently.

Scientists usually talk about 2 branches of chemistry: organic and inorganic. Until a little over a hundred years ago, scientists defined **organic**

chemistry as the study of matter that comes from life processes; that is, it is either alive or once was. **Inorganic chemistry** is the study of matter that is not alive and never was.

There is an easy way to remember this distinction. You may have heard of the old phrase "animal, vegetable, or mineral." It is one way of saying all matter. **Animal** and **vegetable** describe everything that is or was alive. (In addition to obvious examples, this includes a wooden desk, which came from a tree, and the oil in your car—oil was formed millions of years ago from dead plants and animals.) The last part of that phrase, mineral, describes inorganic matter. Rocks and metals are examples of inorganic matter.

This difference between **organic** (living) and **inorganic** (nonliving) matter should be a convenient and useful one for your purposes, but keep in mind that it is not really this simple. Scientists have been able to make many combinations of organic matter in laboratories. So, the distinction between organic and inorganic is much more complicated than the difference between rocks and trees, but it should fit your purposes in most cases as long as you keep in mind that it is a useful working definition rather than one that is 100 percent accurate in a scientific sense.

Another important term is related to matter: **substance**. A substance is a unit or part of matter that has a particular set of qualities that define what it is. Elements and compounds are pure substances. In cosmetology, organic substances are usually used in cosmetics; however, they must also contain an **antioxidant** to prevent them from spoiling.

Substances can be changed in 2 ways. You make a physical change in a substance. If you do this, you may change the way it looks, but you **will not change its makeup**. For example, you may change the way an ice cube looks by letting it sit in the open air, but you will not change its makeup: it will be liquid water instead of frozen water, but it will still be water.

A **chemical change** is different. If you chemically change a substance, you destroy it. You will still have a substance, but it will be a new one. For example, when you combine hydrogen and oxygen, you create hydrogen peroxide, which is very different from either hydrogen or oxygen alone.

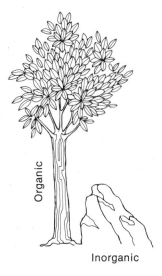

Organic

Inorganic

As you know, chemistry is a science that is concerned with the makeup and changes of both kinds of matter—**organic** and **inorganic**. **Organic chemistry** is concerned with combinations of carbon, especially one type called hydrocarbons, in matter. Most combinations of **carbons are organic**. They can be found in all types of living things (plants and animals) or products from living things, such as soft coal, petroleum, and natural gas. In general, carbons will burn and are soluble only in organic solvents, such as alcohol, not water.

Inorganic chemistry is concerned with the study of matter that does not have carbon in it. The simplest example is minerals. Many occur in nature, and scientists have learned how to make new combinations of inorganic matter. Some examples of inorganic matter would be sodium hydroxide, lead, silver, and water.

Chemistry—Organic and Inorganic

There are a few examples of inorganic matter that contain carbon. One is carbon dioxide, which is what you exhale when you breathe. Two others are diamonds and lead pencil.

Changing the Forms of Matter

Matter appears in nature in many shapes and forms. One of the achievements of science has been the way scientists have been able to show how matter changes and to make up new combinations of matter. There are two basic ways that the form of matter can be changed: physically and chemically.

You have already read about **physical changes** in this chapter. When you opened the window to let a cool breeze into your house, you created a physical change: you lowered the temperature inside the house. Another example of this kind of change is the ice cube in your glass. If your drink sits for awhile, the ice cube will melt. Heat caused the physical change.

Another way to cause a physical change is force, or pressure. If you dropped the ice cube on the floor or you smashed it into little chips, the ice cube's form would be changed: it is not an ice cube anymore.

These changes have one thing in common: the form of the matter is changed but not what makes it up. The ice cube is still water. Only its form has been changed.

Chemical changes are different. Matter is changed chemically when another kind of matter is added to or taken away from it. The result of a chemical change is something new and different. If you think of yourself as a "master chef," there may be many examples of very complicated combinations of chemicals right in your kitchen, in the seasonings you use. But even if you aren't, there is one simple example of a chemical change in almost everyone's kitchen: salt. Salt is made of sodium (a metal) and chlorine (a gas). They are two completely different kinds of substances, but when they are combined, the result is something completely different from either sodium or chlorine: sodium chloride (salt). This is a chemical change: what the substances actually are is changed. As you have probably guessed, the products you will use sometimes are very complicated combinations of chemicals.

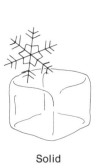
Solid

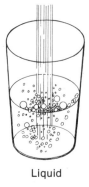
Liquid

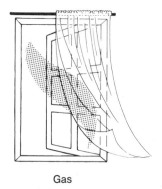
Gas

Heat also plays an important part in chemical changes. Some chemical changes need heat to take place. Others give off heat when they do take place.

There are two kinds of chemical changes: **synthesis** and **decomposition**. You will read more about these changes later in this chapter.

KNOWING SUBOBJECTIVE 2

Elements and Compounds   Salt is a simple combination of chemicals. This kind of combination is called a **compound**. Compounds can be very complicated, but all of them are made from **elements**.

Do you know how many letters there are in the alphabet? Of course, there are 26. And with only 26 letters we can make thousands of words. This is similarly true for elements. Elements are the basic units of substances. Although there are only 105 elements (92 can be found in the natural world; 13 have been created by scientists), they can be combined to form an almost limitless number of compounds.

At one time scientists thought that elements were the smallest kind of matter in creation. But later they learned differently. Elements are made up of atoms, which are much smaller than elements and cannot be seen by the unaided eye. An **atom** is the basic part of an element. An element, such as hydrogen or oxygen, has only **one kind** of atom.

An atom can be broken into smaller parts, but it is no longer an element. For example, if you broke up an atom of sodium, you would no longer have an atom of sodium. You would have a sodium **ion**.

Here is how it works. An atom has, basically, 3 kinds of particles—**protons, electrons, and neutrons**. Protons and electrons have power which scientists call an electrical charge. Protons have a positive (plus) charge and electrons have a negative (minus) charge. The core of the atom sometimes contains neutrons, which do not have a charge. Normally, an atom has the same number of positive and negative charges, so they balance each other off. When the number of protons and electrons is not equal, you have an ion. The number of electrons an atom has is what gives it the ability to combine with other atoms in chemical reactions.

Sometimes an atom gains an electron from an atom of another element. The atom that gained an electron is called a negatively charged ion (it has one more electron—negative charge—than proton). The atom that lost an electron is called a positively charged ion (1 more proton—positive charge—than electron).

This is the chemical process that goes into making a compound. Atoms gain or lose electrons and become joined to each other and form a molecule. This form is a compound. An atom is to an element what a molecule is to a compound. If you break up an atom of an element, you no longer have a compound.

Define elements, compounds, atoms, ions, and molecules.

The earlier example of salt will help you see this. Sodium and chlorine are the 2 elements in this compound. An atom of sodium gives up one of its electrons to an atom of chlorine. The result is 2 ions: 1 sodium, the other chlorine. The sodium ion does not have all of the characteristics of the element sodium because it is not a complete atom. The same thing is true for the chlorine. They form the compound sodium chloride, which is totally different. If you wanted to separate the sodium and chlorine, you would destroy the compound.

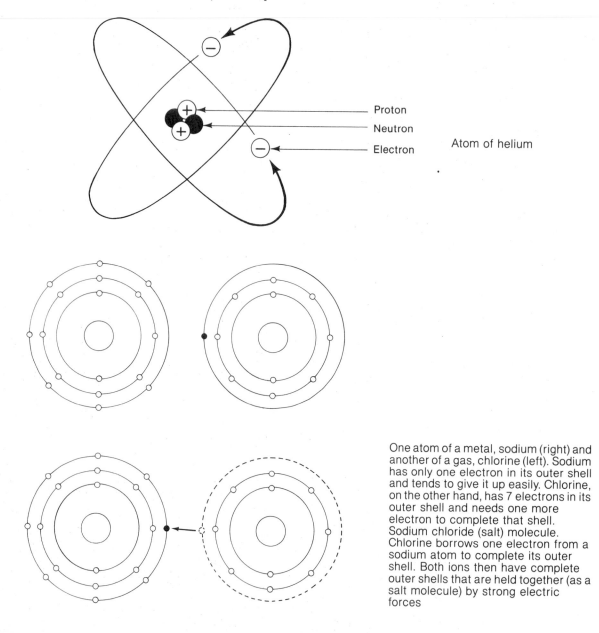

Proton

Neutron

Electron   Atom of helium

One atom of a metal, sodium (right) and another of a gas, chlorine (left). Sodium has only one electron in its outer shell and tends to give it up easily. Chlorine, on the other hand, has 7 electrons in its outer shell and needs one more electron to complete that shell. Sodium chloride (salt) molecule. Chlorine borrows one electron from a sodium atom to complete its outer shell. Both ions then have complete outer shells that are held together (as a salt molecule) by strong electric forces

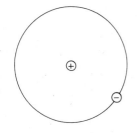

Hydrogen atom

(a)

Water molecule. Another way that atoms combine is by **sharing** electrons. In the water molecule, 2 atoms of hydrogen share their electrons with one atom of oxygen. The oxygen atom then has 8 electrons in its outer shell, and then each hydrogen atom has 2 electrons in its outer shell. In any atom the first shell can hold only 2 electrons and the second can hold only 8 electrons

(a)

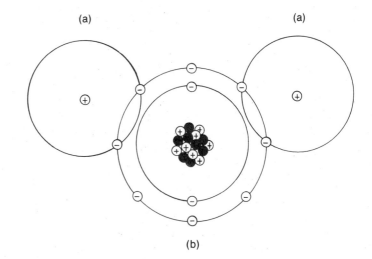

(a)

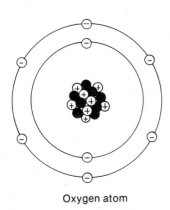

Oxygen atom

(b)

(b)

KNOWING SUBOBJECTIVE 3

The difference between physical and chemical changes is due to the **properties** of substances. The physical state of a substance is one of its properties. Others include its color and odor. Physical changes do not change the chemical makeup of a substance. They can be reversed.

A substance's **chemical properties** are the ways it reacts when it is combined with another substance. One chemical property of hydrogen is its ability to **attract** or draw oxygen atoms from other elements.

There are two kinds of chemical changes: synthesis and decomposition (or analysis). **Synthesis** involves the creation of a compound by combining elements of simpler compounds. **Decomposition** (or analysis) involves breaking down a compound into its parts.

Any chemical change results in a change in chemical energy. A chemical change is often more difficult to observe than a physical change, such as burning wood. But one example is the use of hydrogen peroxide. When you apply it to the hair, it gives up an atom (ion) of oxygen. The chemical formula for peroxide is H_2O_2. When it loses oxygen, it becomes water (H_2O).

Define physical and chemical properties.

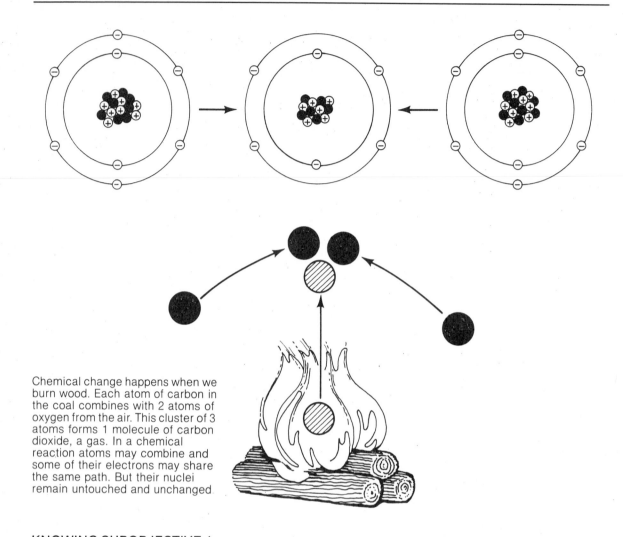

Chemical change happens when we burn wood. Each atom of carbon in the coal combines with 2 atoms of oxygen from the air. This cluster of 3 atoms forms 1 molecule of carbon dioxide, a gas. In a chemical reaction atoms may combine and some of their electrons may share the same path. But their nuclei remain untouched and unchanged.

KNOWING SUBOBJECTIVE 4

Define the kinds of mixtures: solutions, colloids, and suspensions.

Mixtures As you read earlier in this chapter, compounds are combinations of elements that are joined by chemical means. **Mixtures** are combinations of elements or compounds, or both, but there are different kinds of combinations. They are only joined **physically**. This means that the individual parts of a mixture keep their own properties and can be separated easily by physical or mechanical means. Face powders are mixtures. The human skin also has mixtures (the body contains water and various kinds of oils). They can take these forms: solid, liquid, or gas.

Types of Mixtures: Solutions, Colloids, and Suspensions

Because many important cosmetic preparations are mixtures, it is important to know the different kinds of mixtures. There are 3 kinds of mixtures: solutions, colloids, and suspensions.

Solutions   True **solutions** are **homogeneous mixtures** of 2 or more substances or compounds. This means that they have the same proportion of the elements or compounds that are in them throughout the mixture. At any place in a mixture that has 35 percent hydrogen, 35 percent oxygen, and 30 percent formaldehyde, you will find those percentages of ingredients. The particles are so small that they cannot be seen separately by looking at them through a microscope.

Two **examples** of **solutions** in different physical states are: (1) air—gases (oxygen, etc.) dissolved in a gas (nitrogen), and (2) formalin—gas (formaldehyde) dissolved in a liquid (water). Most solutions used in the salon are either liquids dissolved in other liquids or solids dissolved in liquids.

Two terms are important in the use of solutions. The particles are dissolved in the **solvent**. The particles that dissolve are called the **solutes (sahl-yoots)**. Water, alcohol, acetone, and glycerine are the most commonly used solvents in salon products, although many others can be solvents.

There can be 3 kinds of solutions, depending on the amount of solute used. **Dilute** solutions have only a small percentage of solute in them; **concentrated** solutions have a much larger percentage; and **saturated** solutions have as much of a solute as a solvent can dissolve at a particular temperature (heat can affect the ability of a solvent to dissolve a solute).

Colloids   **Colloids** are mixtures containing particles that are larger than those in a solution. They have only a **slight** tendency to settle.

The particles of the colloid are called **colloidal particles**; the substance in which the particles are distributed is called the **dispersing medium**. Colloids can be dispersed in substances in any of 3 physical states. Some colloids include:

1. liquid aerosol—a liquid dispersed in a gas
2. solid aerosol—a solid dispersed in a gas
3. liquid emulsion—a liquid dispersed in a liquid
4. sol—a solid dispersed in a liquid

It is especially important for you to know about **liquid emulsions**, since many preparations are in this form. Emulsions contain tiny droplets of one liquid suspended in another liquid. Salon emulsions are usually oil-in-water mixtures. If emulsions are allowed to stand, the 2 types of ingredients can separate into layers. However, the emulsions sold by cosmetics manufacturers usually contain an **emulsifying agent**, which breaks the oil into very small droplets and keeps them from coming together again. Thus, the agent forms a smoother, more stable mixture. Many salon creams and lotions are emulsions.

Suspensions   **Suspensions** are mixtures of a solid and a liquid or a solid and a gas. The solid particles in suspensions will **settle** out (separate) when the preparation is allowed to stand. Because of the large size of these particles, suspensions have a cloudy appearance.

KNOWING SUBOBJECTIVE 5

Define acids, bases, salts, and pH.

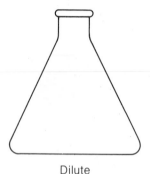

Dilute

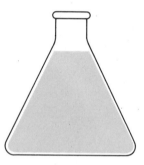

Concentrated

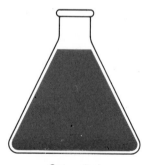

Saturated

Acids, Bases, Salts, and pH **Acids** and **bases** are compounds. They are used in many hair care products because their effects on the hair are predictable.

You can understand how acids and bases work by looking at the structure of compounds. As you read earlier in this chapter, an atom is the basic unit of an element and a molecule—a combination of atoms—is the smallest basic unit of a compound. An ion is a particle that has a charge. An ion has a "positive" or "negative" electric charge, depending on the makeup of the ion.

Cosmetologists are especially concerned with 2 types of ions: hydrogen and hydroxyl (hydroxide). **Hydrogen ions** are positively (+) charged particles (one or a group of atoms) of hydrogen. **Hydroxyl ions** are negatively (−) charged hydrogen ions that also have oxygen (hydroxyl radical). If a solution has more hydrogen ions than hydroxyl ions, it is an acid. If a solution has more hydroxyl ions than hydrogen ions, it is a base.

The term **pH** indicates the **concentration** (percentage) of hydrogen ions in a solution. This concentration determines if the solution has acidity (an acid) or alkalinity (a base). If a solution is not an acid, it is either a base or it is neutral. Solutions that have the **same concentration** of hydrogen and hydroxyl are **neutral** because the acid and the base balance each other.

The pH scale (0-14) shows the degree of acidity or alkalinity of a solution or substance. The middle of the scale, 7, is the neutral point. The numbers 0 to 6.9 indicate acidity; 7.1 to 14 represent alkalinity. (Refer to color plate 4.)

Certain substances, such as litmus paper, are **indicators**. They have a certain color in the presence of an acid and a different color in the presence of a base. You can use them to find out if a solution is alkaline or acid. There are many other kinds of indicators available from dealers.

When acids and bases react, they form a **salt**, plus water. This reaction is called **neutralization**. Salts contain both a metal and a nonmetal because salts are formed by a combination of an acid and a base. Some salts also contain oxygen.

Acid and alkaline products affect the hair differently. **Acid products** shrink and harden the imbrications (scales) of the shaft of hair. They also neutralize the alkalinity of hair products that have a pH over 7 (bases). Acid rinses, for example, are used to neutralize alkaline shampoos.

Alkaline products swell and soften the hair strand, opening the imbrications. Ammonia, for example, is an alkali that is used in permanent hair colors to open the imbrications of the hair so that the color molecules can pass into the inner layer of the hair. Alkaline products can neutralize acid products, but this is not a common application in cosmetology.

Skin and hair are acid. They have a pH of 4.5 to 5.5. Salon products that have a pH of 4.5 to 5.5 are said to be **acid-balanced in respect to skin and hair**. Thus, using an acid-balanced product does not change the natural pH of the skin or hair.

Acid   Any substance that has a pH rating under 7.

Alkaline   Any substance that has a pH rating of over 7.

Antioxidant   An additive to cosmetics which are made from organic substances to prevent spoilage.

Atom   The basic part of an element.

Chemical change   A change in a substance made by adding or removing another kind of matter.

Chemical properties   The way a substance behaves when it reacts to other substances, compounds, or forms of energy.

Chemistry   The study of matter and the way it changes.

Colloid   A mixture containing particles that are larger than those of a solution.

Compound   A chemical combination of elements.

Concentrated solutions   Solutions that have a large percentage of solute in them.

Dilute solutions   Solutions that have only a small percentage of solute in them.

Element   The basic unit of substances which are made up of atoms.

Emulsion   A mixture containing tiny droplets of one liquid suspended in another liquid.

Gas   One form of matter having indefinite shape and indefinite volume.

Inorganic chemistry   A branch of chemistry concerned with the study of matter which does not have carbons in it (inorganic substances).

Inorganic matter   Anything that is not or never has been alive.

Liquid   A form of matter which has definite volume but indefinite shape.

Matter   Anything that has weight and takes up space.

Mixture   A physical combination of elements or compounds or both.

Molecule   A combination of atoms that is the smallest basic unit of a compound.

Organic chemistry   A branch of chemistry concerned with combinations of carbons, especially hydrocarbons.

Organic matter   Anything that is or was once alive.

Physical change   A change in a substance made through the use of physical forces, such as a change in temperature or pressure.

Physical properties   Characteristics such as a substance's physical state, color, and odor.

Salt   A compound formed when acids and bases (alkalis) react.

Saturated solutions   Solutions that have as much of a solute as a solvent can dissolve at a particular temperature.

Solid   A form of matter having definite shape and definite volume.

Solute (SAHL-yoot)   The particles that are dissolved in a solvent, making a solution.

Solution   A homogeneous mixture of two or more substances or compounds.

Solvent   A substance that dissolves particles, making a solution.

Substance   A unit or part of matter that has a particular set of qualities that define what it is.

Suspension   A mixture of a solid and a liquid or a solid and a gas.

QUESTIONS

1. What is something that takes up space and has weight?
2. A rock would be an example of what kind of chemistry?
3. Studying a dead tree limb would be an example of what kind of chemistry?
4. The science concerned with matter and the way it changes is called what?
5. Are carbons organic?
6. Many elements joined chemically make what?
7. What is the science that deals with matter and the way it changes?
8. Does a solid have a definite shape and volume?
9. Does a liquid have a definite volume and a definite shape?
10. True or false. A gas has an indefinite shape and an indefinite volume.
11. Are elements and compounds pure substances?
12. What is made when different elements are added together?
13. What is the smallest and most basic part of an element?
14. Name the three particles found in an atom.
15. True or false. Breaking down a compound into its parts is known as decomposition.
16. True or false. When compounds are physically joined together, the result is called a mixture.
17. Give four examples of solvents used in the beauty salon.
18. Are hydrogen ions positively charged?
19. Are hydroxyl ions negatively charged?

ANSWERS

1. Matter 2. Inorganic 3. Organic 4. Chemistry 5. Yes 6. A compound 7. Chemistry 8. Yes 9. No; indefinite shape 10. True 11. Yes. 12. A compound 13. Atom 14. Protons, electrons, and neutrons 15. True 16. True 17. Water, acetone, alcohol, and glycerine 18. Yes 19. Yes

Anatomy and Physiology in Cosmetology: Bone Structures, Muscles and Nerves

33

Anatomy and physiology concern the structure and functions of the body. Bone structure, muscles, and nerves of the body often are involved in the services you will perform as a cosmetologist, so it is important that you understand the basics of these subjects.

Purpose

Provided with the information contained in this chapter and classroom instruction, define anatomy and physiology, and important bone structures, muscles, and nerves.

Major Objectives

Score 75 percent or better on a multiple-choice exam on the information in this chapter.

Level of Acceptability

1. Define the terms physiology and anatomy, describe physiological cells and tissues, and list systems of the body that affect school and salon services.
2. Define osteology and explain the structure and function of bones, cartilage, ligaments, joints, and synovial fluid.
3. Describe the major bones of the head, neck, trunk, arm, and hand.
4. Define myology; describe the functions of muscles and 3 types of muscles; and explain muscle contraction, origin, and insertion.
5. Describe the muscles of the head, face, trunk, and arm.
6. Define neurological terms and explain the division of the nervous system and the brain.
7. Explain the types and functions of nerves found in the head, face, neck, arm, hand, and fingers, and define the reflex arc.

Knowing Subobjectives

KNOWING SUBOBJECTIVE 1

Define the terms physiology and anatomy, describe physiological cells and tissues, and list systems of the body that affect school and salon services.

The study of the body may be broken into two very broad categories: **physiology**, which is the study of **body function**, and **anatomy**, which is the study of the **structure of the body**.

The study of physiology begins with the smallest, most basic unit of the body: the cell. Cells have several structures that you can see through a microscope. The outside of the cell is called the **cell membrane**. Inside is **cytoplasm** (SIGHT-ah-plaz-uhm), which is a jelly-like substance. The nucleus (NOO-klee-uhs) is like the brain (center) of the cell. It directs the cell's activities. When a cell becomes fully grown, it splits to make 2 cells from 1. The parent cell becomes 2 equal cells. The centrosome (SEN-treh-sohm) of the cell helps the cell divide.

Each cell of the body can take in nutrients (food) and grow. It does this for 3 reasons: for **energy**, for **growth**, and for **storage** to be used later. These functions are called **metabolism** (meh-TAB-eh-liz-uhm). **Anabolism** (ah-NAB-eh-liz-uhm) refers to processes that build up the cell, and the term **catabolism** (keh-TAB-eh-liz-uhm) describes those processes that supply energy.

A **tissue** is made up of thousands of similar cells that work together to accomplish a specialized function. You should be concerned with 4 types of tissue: connective, muscular, nervous, and epithelial.

Connective tissue binds, supports, protects, and nourishes the body. This type includes bone, cartilage, ligament, tendon, blood, and adipose (or fatty) tissue.

Muscular tissue forms the muscular system that gives the body the ability to **move**.

Nervous tissue makes up the nerves and brain. Nerve tissue is the body's communication system.

Epithelial (ep-eh-THEE-lee-ehl) **tissue** lines all the surfaces of the body.

An **organ** is made up of 2 or more different types of tissues **working together** to perform a particular function. The liver is an organ. A **group** of **organs** working together to accomplish a major function is a **system**.

Anatomical terms

superior	above, upper
inferior	below, lower
anterior	in front of, frontal
posterior	in back of, behind
medial	toward the midline of the body
lateral	away from the midline, toward the edge of the body
proximal	closer to center
distal	away from center

The systems of the body that have a **direct effect** on the practice of cosmetology include: **skeletal, muscular, nervous, vascular,** and **endocrine**. There are other systems, but you will not need to know them.

List Some Important
Systems of the Body

KNOWING SUBOJECTIVE 2

Ostelogy (ahs-tee-AHL-eh-jee) is the scientific study of **bone**. The bones of the body as a group are called the **skeletal system**.

The skeletal system is made up of 3 kinds of connective tissue—bone, ligament, and cartilage. The skeleton **protects** the **organs** of the body (such as the rib cage, which protects the heart and lungs), supports the body, and provides the leverage necessary for body movement.

Although bone is considered a living tissue (though it does contain non-living matter), it is both rigid enough to support the body and flexible enough to remain intact despite the jarring of everyday life. Living bone tissue is made up of cancellous and compact tissue.

Cancellous (spongy) tissue can be found at each end of the shafts of the **long bones**, such as the leg bones. It makes up most of the inside of the **flat bones**, such as those of the skull.

Compact, or **dense, bone tissue** makes up the shafts of the long bones and the outsides of the flat bones. Blood vessels pass through canals in this layer.

The **marrow** of the shafts of long bones is yellow, fatty tissue. Cancellous bones contain **red marrow**. All blood cells are produced in this red marrow.

Each bone is covered with a fiber known as the **periosteum** (per-ee-AHS-tee-uhm). It is an outer covering that forms new bone tissue, has blood vessels and nerves that go to the bone, and is where muscles, ligaments, and tendons attach to the bone.

Bones are held together by ligaments, cushioned by cartilage, and lubricated by the synovial fluid.

Cartilage is basically the same as bone tissue, but it does not contain inorganic matter. It has a smooth surface that protects the bones from stress. Bones normally rub together. Cartilage keeps this from being painful. Cartilage also aids in shaping the external features of the face, such as the ends of the nose and ear.

Ligaments (LIG-eh-mehnts) are bands or sheets of connective tissue that hold the bones together. They allow bones to move without slipping out of place.

The place at which 2 or more bones are joined is commonly called a joint. There are 3 kinds of joints: immovable (such as those in the skull), slightly movable (such as the spine), or freely movable (such as the knee).

The **synovial** (seh-NOH-vee-ahl) **fluid** is a special type of tissue that helps to lubricate and cushion the bones at the joints. It cuts down on friction and makes movement easier.

Define osteology and
explain the structure
and function of bones,
cartilage, ligaments,
joints, and synovial
fluid.

KNOWING SUBOBJECTIVE 3

Describe the major bones of the head, neck, trunk, arm, and hand.

The **skull** is the skeleton of the entire head. It protects the brain and gives the head its shape. Its major parts are:

Cranium   The bones that encase the brain. One of the 2 main parts of the skull.

Ethmoid (ETH-moid)   The upper part of the bony structure dividing the nasal cavity in half.

Frontal bone   The front of the skull, including the forehead, and the roof of the eye sockets.

Occipital (ahk-SIP-eh-tehl) bone   The rearmost bone of the skull and cranium.

Parietal (peh-RIGH-eht-ehl) bones   The top and sides of the cranium.

Sphenoid (SFEE-noid) bone   A butterfly-shaped bone located almost at the exact center of the head. It is a connecting bone.

Temporal bones   Form the bony part of the skull above and in front of the ears.

The face is the other main part of the skull. The bones of the face include:

Conchae or Turbinals   Located at the side walls of and protruding into the nasal cavity. Warms and cleans air.

Lacrimals (LAK-rih-mehlz)   On the inner sides of the eye sockets. They form the part of the canal through which the lacrimal **(tear)** duct joins the eye socket with the nasal cavity.

Mandible   Forms the entire lower portion of face and holds the teeth.

Maxillae (mak-SIL-ee)   The hard palate and lower portion of the eye sockets and the upper portion of the jaw.

Nasal bones   Shape the bridge of the nose.

Palatines (PAL-eh-tynes)   Part of the palate that forms the roof of the mouth.

Zygomaticus (zigh-goh-MAT-i-kus) or Malars (MAY-lahrz)   The outer, lower portion of the eye sockets and the cheekbones.

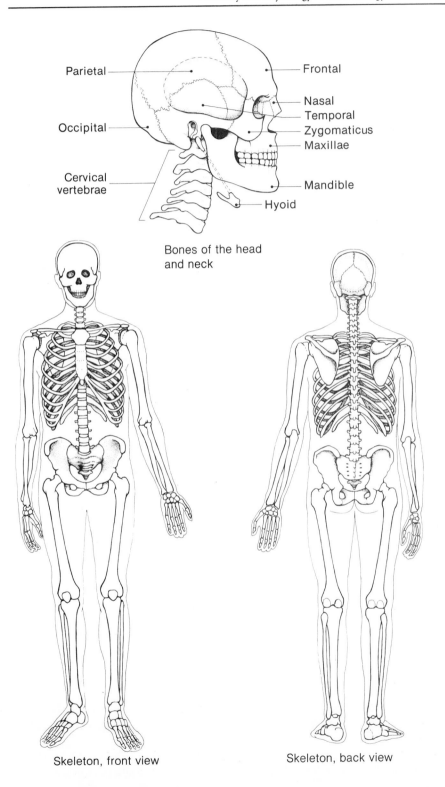

Parietal

Frontal

Occipital

Nasal
Temporal
Zygomaticus
Maxillae

Cervical
vertebrae

Mandible

Hyoid

Bones of the head
and neck

Skeleton, front view

Skeleton, back view

The bones of the neck and trunk are:

Cervical vertebrae (SER-vi-kehl VEHRT-eh-bray)   The first 7 cervical vertebrae are in the neck.

Hyoid (HIGH-oid)   U-shaped bone situated above the larynx (Adam's apple).

Ribs   A bony cage of 24 bones that protects the heart, lungs, and other organs.

Sternum (STEHR-nuhm)   The breastbone. The front attachment for the ribs.

The bones of the arm and hand include:

Carpals (CAHR-puhlz)   The bones of the wrist.

Clavicles (KLAV-i-kehlz)   The collarbones.

Humerus (HYOOM-eh-ruhs)   The large bone of the upper arm.

Metacarpals (met-ah-KAHR-puhlz)   The bones of the palm. They connect the wrist with the fingers in this order: first metacarpal (thumb); second metacarpal (index finger); third metacarpal (middle finger); fourth metacarpal (ring finger); fifth metacarpal (little finger).

Phalanges (FAY-lanj-eez)   The fingers (digits).

Radius (RAY-dee-uhs)   One bone of the forearm. It is on the thumbside.

Scapulae (SKAP-yeh-lee)   The shoulder blades.

Ulna (UHL-nah)   One of the 2 bones of the forearm. It is on the little-finger side.

KNOWING SUBOBJECTIVE 4

Define myology; describe the functions of muscles and 3 types of muscles; and explain muscle contraction, origin, and insertion.

Myology (migh-AHL-eh-jee) is the study of the muscular system, including both the muscles (over 500 of them) and the specialized connective tissue associated with them.

The term **muscle** refers to a bundle of elastic fibers surrounded by a tough membrane known as the **fascia** (FASH-yah). The fascia separates the muscles and helps to hold them in place. Muscles may vary in size, length, and shape according to their function and the area they affect. Muscle pressure on bones causes the body to move or results in body movement.

The cells that make up muscle tissue have: **extensibility** (ability to stretch); **contractibility** (ability to shorten); **elasticity** (ability to return to its original shape); and **excitability** (ability to respond to stimulus). In the muscular system this stimulus is provided by the nerves.

Three different types of muscle tissue are found in the body. They are striated, smooth, and cardiac muscles.

Striated (STRIGH-ayt-ed), also called voluntary muscle and skeletal muscle, looks striped if you look at it under a microscope. Its nerves come from the **cerebrospinal tract** of the **nervous system**. These muscles can be controlled by the individual.

Parts of the body that function automatically, such as the internal organs and the blood vessels, are lined with **smooth** (involuntary) muscles. The nerves in this kind of muscle come from a special branch of the nervous system known as the **autonomic** (awt-eh-NAHM-ik) **nervous system**.

Cardiac muscle tissue is found only in the heart. It has some of the characteristics of both of the other types. It is the **only type** of muscle tissue that can **contract on its own** at regular intervals at all times. It is influenced by the autonomic nervous system.

You cannot move if your muscles do not contract. Absolutely all bodily movements result from the contraction of 1 or more muscles.

Muscle is attached to the skeleton at 2 points. One is called the **origin**, or **proximal**, point; the other is called the **insertion**, or **distal**, point. The proximal point is **closer** to the center of the body than the distal point. When a muscle is relaxed, it has a certain length and width. When it is stimulated, it contracts and becomes shorter and thicker, and the 2 points of the muscle come closer together. When the muscle contracts, the insertion moves much more than the origin. Thus, it contracts from the origin to the insertion, and back again.

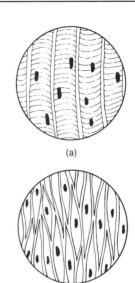

(a)

(b)

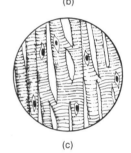

(c)

Types of muscle tissue:
(a) striated, (b) smooth,
(c) cardiac

KNOWING SUBOBJECTIVE 5

When you massage a client's head and face, the following muscles are affected:

Buccinator (BUK-si-nay-tehr)   From the mandible and maxilla to the orbicularis oris muscle and skin of lips. Draws in the cheeks.

Corrugator (kor-uh-GAY-ter)   (Named for its zigzag edge.) On the frontal bone between the eyebrows to middle of the eyebrow. Draws eyebrows together and down.

Depressor anguli (AN-gyoo-ligh) oris triangularis   From the mandible to the lower corner of the mouth.

Describe the muscles of the head, face, trunk, and arm.

Depressor labii inferioris (de-PRES-ehr LAY-bee-eye in-FIHR-ee-or-iss) From the mandible to the lower lip. Lowers the corner of the mouth.

Epicranius (ep-i-KRA-nee-uhs) The epicranius muscle has 2 bellies of muscle joined by a sheet of connective tissue, called an **aponeurosis** (ap-oh-noo-ROH-siss). The 2 bellies are called the **frontalis** and the **occipitalis**.

Frontalis (fruhn-TAL-iss) Along the eyebrows to the aponeurosis. Raises the eyebrows and wrinkles the forehead.

Levator anguli oris ("corner-of-the-mouth raiser") Muscles of the upper lip that raise the angle of the mouth.

Levator labii (le-VAT-ehr LAY-bee-igh) superioris From the maxilla to the upper lip. Raises the upper lip.

Levator palpebrae superioris (li-VAH-tehr PAL-peh-bree soo-PEHR-ee-or-is) The margin of optic foramen to the upper eyelid. Raises the upper eyelid.

Masseter (mah-SEET-ehr) From the bony prominence in front of the ear to the angle of the jaw. Used to clench the teeth.

Mentalis (men-TAL-iss) From the point of the chin to the skin of the chin. Used to pout.

Nasalis (nas-SAL-iss) Muscles of the nose. They can be used to wrinkle the nose.

Occipitalis (ohk-sip-eh-TAL-iss) From the occipital bone to the aponeurosis. Draws the scalp backward.

Orbicularis oculi (or-bik-yool-LAY-riss AHK-yeh-eye) Bands of circular muscle in the eye socket. Closes the eyelids.

Orbicularis oris (or-bik-yoo-LAY-riss OH-riss) Muscles surrounding and running into the lip. Used to pucker.

Platysma (pla-TIZ-mah) From the chest to the entire length of the mandible. Pulls the corner of the mouth down.

Risorius (ri-SAH-ri-uhs) Subcutaneous tissue to the skin at corner of mouth. Used to smile.

Temporalis (tem-peh-RA-liss) The flat part of the side of the head above the ear to the mandible. Used to bite.

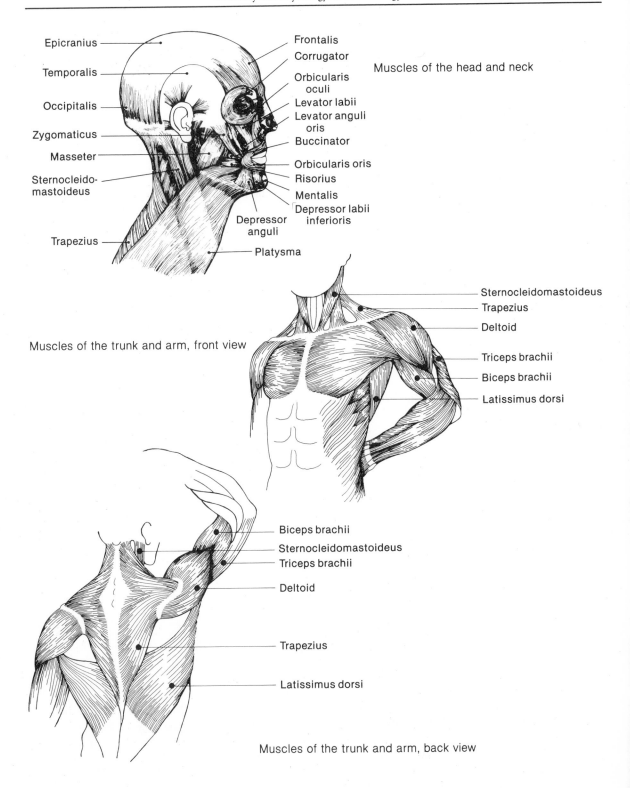

Epicranius

Temporalis

Occipitalis

Zygomaticus

Masseter

Sternocleido-
mastoideus

Trapezius

Frontalis

Corrugator

Orbicularis
oculi

Levator labii

Levator anguli
oris

Buccinator

Orbicularis oris

Risorius

Mentalis

Depressor labii
inferioris

Depressor
anguli

Platysma

Muscles of the head and neck

Muscles of the trunk and arm, front view

Sternocleidomastoideus

Trapezius

Deltoid

Triceps brachii

Biceps brachii

Latissimus dorsi

Biceps brachii

Sternocleidomastoideus

Triceps brachii

Deltoid

Trapezius

Latissimus dorsi

Muscles of the trunk and arm, back view

Zygomaticus (zigh-goh-MAT-i-kuhs) major From the zygomatic bone to the corner of the orbicularis oris muscle. Draws the angle of the mouth back and up.

The trunk muscles include:

Latissimus dorsi (la-TIS-seh-muhs DOR-sigh) Lower half of the thoracic vertebrae, all lumbar vertebrae, illiac crest to the humerus. Draws arm to the body and rotates the arm outward.

Sternocleidomastoideus (ster-noh-KLYE-doh-mas-toyd-ee-ahs) From the clavicle and sternum to the bony prominence behind the ear. Flexes head toward the shoulder of 1 side and turns the face to the opposite side.

Trapezius (tra-PEE-see-uz) Muscles covering occipital bone, vertebrae of neck and throat to the clavicle and scapulae. And rotates should blades and draws head backwards or to one side.

The main muscles of the arm are:

Biceps brachii (BIGH-seps BRAK-ee-igh) From the scapula to the radius and the aponeurosis in the forearm. Flexes the forearm.

Deltoid (DEL-toyd) From the clavicle and scapula to the humerus. Extends and rotates the arm.

Triceps brachii (TRIGH-seps BRAK-ee-igh) From the scapula and back of humerus to the ulna. Extends the forearm.

KNOWING SUBOBJECTIVE 6

Define neurological terms and explain the divisions of the nervous system and the brain.

Neurology (noo-RAHL-eh-jee) describes the study of the nervous system. The nervous system covers all of the body and enables the parts of the body to communicate.

The basic structural unit of the nervous system is called the **neuron (NOO-rahn)**. It is composed of a cell body: the **axon (AK-sahn)**, which carries nervous impulses away from the cell body, and the **dendrite(s) (DEN-dright)**, which carries impulses to the cell body.

A single nerve contains many neurons and may vary in diameter from microscopic to almost the size of a clothesline.

Sensory, or **afferent**, neurons carry nervous impulses such as smell, hearing, sight, taste, and touch toward the brain. **Motor**, or **efferent**, neurons carry nervous impulses away from the brain to the body.

The nervous system is divided into 3 units—**central**, **peripheral**, and **autonomic**.

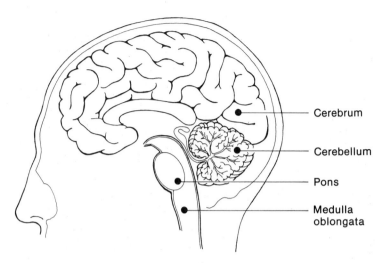

Main parts of the brain

The **central nervous system** is the brain and spinal cord. It carries all of the incoming and outgoing messages of the body.

The **peripheral nervous system** refers to all nerves branching into the body from the central nervous system.

The **autonomic (or automatic) nervous system** controls all automatic processes, such as circulation, digestion, and respiration. Although the autonomic nervous system is physically part of the central and peripheral system, it operates as a separate unit.

The autonomic nervous system is subdivided into the **sympathetic** and the **parasympathetic** nervous systems. The parasympathetic nervous system controls quiet activities, such as digestion, while the sympathetic nervous system controls reactions to stress, such as fear.

The four major parts of the brain are:

Cerebrum (seh-REE-bruhm)   The large, uppermost portion of the brain. It receives and interprets sensory and motor information. It controls memory and reasoning.

Cerebellum (ser-eh-BEL-uhm)   It is inside the occipital bone. It makes coordinated movement possible.

Pons (PAHNZ)   It is a relay station between the spinal cord, the cerebrum, and the cerebellum.

Medulla oblongata   Some of the parasympathetic and sympathetic nerves start here. It regulates some of the activities controlled by the autonomic nervous system.

KNOWING SUBOBJECTIVE 7

Explain the types and functions of nerves found in head, face, neck, arm, hand, and fingers, and define the reflex arc.

In addition to the brain, portions of the nervous system that are of interest to the cosmetologist include the 12 pairs of cranial nerves. The cranial nerves start in the brain. They reach and affect the head, face, and neck. You should be concerned with these:

The **fifth cranial** (also called **trifacial** or **trigeminal** [trigh-JEM-in-nal]) is a mixed nerve; its motor impulses control chewing, while its sensory neurons carry impulses from the face. The major branches of the trigeminal nerve include:

Ophthalmic (ahf-THAL-mik) branch   Sensory to the skin of the forehead, eyes, and nose. The **supratrochlear** (soo-prah-TROK-lee-ar) nerve, which is involved in facial massage, is part of the ophthalmic branch.

Maxillary (MAK-seh-ler-ee) branch   Sensory to the skin covering the maxillae. The **nasal nerve**, which is involved in facial massage, is a subdivision of the maxillary branch.

Mandibular (man-DIB-yeh-lehr) branch   Sensory to the skin covering the mandible and the teeth of the lower jaw, and motor to the muscles of chewing. The **auriculotemporal** (aw-RIK-yeh-loh-TEM-peh-rehl) and **mental nerves**, which are involved in facial massage, are part of this branch.

The **seventh** cranial, or facial, nerve is the main motor nerve of the face. It is sensory to **taste**.

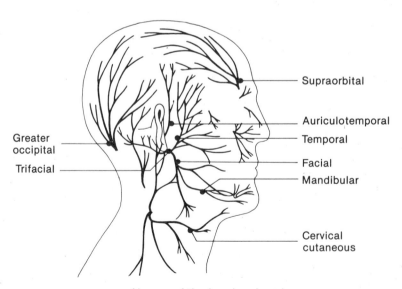

Nerves of the head and neck

The **eleventh** cranial nerve (or **accessory**, or **spinal accessory** is the motor nerve that serves the sternocleidomastoideus and the trapezius muscles, both of which are found in the trunk.

Supplying nerves to the back of the head and neck are the cervical nerves emerging at the neck.

The nerves that supply the arm and hand include the:

Ulnar   It starts on the little-finger side of the forearm and goes to that side of the hand and forearm.

Radial   It starts on the thumb side of the arm and goes to the back of the arm and the back and lateral sides of the forearm and hand.

Median   It is very deep in the arm and goes to the middle portion of the forearm and hand.

Musculocutaneous (MUHS-kyoo-loh-kyoo-TAY-nee-uhs)   It is in the muscles of the anterior arm and goes to those muscles (i.e., the biceps, etc.) that flex the forearm.

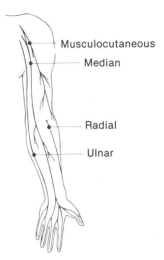

Nerves of the arm and hand—anterior view, palm

Branches of the nerves supply the **phalanges** (fingers), at which point they are called the **digital nerves**.

The simplest nerve pathway an impulse can travel is the **reflex arc**. It brings together information to which one responds automatically. For example, the reflex arc causes you to pull away from a hot stove.

Afferent (AF-eh-rent) neurons   See **Sensory neurons**.

Anabolism (ah-NAB-eh-liz-uhm)   The processes of building up the cell.

Anatomy   The study of the structure of the body.

Aponeurosis (ap-oh-nyoo-ROH-siss)   A connective tissue that joins two muscles.

Auriculotemporal (aw-RIK-yeh-loh-TEM-peh-rehl)   A subdivision of the mandibular branch of the fifth cranial nerve involved in facial massage.

Autonomic (aw-teh-NAHM-ik) nervous system   The portion of the nervous system that controls a person's automatic functions, such as breathing, heartbeat, etc.

Axon (AK-sahn)   The part of the neuron that carries impulses away from the cell body.

Biceps brachii (BIGH-seps BRAK-ee-igh)   A muscle that flexes the forearm.

Buccinator (BUK-si-nay-tehr)   A muscle that draws the cheeks in and is used to suck.

Cancellous (KAN-seh-luhs) tissue   The spongy tissue found at each end of the shafts of the long bones and inside the flat bones.

Carpals (KAHR-puhlz)   The bones of the wrist.

Cartilage (KAHR-tah-lij)   A tissue similar to bone tissue that protects the bones from stress; acts like a cushion for bones.

Catabolism (keh-TAB-eh-liz-uhm)   The processes that supply energy to the body.

Cell   The basic unit of the body. The entire body structure is made of cells.

Cell membrane   The outside of the cell.

Central nervous system   The brain and the spinal cord.

Centrosome (SEN-treh-sohm)   The part of the cell that helps the cell divide and reproduce.

Cerebellum (ser-eh-BEL-uhm)   The portion of the brain inside the occipital bone that makes coordinated movement possible.

Cerebrum (seh-REE-bruhm)   The large, uppermost portion of the brain that receives and interprets sensory and motor information and controls memory and reasoning.

Cervical vertebrae (SER-vi-kehl VEHRT-eh-bray)   The 7 bones in the back of the neck. The first 2 of these enable the head to move.

Clavicles (KLAV-i-kehlz)   The 2 bones commonly called the collar-bones.

Compact bone tissue   The tissue that makes up the shafts of long bones and the outside of flat bones. Blood vessels are contained in this layer.

Conchae   The bones located at the side walls of the nasal cavity and protrude into it.

Connective tissue   Tissue that binds, supports, or helps protect the body, such as bone, cartilage, ligament, tendon and fat tissue.

Corrugator (kor-uh-GAY-tehr)   The muscle between the eyebrows that draws the eyebrows down and together.

Cranial nerves   The 12 pairs of nerves that start in the brain and reach and affect the head, face, and neck.

Cranium   The bones that encase the brain.

Cytoplasm (SIGHT-ah-plaz-uhm)   A jelly-like substance within the cell membrane that contains the nucleus of the cell.

Deltoid (DEL-toyd)   A muscle that extends and rotates the arm.

Dendrite (DEN-dright)   The part of the neuron that carries impulses to the cell body.

Depressor anguli oris (di-PRES-ehr AN-gyoo-ligh OR-iss)   A muscle that depresses the corner of the mouth and is used to frown. Also called the triangularis.

Depressor labii inferioris (di-PRES-ehr LAY-bee-igh in-FIHR-ee-or-iss)   The muscle that lowers the lower lip.

Digital nerves   Branches of the arm nerves that serve the fingers.

Distal point   See **Insertion.**

Efferent (EF-eh-rent) neurons   See Motor neurons.

Eleventh cranial nerve   The motor nerve that serves the sternocleidomastoideus and trapezius muscles. Also called the accessory or spinal accessory.

Epicranius (ep-i-KRA-nee-uhs)   A two-part muscle joined by a sheet of connective tissue. The two parts are the frontalis and the occipitalis.

Epithelial (ep-eh-THEE-lee-ehl) tissue   The tissue that lines all the surfaces of the body.

Ethmoid (ETH-moid) bone   The bone that forms the upper part of the bony structure dividing the nasal cavity in half.

Facial nerve   See **Seventh cranial nerve.**

Fascia (FASH-yah)   A tough membrane that separates the muscles and helps to hold them in place.

Fifth cranial nerve   The nerve that controls chewing and carries impulses from the face. Also called the trifacial or trigeminal nerve.

Frontal bone   The bone that forms the front of the skull.

Frontalis (fruhn-TAL-iss)   The muscle along the eyebrows that raises the brows and wrinkles the forehead. Part of the epicranius muscle.

Humerus (HYOOM-eh-ruhs)   The large bone of the upper arm.

Hyoid (HIGH-oid)   The U-shaped bone above the larynx to which the muscles of the tongue are attached.

Insertion   The point of muscle attachment that is farthest away from the center of the body. Also called the distal point.

Joint   The place where two or more bones are joined.

Lacrimal (LAK-ri-mehl) bones   The 2 bones on the inner sides of the eye sockets.

Latissimus dorsi (la-TIS-seh-muhs DOR-sigh)   A muscle that draws the arm in toward the body, extends the elbow to the back, and rotates the arm outward.

Levator anguli oris (li-VAT-ehr AN-gyoo-ligh OR-iss)   The muscle that raises the corner of the mouth.

Levator labii superioris (li-VAT-ehr LAY-bee-igh soo-PIHR-ee-or-iss)   The muscle that raises the upper lip.

Levator palpebrae superioris (li-VAT-ehr PAL-peh-bree soo-PIHR-ee-or-iss)   The "upper-eyelid raiser."

Ligaments (LIG-eh-mehnts)   Bands or sheets of connective tissue that hold the bones together.

Malar (MAY-lahr) bones   See **Zygomatic bones.**

Mandible (MAN-deh-behl)   The jawbone.

Mandibular (man-DIB-yeh-lehr) nerve branch   A part of the fifth cranial nerve that is sensory to the skin covering the mandible and the teeth of the lower jaw, and motor to the muscles of chewing.

Marrow   A yellow or red fatty tissue found in the shafts of long bones that produces the blood cells.

Masseter (mah-SEET-ehr)   A muscle of the jaw used to clench the teeth.

Maxillae (mak-SIL-ee)   The 2 bones that, together with the palatines, form the hard palate. They also form the lower portion of the eye sockets and the upper portion of the jaw.

Maxillary (MAK-seh-ler-ee) nerve branch   A branch of the fifth cranial nerve sensory to the skin covering the maxillae.

Median nerve   One of the nerves of the forearm and hand.

Medulla oblongata (meh-DUHL-ah ahb-lon-GAHT-ah)   The part of the brain that regulates some of the activities controlled by the autonomic nervous system.

Mentalis (men-TAL-iss)   A chin muscle that makes the lower lip protrude; used to frown.

Metabolism (meh-TAB-eh-liz-uhm)   The processes of taking in nutrients and processing them for use in the body.

Metacarpals (met-ah-KAHR-puhlz)   The 5 bones of the palm.

Motor neurons   The neurons that carry impulses away from the brain. Also called efferent neurons.

Muscular tissue   The tissue that forms the muscles.

Muscle   A bundle of elastic fibers surrounded by fascia that enables the body to move.

Musculocutaneous (MUHS-kyoo-loh-kyoo-TAY-nee-uhs)   One of the nerves of the arm.

Myology (migh-AHL-eh-jee)   The study of the muscular system.

Nasal bones   The 2 bones that shape the bridge of the nose.

Nasal nerve   A part of the maxillary branch of the fifth cranial nerve involved in facial massage.

Neurology (noo-RAHL-eh-jee)   The study of the nervous system.

Neuron (NOO-rahn)   The basic structural unit of the nervous system composed of the axon and the dendrite(s).

Nervous tissue   The tissue that makes up the nerves and brain.

Nucleus (NOO-klee-uhs)   The center of the cell. The portion of the cell that directs the cell's activities.

Occipital (ohk-SIP-eh-tehl)   The rearmost bone of the skull.

Occipitalis (ohk-sip-eh-TAL-iss)   The muscle that draws the scalp backward. Part of the epicranius muscle.

Ophthalmic (ahf-THAL-mik) nerve branch   A branch of the fifth cranial nerve sensory to the skin of the forehead, eyes, and nose.

Orbicularis oculi (or-bik-you-LAY-riss AHK-yeh-lye)   The bands of circular muscle in the eye socket that close the eyelids.

Orbicularis oris (or-bik-yoo-LAY-riss OH-riss)   A circular band of muscle surrounding the mouth that causes the lips to pucker.

Origin   The point of muscle attachment that is closest to the center of the body. Also called the proximal point.

Osteology (ahs-tee-AHL-eh-jee)   The scientific study of bone.

Palatines (PAL-eh-tynes)   The 2 bones that form part of the hard palate, which is the back portion of the roof of the mouth.

Parasympathetic (par-eh-sim-peh-THET-ik) nervous system   The part of the autonomic nervous system that controls quiet activities, such as digestion.

Peripheral (peh-RIF-eh-rehl) nervous system   All nerves branching into the body from the central nervous system.

Parietal (peh-RIGH-eh-tull)   The bones that form the top and sides of the skull.

Periosteum (per-ee-AHS-tee-uhm)   The outer fiber covering of the bone that connects the bone to muscles, ligaments, and tendons.

Phalanges (FAY-lanj-ez)   The bones of the fingers.

Physiology   The study of body function.

Pia mater (PYE-ah MAYT-ehr)   One of the three membrane layers that cover the brain; the layer in direct contact with the brain.

Platysma (pla-TIZ-mah)   A muscle that pulls the corner of the mouth down; used to frown.

Pons (Pahnz)   The part of the brain that serves as a relay station between the spinal cord, the cerebrum, and the cerebellum.

Pronate (PROH-nayt)   To rotate outward.

Proximal point   See **Origin**.

Radial nerve   One of the nerves of the arm.

Radius (RAYD-ee-uhs)   The bone of the forearm located on the thumb side.

Reflex arc   The simplest of the nerve pathways a nerve impulse can travel.

Ribs   The 24 bones of the chest that protect the heart, lungs, and other internal organs.

Risorius (ri-SAH-ri-uhs)   A mouth muscle that is used to smile.

Scapulae (SKAP-yeh-lee)   The 2 bones that, with the clavicles, hold the arm in place. Commonly called the shoulder blades.

Sensory neurons   The neurons that carry impulses toward the brain. Also called afferent neurons.

Seventh cranial nerve   The main motor nerve to the face, also sensory to taste.

Skeletal system   All the bones in the body.

Smooth muscles   The type of muscle tissue that makes up the involuntary muscle system and is not under control of the individual, such as the muscles of internal organs. Called smooth because under a microscope this tissue looks smooth.

Sphenoid (SFEE-noid) bone   A butterfly-shaped bone located almost at the center of the head.

Sternocleidomastoideus (ster-noh-KLYE-doh-mas-toid-ee-uhs)   A muscle that flexes the head toward the shoulder on the same side and turns the face to the opposite side.

Sternum (STEHR-nehm)   The breastbone, located in the center of the chest.

Striated (STRIGH-ay-tehd) muscle   Muscle that is controlled by the individual, such as the arm or leg muscles. Called striated because under the microscope this tissue looks striped.

Supinate (SOO-pih-nayt)   To rotate inward.

Supratrochlear (soo-pra-TROK-lee-ar) nerve   A nerve that is part of the ophthalmic branch of the fifth cranial nerve and is involved in facial massage.

Sympathetic (sim-peh-THET-ik) nervous system   The part of the autonomic nervous system that reacts to stress, such as fear.

Synovial (seh-NOH-vee-ahl) fluid   A tissue that helps lubricate and cushion the joints.

System   A group of organs working together to accomplish a major function of the body.

Temporal bones   The bones that form the bony part of the skull around the ears.

Temporalis (tem-peh-RAH-liss)   A muscle on the side of the head used for biting.

Tissue   A group of similar cells that work together to accomplish a specialized function.

Trapezius (tra-PEE-zee-uhs) A muscle that draws the head back and to the side, raises the shoulder, and rotates the shoulder blades.

Triceps brachii (TRIGH-seps BRAK-ee-eye) A muscle that extends the forearm.

Trifacial nerve See **Fifth cranial nerve.**

Trigeminal (trigh-JEM-i-nal) nerve See **Fifth cranial nerve.**

Turbinals See **Conchae.**

Ulna (UHL-nah) The bone of the forearm on the little-finger side.

Ulnar nerve One of the nerves of the arm.

Zygomatic (zigh-goh-MAT-ik) bones The 2 bones that form the outer, lower portion of the eye sockets and the cheekbones.

Zygomaticus (zigh-goh-MAT-i-kuhs) major A muscle that draws the angle of the mouth backward and upward.

QUESTIONS

1. Define physiology.
2. Name the term that describes the overall structure of the body.
3. What is the outside of the cell called?
4. Define cytoplasm.
5. The cycle of cell energy, growth and storage is called what?
6. What is tissue?
7. Can you define connective tissue?
8. What is epithelial tissue?
9. When two or more different types of tissues work together to do a certain function, what term applies here?
10. When a group of organs work together to do a major function, what term applies?
11. What is the scientific name for the study of bones?
12. Is the cranium located in the head?
13. Does synovial fluid lubricate body joints where the bones meet?
14. Does the mandible form the lower jaw?
15. What is the scientific study of muscles called?
16. Is the deltoid muscle located in the forehead?
17. Where is the occipital bone located?

ANSWERS

1. Physiology is the study of the function of the body. 2. Anatomy. 3. Cell membrane. 4. Cytoplasm is the jelly-like inside of the cell. 5. Metabolism. 6. Tissue is a group of similar cells that perform a specialized function. For example, muscle tissue is made up of the same cells. 7. Connective tissue binds, supports, protects, and nourishes the body. 8. The tissue that covers the surfaces (outside coverings) of the body. 9. Organ. 10. System. 11. Osteology. 12. Yes. 13. Yes. 14. Yes. 15. Myology. 16. No; the arm. 17. The head.

Anatomy and Physiology in Cosmetology: The Vascular System and the Endocrine System

34

Blood circulates through the body through the **vascular system**. Services involving massage, heat, chemicals, and light therapy increase blood circulation, so it is important to have a basic knowledge of this system.

Purpose

Provided with the information in this chapter and classroom instruction, define, describe, and classify the parts of the vascular system of the body.

Major Objective

Score 75 percent or better on the information in this chapter.

Level of Acceptability

1. Define angiology and identify the 3 subdivisions of the vascular system, the parts and functions of the heart and blood vessels, and the function of pulmonary circulation.
2. Identify arteries and veins of the head, face, neck, arm, and hand, and describe the composition of blood and the lymphatic system.
3. Define the endocrine system and its 5 major glands.

Knowing Subobjectives

KNOWING SUBOBJECTIVE 1

Define angiology and identify the 3 subdivisions of the vascular system, the parts and functions of the heart and blood vessels, and the function of pulmonary circulation.

Angiology (an-jee-AHL-eh-jee) is the study of the vascular system, which includes the **circulatory system** and the **lymphatic system**.

The **circulatory system** consists of the **heart** and **blood vessels**. It brings food and oxygen to all cells of the body, removes the waste and carbon dioxide from the cells, guards the body against infection, and regulates body temperature.

Unlike the circulatory system, the **lymphatic** (lim-FAT-ik) **system** circulates fluids in only one direction—from the tissues **toward the heart**. The open-ended vessels of the lymphatic system collect a fluid that comes from the blood and returns it to the general circulation.

The heart is a major part of the circulatory system. It is made up of cardiac muscle tissue and is about the size of a closed fist. It is located in the chest cavity, between the lungs, and is surrounded by a tough membranous sac called the **pericardium** (per-eh-KAHRD-ee-uhm), meaning **surrounding the heart**.

The heart is divided into four chambers—two upper chambers, or **auricles** (AWR-i-kehlz), which receive the blood, and two lower chambers, or **ventricles** (VEN-tri-kehlz), from which the blood is sent to the body. The heart has four major valves, two of which separate the auricles from the ventricles. These are known as the **bicuspid** (bigh-KUHS-pehd) and **tricuspid** (trigh-KUHS-pehd) valves. The other two valves separate the ventricles from the arteries, which carry blood away from the heart. Normally, these valves close very tightly, allowing no blood to seep from the auricles to ventricles or from ventricles to arteries, which causes a great buildup of pressure that helps the heart pump blood through the body.

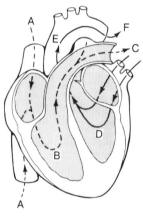

Flow of blood through the heart. (A) Blood is received in the right auricle from the veins; (B) blood then passes through valve into right ventricle; (C) blood is pumped through the pulmonary artery into lungs; (D) blood is received in the left auricle from the lungs; (E) blood passes through valve into left ventricle and then pumped into aorta; (F) and from the aorta the blood is distributed throughout the body

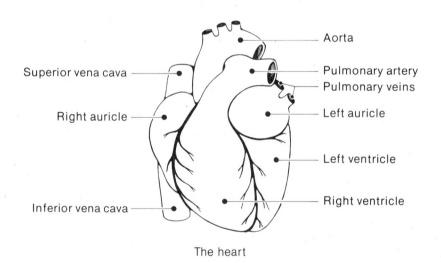

The heart

Arteries are the vessels that carry blood **from the heart** to the body. The arteries vary in size. Arteries have three layers of tissue—an outer layer, an inner layer, and a middle layer of smooth muscle, which can make the artery larger or smaller.

From the arteries, the blood moves into the **capillaries**. They are made up of just one layer of tissue, and can be seen only with the aid of a microscope. They take nutrients (food) and oxygen to the cells and take waste products and carbon dioxide away.

There are two methods by which this exchange is accomplished. One is **pressure**. The force of blood flow (the pulse) pushes food through the capillary walls at the arterial end of the capillary bed.

The other method by which material is exchanged is **osmosis** (ahz-MOH-siss). Simply stated, osmosis involves the tendency of substances (in this case, the nutrients) to equalize on either side of a membrane (the capillary wall).

After the blood leaves the capillaries, it goes on to the **veins**, which will carry it back **to the heart**. The veins are only two layers thick. They carry the used blood, waste products, and carbon dioxide to a point of removal. The kidneys and liver remove the metabolic waste products, excess water, salts, and dead cells. The lungs rid the body of carbon dioxide.

The blood is sent back **to the heart** primarily by the activity of the contracting skeletal muscles. The veins also help keep the blood moving to the heart.

Pulmonary (PUHL-mah-ner-ee) **circulation** is how carbon dioxide is removed from the blood and replaced by oxygen. The pulmonary artery carries blood that has carbon dioxide in it through the veins from the body to the heart. Then the heart sends it through the pulmonary arteries to the lungs, where carbon dioxide is replaced with oxygen. The fresh blood (that contains oxygen) comes back from the **lungs to the heart** in the pulmonary veins. Then the heart sends this fresh blood to the rest of the body.

KNOWING SUBOBJECTIVE 2

The arterial blood supply to the head, face, and neck is as follows.

Immediately off the heart is the **aorta** (ay-ORT-ah), **the largest artery in the body**. Branching from the aorta is the **common carotid** (keh-RAHT-ehd) **artery**, which is the main supplier of blood to the head, face, and neck, and to the area on either side of the throat. The common carotid branches into the **internal and external carotid arteries**. The **internal carotid artery** supplies the brain and the eye sockets, eyelids, and forehead via the **ophthalmic** (ahf-THAL-mik) **artery**. The **external carotid artery** supplies blood to the superficial tissues of the head, face, and neck. Its branches include the **facial (or external maxillary)** (MAK-seh-ler-ee) **artery**, which supplies the lower portion of the face, the mouth, and the nose; the **occipital** (ahk-SIP-eh-tahl) **artery**, which supplies the scalp and the back of the

Identify arteries and veins of the head, face, neck, arm, and hand, and describe the composition of blood and the lymphatic system.

head up to the crown; the **posterior auricular artery**, which is the source of blood for the scalp behind and above the ear; and the **transverse facial artery**, which supplies the muscles, skin, and scalp of the sides, front, and top of the head.

The veins in these regions follow the arteries and have the same names. For instance, the **transverse facial vein** is near the **transverse facial artery**. There is one exception to the rule. The veins that drain the area supplied by the internal and external carotid arteries are called the **internal** and **external jugular** (JUHG-yeh-lehr) **veins**.

The **brachial** (BRAK-ee-ehl) **artery** supplies the arm and hand. It comes from the aorta and divides into the **radial** and **ulnar arteries.**

The veins in the deeper body tissues follow the same pattern and have the same names as the arteries, but the superficial (close to the surface) veins do not. They are on the anterior side of the forearm (inner arm).

To understand how waste is removed and nutrition given to the body at the same time, you must look at the blood itself.

The body contains 8 to 10 pints of **blood**, one-half to two-thirds of which is held by the skin. The temperature of blood is approximately 98.6 degrees Fahrenheit. The color of blood can be **bright red or scarlet in the arteries** and a **deep red, almost purple, in the veins**. It is considered a specialized connective tissue. Its main components follow.

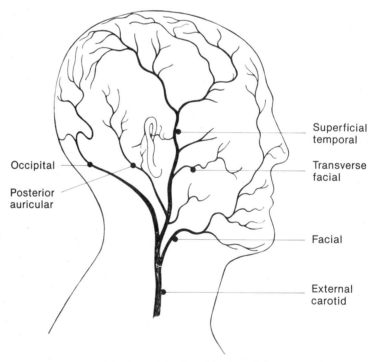

Arteries of the head and neck

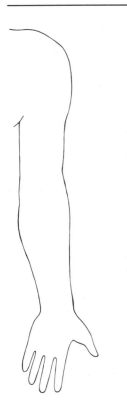

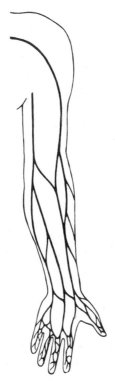

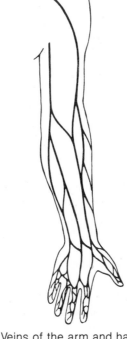

Veins of the arm and hand

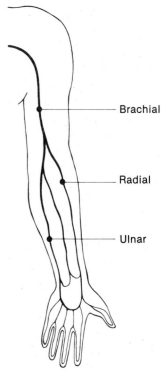

Arteries of the arm and hand

— Brachial

— Radial

— Ulnar

Plasma (PLAZ-mah) is a **yellow liquid** that accounts for approximately two-thirds of the volume of blood. Plasma is mostly water, but it does contain food elements, waste products, and dissolved salts.

Red blood cells (or **erythrocytes** [i-RITH-rah-sights]) give blood its color. They are shaped like discs, have exceptional flexibility, and contain a substance called **hemoglobin** (HEE-mah-gloh-behn). They exchange oxygen for carbon dioxide in the body. They are manufactured primarily by the marrow of flat bones in adults.

White blood cells (or **leukocytes** [LOO-koh-sights]) are much larger than red blood cells. They fight infection in the body.

Blood platelets (or **thrombocytes**) are colorless cells. They **help blood clot** and thus form a scab over a wound. This process, together with the activity of the **leukocytes**, is how the circulatory system **protects the body against disease**.

The **lymphatic** (lim-FAT-ik) **system** is closely related to the circulatory system. It is a one-directional vascular system that collects excess fluid from the spaces between the cells and puts it back into the body's circulation.

Lymph (LIMF) itself is a colorless liquid that comes from plasma. It contains white blood cells and a few red blood cells. It gets leukocytes from the blood and makes its own kind of leukocytes called **lymphocytes** (LIM-feh-sights) at the lymph nodes.

The lymphatic system has only one kind of vessel, which varies in size. It can be as small as the lymphatic (the minute vessel that collects the excess fluid) to the larger vessels that eventually empty into the **vena cava** (VAY-nah KAY-vah—the large vein that empties into the right auricle of the heart itself).

There is, however, a specialized set of lymphatic vessels called **lacteals** (LAK-tee-ehls). They absorb fat (**chyle**) from the intestine and carry it to the main lymphatic vessel, which in turn drains into the veins.

KNOWING SUBOBJECTIVE 3

Define the endocrine system and its 5 major glands.

The **endocrine** (EN-deh-krehn) **system** is a system of **ductless glands** that release chemicals called **hormones** (HOR-mohnz) into the blood. The hormones affect, among other things, the skin, hair, and scalp. The endocrine system helps control such bodily functions as growth, general health, and reproduction.

The major glands of the endocrine system are:

Pituitary (peh-TYOO-eh-ter-ee) gland   It is located **at the base of the brain**. It **regulates** the functions of **all other endocrine glands** and also regulates the water balance in the body. The **hypothalamus** (high-poh-THAL-eh-muhs) (the part of the brain to which the pituitary is connected) regulates the activities (secretions) of the pituitary gland. The hypothalamus, in turn, can be regulated by higher centers in the brain.

Thyroid (THIGH-roid) gland   The thyroid gland located **on either side of the larynx (throat) controls** the body's **metabolism**, which affects the weight of the body. An underactive thyroid results in a condition known as hypothyroidism that is characterized by excessive weight gain. An overactive thyroid results in hyperthyroidism, which involves severe weight loss.

Pancreas (PAN-kree-uhs)   It is located **behind the stomach**. It **affects the amount of sugar used** by the **body**. Specialized cells in the pancreas produce the **hormone insulin** (IN-suh-lehn). If the pancreas does not produce enough insulin, diabetes results.

Adrenal (ah-DREEN-l) glands   They are located just **above the kidneys**. They **produce** the hormone **adrenaline**, which supports the body's ability to withstand stress.

Reproductive glands   The reproductive glands include both **ductless (endocrine)** and **ducted (exocrine)** glands.

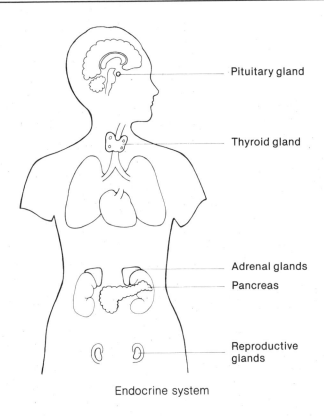

Pituitary gland

Thyroid gland

Adrenal glands

Pancreas

Reproductive glands

Endocrine system

Adrenal (ah-DREEN-l) glands   Endocrine glands located just above the kidney that help the body cope with stress by producing the hormone adrenaline.

Angiology (an-jee-AHL-eh-jee)   The study of the vascular system, which includes the circulatory system and the lymphatic system.

Aorta (ay-ORT-ah)   The largest artery in the body.

Arteries (AHRT-eh-reez)   The vessels that carry blood from the heart to the body.

Auricles (AWR-i-kehlz)   The two upper chambers of the heart.

Bicuspid (bye-KUHS-pehd)   One of the major valves of the heart that separates the auricles from the ventricles.

Blood platelets (PLAYT-lehts)   Colorless cells in the blood that help the blood clot.

Brachial (BRAK-ee-ehl) artery   The artery that supplies blood to the arms and hands. It comes from the aorta and divides into the radial and ulnar arteries.

Capillaries (KAP-eh-ler-eez)   The microscopic blood vessels that take nutrients and oxygen to the cells from the arteries and take waste products to the veins.

Chyle (KYLE)   The fat in the intestine absorbed by the lacteals.

Circulatory system   The heart and the blood vessels. This system brings food and oxygen to all the cells of the body, removes the waste and carbon dioxide from the cells, guards the body against infection, and regulates body temperature.

Common carotid artery   The artery that is the main supplier of blood to the head, face, and neck, and to the area on either side of the throat.

Endocrine (EN-deh-krehn) system   A system of ductless glands that release hormones into the blood.

Erythrocytes (i-RITH-rah-sights)   See **Red blood cells**.

External carotid artery   The artery that supplies blood to the superficial tissues of the head, face, and neck.

External maxillary (MAX-seh-ler-ee) artery   See **Facial artery**.

Facial artery   A branch of the external carotid artery that supplies the lower portion of the face, the mouth, and the nose. Also called the external maxillary artery.

Hemoglobin (HEE-mah-gloh-behn)   A substance found in red blood cells.

Hormones (HOR-mohnz)   The chemicals that help control growth, general health, and reproduction.

Hypothalamus (high-poh-THAL-eh-muhs)   The part of the brain that regulates the activities of the pituitary gland.

Insulin (IN-suh-lehn)   The hormone produced by the pancreas that affects the amount of sugar used by the body.

Internal carotid artery   The artery that supplies the brain, eye sockets, eyelids, and head via the ophthalmic artery.

Jugular (JUGH-yeh-lehr) veins   The veins that drain the area supplied by the internal and external carotid arteries.

Lacteals (LAK-tee-ehlz)   A specialized set of lymphatic vessels that absorb fat from the intestine and carry it to the main lymphatic vessel, which drains into the veins.

Leukocytes (LOO-koh-sights)   See **White blood cells**.

Lymph (LIMF)   A colorless liquid that comes from plasma that makes lymphocytes.

Lymphatic (lim-FAT-ik) system   The part of the circulatory system that collects excess fluid from the spaces between the cells and puts it back into the body's circulation.

Lymphocytes (LIM-feh-sights)   A white blood cell manufactured by the lymph nodes.

Occipital (ahk-SIP-eh-tehl) artery   The artery that supplies blood to the scalp and the back of the head up to the crown.

Ophthalmic (ahf-THAL-mik) artery   A subdivision of the internal carotid artery.

Osmosis (ahz-MOH-sis)   A process of exchange in the capillary that provides nutrients to the cells and removes waste products from the cells.

Pancreas (PAN-kree-us)   An endocrine gland located behind the stomach that affects the amount of sugar used by the body by producing the hormone insulin.

Pericardium (per-eh-KAHRD-ee-uhm)   The tough membrane that surrounds the heart.

Pituitary (peh-TOO-eh-ter-ee) gland A gland located at the base of the brain that regulates the functions of all other endocrine glands and regulates the water balance in the body.

Plasma (PLAZ-mah) A yellow liquid found in the blood that contains water, food elements, waste products, and dissolved salts.

Posterior auricular (pah-STIR-ee-ehr aw-RIK-yeh-lehr) artery The artery that supplies blood to the scalp behind and above the ear.

Pulmonary (PUHL-mah-ner-ee) circulation The process of removing carbon dioxide from the blood and replacing it with oxygen.

Radial (RAY-dee-ehl) artery A subdivision of the brachial artery.

Red blood cells Red, disc-shaped cells in the blood that give blood its color and exchange oxygen for carbon dioxide in the body.

Thyroid (THIGH-roid) The endocrine glands located on either side of the throat that control the body's metabolism.

Transverse facial artery The artery that supplies blood to the masseter muscle.

Tricuspid (try-KUHS-pehd) One of the major valves of the heart that separates the auricles from the ventricles.

Ulnar (UHL-nahr) artery A subdivision of the brachial artery.

Veins The blood vessels that carry blood, waste products, and carbon dioxide to a point of removal.

Vena cava (VAY-nah KAY-vah) The large vein that empties into the right auricle of the heart.

Ventricles (VEN-tri-kehlz) The two lower chambers of the heart.

White blood cells Large, white blood cells that fight infection in the body. See Leukocytes.

QUESTIONS

1. In brief, what is angiology the study of?
2. What is another name for the vascular system?
3. What is another name for the cardiac muscle tissue that surrounds the heart?
4. What is the function of the circulatory system?
5. In what part of the body is the heart located?
6. Are the upper chambers of the heart called auricles?
7. Are the lower chambers of the heart called ventricles?
8. Do arteries carry blood from the heart?
9. Do veins carry blood to the heart?
10. Are capillaries large or small blood vessels?
11. If you were looking for the flow of pulmonary blood vessels, in which organs would they be found?

ANSWERS

1. Blood. 2. The circulatory system. 3. Pericardium. 4. To bring food and oxygen to the body, and remove waste and carbon dioxide from the blood cells. 5. The chest cavity. 6. Yes. 7. Yes. 8. Yes. 9. Yes. 10. Small, and can only be seen with aid of microscope. 11. The lungs.

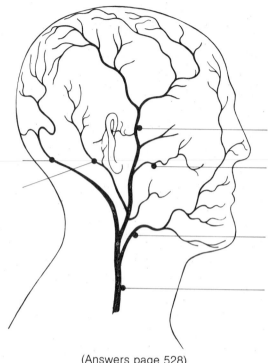

(Answers page 528)

QUESTIONS SUBOBJECTIVE 2

1. Which is the largest artery in the human body?
2. What artery in the neck is a major branch of the aorta?
3. What main artery divides into two branches to become the radial and ulnar arteries?
4. How many pints of blood are contained in the human body?
5. Would blood in an artery look bright red or scarlet?
6. Are red blood cells called erythrocytes?
7. What are white blood cells called?
8. What special part of blood causes it to clot?

ANSWERS

1. The aorta. 2. Carotid. 3. Brachial. 4. 8-10 pints. 5. Yes. 6. Yes. 7. Leukocytes. 8. Platelets.

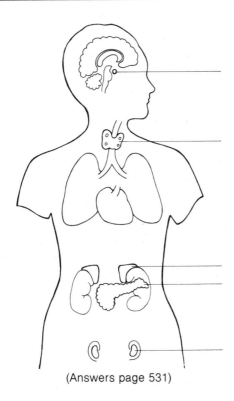

(Answers page 531)

QUESTIONS SUBOBJECTIVE 3

1. Is it true that the endocrine system is made up of ductless glands?
2. Does the endocrine system have something to do with hormones in the body?
3. Where is the pituitary gland located?
4. Does the pituitary gland regulate all other endocrine glands?
5. Does the hypothalamus regulate the pituitary gland?
6. What gland located in the throat regulates body metabolism?
7. What gland makes insulin in the body?

ANSWERS

1. Yes. 2. Yes. 3. The base of the brain. 4. Yes. 5. Yes. 6. The thyroid gland. 7. The pancreas.

Using the Glossaries in this Book   The terms in the glossaries at the end of each chapter are defined only as they relate to the practice of cosmetology.

Entries are alphabetized in the letter-by-letter rather than word-by-word system. This means that the first order of alphabetizing has been followed through the first mark of punctuation, disregarding hyphens and spaces between words. For example:

Acid
Acid-balanced
Acidity
Acid rinse

Prepositions have been ignored in alphabetizing the index entries.

Pronunciations are indicated by respellings, according to sounds shown in familiar words. See Pronunciation Key. The syllable which is accented (stressed) is shown in capital letters.

PRONUNCIATION KEY

SYMBOL FOR A SOUND	KEY WORD AND RESPELLING	SYMBOL FOR A SOUND	KEY WORD AND RESPELLING
a	sat (SAT), paddle (PAD-l)	n	notice (NOH-tiss)
*ah	bar (BAHR)	ng	ring (RING), singer (SING-gehr)
ai	pair (PAIR)	o	dot (DOT)
ar	fare (FARE)	oh	goat (GOHT), go (GOH)
aw	saw (SAW)	oi	soil (SOIL)
ay	day (DAY)	oo	scoot (SKOOT)
b	bob (BOB)		yule (YOOL), leukemia (loo-KEE-mee-ah)
ch	chin (CHIN)		
d	did (DID)	or	nor (NOR)
e	set (SET)	ow	tower (TOW-ehr)
ee	see (SEE)	p	pep (PEP)
ehr	merry (MEHR-ee)	ph	phy (fee), phone (fone)
er	fern (FERN), turn (TURN)	r	reed (REED)
f	fifty (FIF-tee)	s	sips (SIPS)
g	gig (GIG)	sh	ship (SHIP)
h	hat (HAT)	ss	base (BAYSS)
hw	wheel (WHEEL)	t	tent (TENT)
i	sit (SIT)	th	thank (THANK)
igh	might (MIGHT)	*th*	than (*THAN*)
ihr	tier (TIHR)	u	shut (SHUT), hook (HUK)
ism	organism (OR-gehn-iz-uhm), patriotism (PAY-tree-ah-tiz-uhm)	*uh	but (BUHT)
		v	vivid (VIV-id)
		w	wag (WAG)
j	jam (JAM)	y	yes (YESS)
k	kid (KID)	The y sometimes replaces (igh); example: childish (CHYL-dish).	
ks	six (SIKS)		
kw	quack (KWAK)		
l	let (LET), battle (BAT-l)	z	zoos (ZOOZ)
m	mom (MOM)	zh	measure (MEZH-ehr)

*The symbols ah, eh, and uh sometimes show syllables containing vowel sounds which are muted (stressed very little).

Glossary Index

Subject Index

543